AHA Hospital Statistics™

2008 Edition

D1609600

AHA Institutional Members $175
Nonmembers $235
AHA Catalog NUMBER 082008
Telephone ORDERS 1-800-AHA-2626

ISSN 0090-6662
ISBN-10: 0-87258-831-9
ISBN-13: 978-0-87258-831-8

Contents

Acknowledgements & Advisements

Acknowledgments

The 2008 edition of AHA Hospital Statistics is published by Health Forum an affiliate of the American Hospital Association, Richard J. Umbdenstock, President and CEO.

Advisements

The data published here should be used with the following advisements: The data are based on replies to an annual survey that seeks a variety of information, not all of which is published in this book. The information gathered by the survey includes specific services, but not all of each hospital's services. Therefore, the data do not reflect an exhaustive list of all services offered by all hospitals. For information on the availability of additional data, please contact Health Forum, (800) 821-2039.

Health Forum does not assume responsibility for the accuracy of information voluntarily reported by the individual institutions surveyed. The purpose of this publication is to provide basic data reflecting the delivery of health care in the United States and associated areas, and is not to serve an official and all-inclusive list of services offered by individual hospitals.

Trends:
a look ahead

The Wave of Baby Boomers is Coming: Are Hospitals Ready?

AHA Hospital Statistics is a comprehensive compilation of data on trends in the hospital field through 2006 based on the results of the American Hospital Association's (AHA) Annual Survey of Hospitals. Overall, Hospital Statistics identifies both long-standing and emerging trends and offers insights into what the future may hold for hospitals. This introduction focuses on an area of increasing concern: caring for aging Baby Boomers.

Caroline Rossi Steinberg
Vice President, Trends Analysis
American Hospital Association

The Wave of Baby Boomers is Coming: Are Hospitals Ready?

Born between 1946 and 1964, the 78 million Baby Boomers have had a tremendous cultural and economic impact on the United States. As they have entered each stage of their lives, this dynamic generation has driven the need for schools and housing, altered the labor market and introduced lifestyle changes. The first Baby Boomers recently hit 60 – an age where use of health care services begins to increase dramatically. By 2030, Baby Boomers will lead to a doubling of the over-65 population (Chart 1). Are hospitals ready to meet this challenge?

People Use More Health Care Services as They Age

As people age, they tend to use more health care services and the Baby Boomers will be no exception. Today someone 75 or older has 5 times more hospital stays as someone between 18 and 44 (Chart 2).[1] But the health profile of the elderly population is changing. Advances in health care are keeping people alive who would have died of heart disease, cancer, diabetes or other diseases a generation ago. With the help of surgical techniques, advanced diagnostics, drugs and

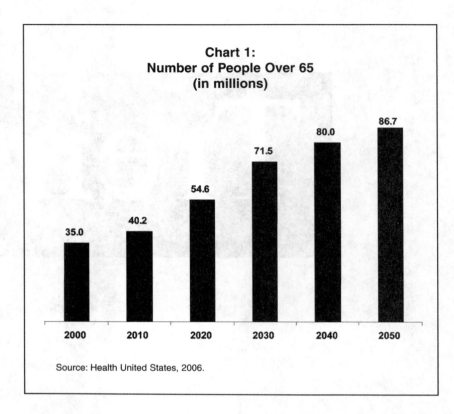

Chart 1:
Number of People Over 65
(in millions)

Source: Health United States, 2006.

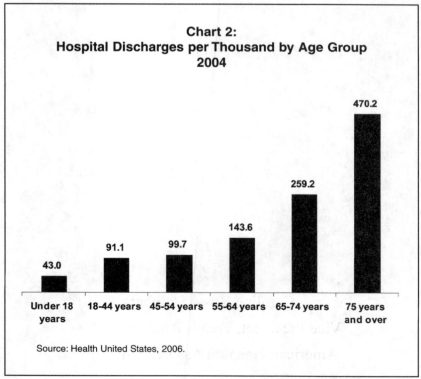

Chart 2:
Hospital Discharges per Thousand by Age Group
2004

Source: Health United States, 2006.

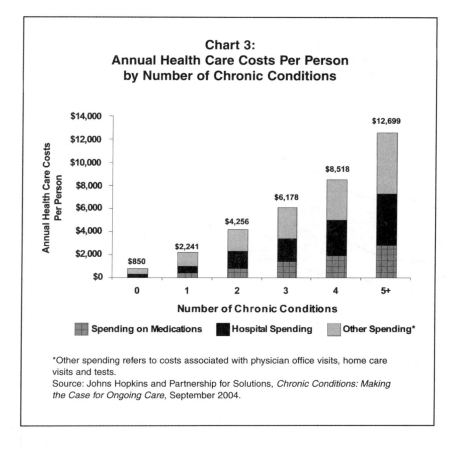

Chart 3:
Annual Health Care Costs Per Person
by Number of Chronic Conditions

*Other spending refers to costs associated with physician office visits, home care visits and tests.
Source: Johns Hopkins and Partnership for Solutions, *Chronic Conditions: Making the Case for Ongoing Care*, September 2004.

devices, people are living longer with disease. And, while advances in medicine improve the length and quality of life for the elderly population, these same advances generate increased demand for health care services.

Aging Baby Boomers Will Contribute to Increased Rates of Chronic Illness

Sixty-two percent of individuals between 50 and 64 have at least one of six chronic conditions (heart disease, hypertension, diabetes, arthritis, high cholesterol or cancer).[2] Chronic diseases generally require continual medical management. Consequently, people with chronic conditions tend to use significantly more health care services. Not surprisingly, resource use increases with the number of chronic diseases (Chart 3). An estimated 8.6 million Baby Boomers have more than one chronic condition, but by 2030, this number is expected to increase to 37 million.[3] This trend will place a significant burden on our health care system.

The number of Americans with diabetes is rising at an alarming rate. Thirty million people have diabetes today, but by 2030 that number is expected to increase by more than 50 percent to nearly 46 million people.[4] Diabetes requires careful medical management to avoid complications such as heart, eye, kidney and nerve disease. If care guidelines are followed, each diabetes patient should receive regular lab tests such as lipid profiles, protein screenings and hemoglobin A1c tests. People with diabetes also require regular eye and foot exams. Without these services, diabetics are more likely to end up in the emergency department or in a hospital bed.

The number of people with arthritis is expected to increase from 46 million to 67 million by 2030.[5] People with arthritis can experience limitations in daily activities, require pain medication or seek joint replacements.

Baby Boomers also are more likely to be obese than prior generations (Chart 4). Today an estimated 28 percent of 50-to-64-year-olds are considered obese. Rates of obesity are expected to continue to rise, with one of every three Baby Boomers likely to be considered obese by 2030.[6] Research shows that obesity increases the risk of diabetes, heart disease, many forms of cancer and other serious illnesses. Rising rates of obesity will strain our nation's health care resources; obese beneficiaries cost Medicare about 34 percent more than those of a healthy weight.[7]

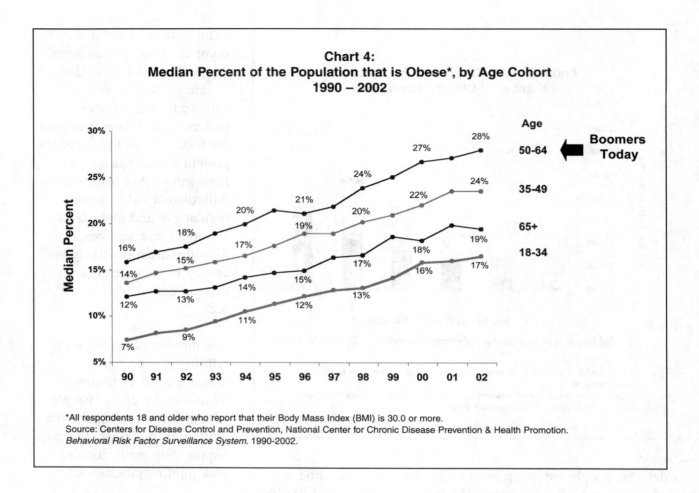

Chart 4:
Median Percent of the Population that is Obese*, by Age Cohort
1990 – 2002

Age

Boomers Today → 50-64

35-49

65+

18-34

Y-axis: Median Percent (5% to 30%)
X-axis: 90 91 92 93 94 95 96 97 98 99 00 01 02

50-64: 16%, 18%, 20%, 21%, 24%, 27%, 28%
35-49: 14%, 15%, 17%, 19%, 20%, 22%, 24%
65+: 12%, 13%, 14%, 15%, 17%, 18%, 19%
18-34: 7%, 9%, 11%, 12%, 13%, 16%, 17%

*All respondents 18 and older who report that their Body Mass Index (BMI) is 30.0 or more.
Source: Centers for Disease Control and Prevention, National Center for Chronic Disease Prevention & Health Promotion.
Behavioral Risk Factor Surveillance System. 1990-2002.

The rise in chronic disease will not only increase the demand for health care services, it also will create the need for changes in how care is delivered. Addressing chronic disease will require a multi-disciplinary approach where services are more coordinated across hospitals, physicians, home care and other providers. Information technology that facilitates the sharing of information across provider types and with the patient will be critical to effective, efficient care management.

Demographics Will Influence Demand for Health Services

Baby Boomers differ from prior generations in ways that influence their expectations of health care including: How much health care they demand, where they receive health care services and how those services are provided.

Baby Boomers have more education and disposable income than prior generations (Chart 5).[8,9] Both of these factors are linked to increased use of health care services. Baby Boomers tend to lead a more active lifestyle than their parents and look to innovations like joint replacements and new pain medications to keep them active.

Where Baby Boomers choose to retire will influence future hospital capacity needs. Today the states cited by Baby Boomers as the most preferred locations for retirement include Florida (14 percent), Arizona (12 percent), North Carolina (10 percent), California (8 percent) and Texas (5 percent). By 2020, the Census Bureau projects that Florida will replace New York as the third most populous state.[10]

7. Registered nurse supervision and other nursing services are continuous.

8. A current and complete‡ medical record shall be maintained by the institution for each patient and shall be available for reference.

9. Pharmacy service shall be maintained in the institution and shall be supervised by a registered pharmacist.

10. The institution shall provide patients with food service that meets their nutritional and therapeutic requirements; special diets shall also be available.

Types of Hospitals
In addition to meeting these 10 general registration requirements, hospitals are registered as one of four types of hospitals: general, special, rehabilitation and chronic disease, or psychiatric. The following type of hospital and special requirements for registration are employed:

General
The primary function of the institution is to provide patient services, diagnostic and therapeutic, for a variety of medical conditions. A general hospital also shall provide:

- diagnostic x-ray services with facilities and staff for a variety of procedures
- clinical laboratory service with facilities and staff for a variety of procedures and with anatomical pathology services regularly and conveniently available
- operating room service with facilities and staff.

Special
The primary function of the institution is to provide diagnostic and treatment services for patients who have specified medical conditions, both surgical and nonsurgical. A special hospital also shall provide:

- such diagnostic and treatment services as may be determined by the Executive Committee of the Board of Trustees of the American Hospital Association to be appropriate for the specified medical conditions for which medical services are provided shall be maintained in the institution with suitable facilities and staff. If such conditions do not normally require diagnostic x-ray service, laboratory service, or operating room service, and if any such services are therefore not maintained in the institution, there shall be written arrangements to make them available to patients requiring them.
- clinical laboratory services capable of providing tissue diagnosis when offering pregnancy termination services.

Rehabilitation and Chronic Disease
The primary function of the institution is to provide diagnostic and treatment services to handicapped or disabled individuals requiring restorative and adjustive services. A rehabilitation and chronic disease hospital also shall provide:

- arrangements for diagnostic x-ray services, as required, on a regular and conveniently available basis
- arrangements for clinical laboratory service, as required on a regular and conveniently available basis
- arrangements for operating room service, as required, on a regular and conveniently available basis
- a physical therapy service with suitable facilities and staff in the institution
- an occupational therapy service with suitable facilities and staff in the institution
- arrangements for psychological and social work services on a regular and conveniently available basis

---

* Physician–Term used to describe an individual with an M.D. or D.O. degree who is fully licensed to practice medicine in all its phases.

‡ The completed records in general shall contain at least the following: the patient's identifying data and consent forms, medical history, record of physical examination, physicians' progress notes, operative notes, nurses' notes, routine x-ray and laboratory reports, doctors' orders, and final diagnosis.

- arrangements for educational and vocational services on a regular and conveniently available basis
- written arrangements with a general hospital for the transfer of patients who require medical, obstetrical, or surgical services not available in the institution.

Psychiatric

The primary function of the institution is to provide diagnostic and treatment services for patients who have psychiatric-related illnesses. A psychiatric hospital also shall provide:

- arrangements for clinical laboratory service, as required, on a regular and conveniently available basis
- arrangements for diagnostic x-ray services, as required on a regular and conveniently available basis
- psychiatric, psychological, and social work service with facilities and staff in the institution
- arrangements for electroencephalograph services, as required, on a regular and conveniently available basis.
- written arrangements with a general hospital for the transfer of patients who require medical, obstetrical, or surgical services not available in the institution.

The American Hospital Association may, at the sole discretion of the Executive Committee of the Board of Trustees, grant, deny, or withdraw the registration of an institution.

Data Comparability

The economic climate, demographic characteristics, personnel issues, and health care financing and payment policies differ by region, state, and city across the country. *Differences in these factors must be taken into account when using the data.* In addition, the profiles of hospitals across comparison groups vary. For example, states will differ in terms of the number and percentage of hospitals by size, ownership, services provided, types of patients treated, and so forth. *Differences in these variables must also be taken into consideration when doing a comparative analysis.*

The 2008 edition of *AHA Hospital Statistics™* draws its data from the 2006 AHA Annual Survey of Hospitals. It is the statistical complement to the 2008 edition of the *AHA Guide®*, which contains selected data about individual hospitals.

The AHA Survey was mailed to all hospitals, both AHA-registered and nonregistered, in the U.S. and its associated areas: American Samoa, Guam, the Marshall Islands, Puerto Rico, and the Virgin Islands. U.S. government hospitals located outside the U.S. were not included. Overall, the average response rate over the past five years has been approximately 85 percent.

Reporting Period

In completing the survey, hospitals were requested to report data for a full year, in accord with their fiscal year, ending in 2006. The statistical table present data reported or estimated for a 12-month period, except for data on personnel, which represent situations as they existed at the end of the reporting period.

Respondents

Data for Tables 1 and 2 include 5,747 AHA-registered hospitals in the U.S. Data on community hospitals (nonfederal, short-term general and other special hospitals) only are presented in Tables 3-6, and Table 8.

It is important to note that the AHA-registered hospitals included in *AHA Hospital Statistics* are not necessarily identical to those included in *AHA Guide*. The institutions listed in the 2006 edition of *AHA Guide* include all of those institutions registered as of April 2006. Tables 1-6 in *AHA Hospital Statistics* present data for AHA-registered hospitals that were in operation during the 12-month reporting period ending 2006.

Estimates

Estimates were made of data for nonreporting hospitals and for reporting hospitals that submitted incomplete AHA Annual Survey questionnaires. Estimates were not made for beds, bassinets and facilities and services. Data for beds and bassinets of nonreporting hospitals were based on the most recent information from those hospitals. (Note that in all statistical tables, whenever bed-size categories are listed, all eight categories appear, whether or not there are hospitals in every category.)

Missing revenue, expenses, admissions, births, inpatient days, surgical operations, outpatient visits, and full-time-equivalent personnel values are estimates from regression models. For all other variables the estimates were based on ratios such as per bed averages derived from data reported by hospitals similar in size, control, major service provided, length of stay, and geographical characteristics to the hospitals that did not report this information.

Tables 1–2

Table

1

Historical Trends in Utilization, Personnel, and Finances for Selected Years from 1946 through 2006

Data are for all AHA-registered hospitals in the United States. Data are estimated for nonreporting hospitals with the exception of newborn and outpatient data before 1972. Personnel data exclude residents, interns, and students from 1952 on; personnel data include full-time personnel and full-time equivalents for part-time personnel from 1954 on. As a result of the AHA Annual Survey validation process, the New York state expense data from 1976 were revised after the 1977 edition was published. The revised figures are included below. In order to provide trend data on a consistent basis, the 1970 and 1971 psychiatric and long-term data have been slightly modified. The 1982 FTE figures have been updated to provide the most accurate data possible.

CLASSIFICATION: Total United States

YEAR	HOSPITALS	BEDS (in thousands)	ADMISSIONS (in thousands)	AVERAGE DAILY CENSUS (in thousands)	ADJUSTED AVERAGE DAILY CENSUS (in thousands)	AVERAGE STAY (days)	OUTPATIENT VISITS (in thousands)	NEWBORNS Bassinets	NEWBORNS Births	FTE PERSONNEL Number (in thousands)	FTE PERSONNEL Per 100 Adjusted Census	TOTAL EXPENSES Amount (In Millions of dollars)	TOTAL EXPENSES Adjusted per Inpatient Stay (dollars)	TOTAL EXPENSES Adjusted per Inpatient Day (dollars)
1946	6,125	1,436	15,675	1,142	—	—	—	85,585	2,135,327	830	—	$1,963	—	—
1950	6,788	1,456	18,483	1,253	—	—	—	90,101	2,742,780	1,058	—	$3,651	—	—
1955	6,956	1,604	21,073	1,363	—	—	—	98,823	3,476,753	1,301	—	$5,594	—	—
1960	6,876	1,658	25,027	1,402	—	—	—	102,764	3,835,735	1,598	—	$8,421	—	—
1965	7,123	1,704	28,812	1,403	—	—	125,793	101,287	3,565,344	1,952	—	$12,948	—	—
1970	7,123	1,616	31,759	1,298	—	—	181,370	97,128	3,537,000	2,537	—	$25,556	—	—
1971	7,097	1,556	32,664	1,237	—	—	199,725	94,344	3,464,513	2,589	—	$28,812	—	—
1972	7,061	1,550	33,265	1,209	—	—	219,182	92,960	3,231,875	2,671	—	$32,667	—	—
1973	7,123	1,535	34,352	1,189	—	—	233,555	90,071	3,087,210	2,769	—	$36,290	—	—
1974	7,174	1,513	35,506	1,167	—	—	250,481	88,269	3,043,386	2,919	—	$41,406	—	—
1975	7,156	1,466	36,157	1,125	—	—	254,844	86,875	3,091,629	3,023	—	$48,706	—	—
1976	7,082	1,434	36,776	1,090	—	—	270,951	85,284	3,067,063	3,108	—	$56,005	—	—
1977	7,099	1,407	37,060	1,066	—	—	263,775	83,193	3,223,699	3,213	—	$63,630	—	—
1978	7,015	1,381	37,243	1,042	—	—	263,606	80,650	3,250,373	3,280	—	$70,927	—	—
1979	6,988	1,372	37,802	1,043	—	—	262,009	79,720	3,376,467	3,382	—	$79,796	—	—
1980	6,965	1,365	38,892	1,060	—	—	262,951	79,842	3,500,043	3,492	—	$91,886	—	—
1981	6,933	1,362	39,169	1,061	—	—	265,332	78,823	3,558,274	3,661	—	$107,146	—	—
1982	6,915	1,360	39,095	1,053	—	—	313,667	77,998	3,615,751	3,746	—	$123,219	—	—
1983	6,888	1,350	38,887	1,028	—	—	273,168	77,837	3,596,146	3,707	—	$136,315	—	—
1984	6,872	1,339	37,938	970	—	—	276,566	77,845	3,563,106	3,630	—	$144,114	—	—
1985	6,872	1,318	36,304	910	—	—	282,140	77,202	3,630,961	3,625	—	$153,327	—	—
1986	6,841	1,290	35,219	883	—	—	294,634	76,002	3,680,178	3,647	—	$165,194	—	—
1987	6,821	1,267	34,439	873	—	—	310,707	74,770	3,698,294	3,742	—	$178,662	—	—
1988	6,780	1,248	34,107	863	—	—	336,208	72,568	3,794,369	3,839	—	$196,704	—	—
1989	6,720	1,226	33,742	853	—	—	352,248	71,491	3,920,384	3,937	—	$214,886	—	—
1990	6,649	1,213	33,774	844	—	—	368,184	70,539	4,046,704	4,063	—	$234,870	—	—
1991	6,634	1,202	33,567	827	—	—	387,675	69,464	4,047,504	4,165	—	$258,508	—	—
1992	6,539	1,178	33,536	807	—	—	417,874	69,052	4,007,179	4,236	—	$282,531	—	—
1993	6,467	1,163	33,201	783	—	—	435,619	67,911	3,949,788	4,289	—	$301,538	—	—
1994	6,374	1,128	33,125	745	—	—	453,584	67,311	3,886,667	4,270	—	$310,834	—	—
1995	6,291	1,081	33,282	710	—	—	483,195	66,256	3,833,132	4,273	—	$320,252	—	—
1996	6,201	1,062	33,307	685	—	—	505,455	65,138	3,790,678	4,276	—	$330,531	—	—
1997	6,097	1,035	33,624	673	—	—	520,600	64,649	3,811,522	4,333	—	$342,334	—	—
1998	6,021	1,013	33,766	662	—	—	545,481	63,485	3,795,212	4,407	—	$355,450	—	—
1999	5,890	994	34,181	657	—	—	573,461	62,714	3,829,881	4,369	—	$372,933	—	—
2000	5,810	984	34,891	650	—	—	592,673	61,915	3,940,017	4,454	—	$395,391	—	—
2001	5,801	987	35,644	658	—	—	612,276	61,527	3,929,733	4,535	—	$426,849	—	—
2002	5,794	976	36,326	662	—	—	640,515	62,151	3,934,421	4,610	—	$462,222	—	—
2003	5,764	965	36,611	657	—	—	648,560	60,699	3,976,886	4,651	—	$498,104	—	—
2004	5,759	956	36,942	658	—	—	662,131	59,660	3,965,906	4,696	—	$533,853	—	—
2005	5,756	947	37,006	656	—	—	673,689	59,073	4,048,442	4,791	—	$570,534	—	—
2006	5,747	947	37,189	653	—	—	690,425	58,670	4,126,598	4,907	—	$607,355	—	—

Table 1 (Continued)

Classification: Total nonfederal short-term general and other special

YEAR	HOSPITALS	BEDS (in thousands)	ADMISSIONS (in thousands)	AVERAGE DAILY CENSUS (in thousands)	ADJUSTED AVERAGE DAILY CENSUS (in thousands)	AVERAGE LENGTH OF STAY (days)	OUTPATIENT VISITS (in thousands)	NEWBORNS Bassinets	NEWBORNS Births	FTE PERSONNEL Number (in thousands)	FTE PERSONNEL Per 100 Adjusted Census	EXPENSES Amount (In Millions of dollars)	EXPENSES Adjusted per Inpatient Stay (dollars)	EXPENSES Adjusted per Inpatient Day (dollars)
1946	4,444	473	13,655	341	—	9.1	—	80,987	2,087,503	505	—	$1,169	—	—
1950	5,031	505	16,663	372	—	8.1	—	86,019	2,660,982	662	—	$2,120	—	—
1955	5,237	568	19,100	407	—	7.8	—	93,868	3,304,451	826	—	$3,434	—	—
1960	5,407	639	22,970	477	—	7.6	—	98,127	3,678,051	1,080	—	$5,617	—	—
1965	5,736	741	26,463	563	620	7.8	92,631	96,782	3,413,370	1,386	224	$9,147	$316.37	$40.56
1970	5,859	848	29,252	662	727	8.2	133,545	93,079	3,403,064	1,929	265	$19,560	$604.59	$73.73
1971	5,865	867	30,142	665	736	8.0	148,423	90,444	3,337,605	1,999	272	$22,400	$667.44	$83.43
1972	5,843	884	30,777	664	739	7.9	166,983	89,315	3,119,446	2,056	278	$25,549	$747.42	$94.61
1973	5,891	903	31,761	681	768	7.8	178,939	86,851	2,987,089	2,149	280	$28,496	$793.88	$101.78
1974	5,977	931	32,943	701	793	7.8	194,838	85,208	2,947,342	2,289	289	$32,751	$883.04	$113.21
1975	5,979	947	33,519	708	806	7.7	196,311	83,834	2,998,590	2,399	298	$39,110	$1,024.72	$133.08
1976	5,956	961	34,068	715	816	7.7	207,725	82,307	2,962,305	2,483	304	$45,402	$1,172.25	$152.24
1977	5,973	974	34,353	717	820	7.6	204,238	80,228	3,117,756	2,581	315	$51,832	$1,316.70	$173.25
1978	5,935	980	34,575	720	841	7.6	204,461	78,090	3,156,570	2,662	323	$58,348	$1,470.13	$193.81
1979	5,923	988	35,160	729	841	7.6	203,873	77,277	3,287,157	2,762	328	$66,184	$1,631.16	$215.75
1980	5,904	992	36,198	748	861	7.6	206,752	77,539	3,408,699	2,879	334	$76,970	$1,844.19	$244.44
1981	5,879	1,007	36,494	764	876	7.6	206,729	76,567	3,465,683	3,039	347	$90,739	$2,167.70	$283.94
1982	5,863	1,015	36,429	763	882	7.6	250,888	75,739	3,514,761	3,110	353	$105,094	$2,493.09	$326.68
1983	5,843	1,021	36,201	750	869	7.6	213,995	75,471	3,490,629	3,102	357	$116,632	$2,775.55	$368.01
1984	5,814	1,020	35,202	703	824	7.3	216,474	75,587	3,456,467	3,023	367	$123,550	$2,984.00	$409.85
1985	5,784	1,003	33,501	650	780	7.1	222,773	74,899	3,521,296	3,003	385	$130,700	$3,238.94	$459.57
1986	5,728	982	32,410	631	774	7.1	234,270	73,688	3,584,530	3,032	392	$140,907	$3,529.60	$499.19
1987	5,659	961	31,633	624	780	7.2	247,704	72,516	3,602,416	3,120	400	$152,909	$3,848.79	$536.96
1988	5,579	949	31,480	622	795	7.2	271,436	70,361	3,706,748	3,209	404	$168,941	$4,194.39	$581.08
1989	5,497	936	31,141	619	805	7.3	287,909	69,436	3,831,051	3,307	411	$185,204	$4,572.23	$630.59
1990	5,420	929	31,203	620	820	7.3	302,691	68,443	3,958,646	3,423	417	$203,927	$4,929.93	$681.52
1991	5,370	926	31,084	612	828	7.2	323,202	67,440	3,965,489	3,539	427	$225,230	$5,345.63	$745.37
1992	5,321	923	31,053	606	832	7.1	349,397	67,095	3,925,024	3,624	436	$248,318	$5,788.52	$815.99
1993	5,289	921	30,770	593	834	7.0	368,358	66,060	3,870,392	3,681	441	$266,382	$6,120.94	$874.98
1994	5,256	904	30,739	569	814	6.8	384,880	65,728	3,809,367	3,697	454	$276,148	$6,230.33	$929.65
1995	5,220	874	30,966	549	811	6.5	415,710	64,742	3,764,756	3,718	458	$286,073	$6,220.54	$966.79
1996	5,160	864	31,116	531	800	6.2	440,845	63,646	3,723,907	3,728	466	$293,920	$6,225.95	$1,005.45
1997	5,082	855	31,595	529	813	6.1	450,907	63,247	3,742,240	3,794	467	$306,088	$6,266.24	$1,031.68
1998	5,039	842	31,830	527	821	6.0	474,366	62,162	3,726,234	3,835	467	$319,035	$6,387.53	$1,064.93
1999	4,977	831	32,377	527	835	5.9	495,850	61,534	3,760,295	3,840	460	$335,405	$6,512.44	$1,101.47
2000	4,934	825	33,102	527	850	5.8	522,970	60,845	3,880,166	3,916	461	$356,757	$6,650.68	$1,147.99
2001	4,927	828	33,834	534	866	5.8	539,316	60,454	3,873,395	3,990	461	$383,911	$6,979.29	$1,216.04
2002	4,949	823	34,501	541	887	5.7	557,336	59,974	3,870,191	4,072	459	$416,791	$7,353.17	$1,288.63
2003	4,918	815	34,800	540	895	5.7	563,804	59,662	3,915,842	4,112	459	$450,403	$7,798.19	$1,378.78
2004	4,942	810	35,098	542	910	5.6	573,126	58,710	3,931,508	4,151	456	$481,517	$8,168.06	$1,449.90
2005	4,956	804	35,265	542	930	5.6	587,296	58,195	3,987,766	4,260	458	$516,172	$8,538.30	$1,521.58
2006	4,947	805	35,403	540	940	5.6	599,597	57,832	4,075,193	4,347	462	$552,276	$8,972.85	$1,610.76

Table 1 (Continued)

CLASSIFICATION / YEAR	HOSPITALS	BEDS (in thousands)	ADMISSIONS (in thousands)	AVERAGE DAILY CENSUS (in thousands)	ADJUSTED AVERAGE DAILY CENSUS (in thousands)	AVERAGE LENGTH OF STAY (days)	OUTPATIENT VISITS (in thousands)	NEWBORNS Bassinets	NEWBORNS Births	FTE PERSONNEL Number (in thousands)	FTE PERSONNEL Per 100 Adjusted Census	EXPENSES Amount (In Millions of dollars)	EXPENSES Adjusted per Inpatient Stay (dollars)	EXPENSES Adjusted per Inpatient Day (dollars)
Total community hospitals														
1975	5,875	942	33,435	706	798	7.7	190,672	83,829	2,998,552	2,392	300	$38,962	$1,030.34	$133.81
1976	5,857	956	33,979	713	810	7.7	201,247	82,296	2,962,216	2,475	306	$45,240	$1,176.25	$152.76
1979	5,842	984	35,099	727	833	7.6	198,778	77,266	3,287,012	2,756	331	$66,004	$1,641.67	$217.34
1980	5,830	988	36,143	747	857	7.6	202,310	77,522	3,408,482	2,873	335	$76,851	$1,851.04	$245.12
1981	5,813	1,003	36,438	763	873	7.6	202,768	76,561	3,465,401	3,033	347	$90,572	$2,171.20	$284.33
1982	5,801	1,012	36,379	762	878	7.6	248,124	75,733	3,514,457	3,103	353	$104,876	$2,500.52	$327.37
1983	5,783	1,018	36,152	749	864	7.6	210,044	75,465	3,490,254	3,096	358	$116,438	$2,789.18	$369.49
1984	5,759	1,017	35,155	702	820	7.3	211,961	75,581	3,456,308	3,017	368	$123,336	$2,995.38	$411.10
1985	5,732	1,001	33,449	649	777	7.1	218,716	74,893	3,521,135	2,997	386	$130,499	$3,244.74	$460.19
1986	5,678	978	32,379	629	770	7.1	231,912	73,682	3,584,408	3,025	393	$140,654	$3,532.51	$500.81
1987	5,611	958	31,601	622	776	7.2	245,524	72,510	3,602,296	3,114	401	$152,585	$3,850.16	$538.96
1988	5,533	947	31,453	620	787	7.2	269,129	70,325	3,706,402	3,205	407	$168,722	$4,206.73	$586.33
1989	5,455	933	31,116	618	796	7.2	285,712	69,405	3,830,615	3,303	415	$184,898	$4,587.87	$636.96
1990	5,384	927	31,181	619	813	7.2	301,329	68,412	3,958,263	3,420	421	$203,693	$4,946.68	$686.83
1991	5,342	924	31,064	611	820	7.2	322,048	67,434	3,965,396	3,535	431	$225,023	$5,359.56	$752.10
1992	5,292	921	31,034	604	827	7.1	348,522	67,089	3,924,944	3,620	437	$248,095	$5,794.43	$819.83
1993	5,261	919	30,748	592	828	7.0	366,885	66,054	3,870,376	3,677	444	$266,089	$6,132.06	$880.52
1994	5,229	902	30,718	568	812	6.7	382,924	65,722	3,809,367	3,692	455	$275,779	$6,229.83	$930.71
1995	5,194	873	30,945	548	809	6.5	414,345	64,736	3,764,698	3,714	459	$285,588	$6,215.51	$967.69
1996	5,134	862	31,099	531	799	6.2	439,863	63,640	3,723,871	3,725	466	$293,755	$6,224.94	$1,006.14
1997	5,057	853	31,577	528	811	6.1	450,140	63,241	3,742,191	3,790	467	$305,763	$6,261.93	$1,032.70
1998	5,015	840	31,812	525	819	6.0	474,193	62,156	3,726,233	3,831	468	$318,834	$6,385.99	$1,066.96
1999	4,956	830	32,359	526	833	5.9	495,346	61,528	3,760,295	3,838	461	$335,246	$6,511.72	$1,102.61
2000	4,915	824	33,089	533	849	5.8	521,404	60,839	3,880,166	3,911	461	$356,564	$6,648.82	$1,149.40
2001	4,908	826	33,814	540	865	5.7	538,480	60,448	3,873,395	3,987	459	$383,735	$6,979.53	$1,217.27
2002	4,927	821	34,478	539	886	5.7	556,404	59,974	3,870,191	4,069	460	$416,591	$7,354.60	$1,289.87
2003	4,895	813	34,783	541	894	5.7	563,186	59,662	3,915,842	4,109	460	$450,124	$7,796.41	$1,379.48
2004	4,919	808	35,086	540	909	5.6	571,569	58,710	3,931,508	4,148	456	$481,247	$8,165.55	$1,450.35
2005	4,936	802	35,239	540	929	5.6	584,429	58,195	3,987,766	4,257	458	$515,740	$8,534.90	$1,522.42
2006	4,927	803	35,378	538	939	5.6	599,553	57,832	4,075,193	4,343	463	$551,835	$8,970.31	$1,612.23
Nongovernment not-for-profit community hospitals														
1975	3,339	658	23,722	510	574	7.8	131,435	57,496	2,131,057	1,712	298	$27,938	$1,040.21	$133.36
1976	3,345	670	24,082	517	586	7.9	140,914	56,442	2,100,917	1,791	306	$32,764	$1,208.23	$152.94
1979	3,330	690	24,874	528	603	7.7	139,565	52,859	2,308,548	1,999	332	$47,937	$1,684.40	$218.06
1980	3,322	692	25,566	542	621	7.7	142,156	52,659	2,389,478	2,086	336	$55,780	$1,901.64	$245.74
1981	3,340	706	25,945	555	636	7.8	143,380	52,302	2,455,033	2,213	399	$66,267	$2,225.17	$285.64
1982	3,338	712	25,898	553	637	7.8	176,245	51,566	2,483,345	2,265	355	$76,806	$2,572.93	$330.41
1983	3,347	718	25,827	544	629	7.7	150,839	51,649	2,465,604	2,270	362	$85,637	$2,868.80	$373.78
1984	3,351	716	25,236	512	598	7.4	153,281	51,491	2,446,540	2,222	372	$90,814	$3,072.51	$415.04
1985	3,349	707	24,179	476	569	7.2	158,953	51,424	2,507,288	2,216	389	$96,150	$3,307.41	$462.69
1986	3,323	689	23,483	460	563	7.2	167,633	50,885	2,547,170	2,241	398	$103,524	$3,589.64	$503.64
1987	3,274	673	22,937	455	566	7.2	177,413	50,133	2,557,294	2,298	406	$112,325	$3,914.23	$543.67
1988	3,242	668	22,939	456	577	7.3	195,363	48,828	2,653,794	2,373	412	$124,703	$4,272.95	$591.13
1989	3,220	661	22,792	455	584	7.3	209,191	48,305	2,751,426	2,454	420	$136,889	$4,649.22	$642.45
1990	3,191	657	22,878	455	596	7.3	221,073	47,441	2,833,204	2,533	424	$150,673	$5,001.24	$692.36
1991	3,175	656	22,964	451	603	7.2	238,204	47,229	2,845,995	2,624	435	$166,806	$5,393.30	$758.21
1992	3,173	656	23,056	445	606	7.1	257,887	47,185	2,846,386	2,692	443	$183,793	$5,808.80	$828.44
1993	3,154	651	22,749	432	602	6.9	270,138	46,214	2,802,164	2,711	451	$197,187	$6,177.69	$897.70
1994	3,139	637	22,704	413	589	6.6	282,653	46,381	2,792,116	2,719	462	$204,219	$6,256.72	$950.31
1995	3,092	610	22,557	393	578	6.4	303,851	45,198	2,725,641	2,702	468	$209,614	$6,279.17	$994.39
1996	3,045	598	22,542	379	567	6.1	320,746	44,650	2,683,750	2,711	478	$215,950	$6,344.05	$1,042.04
1997	3,000	591	22,905	376	575	6.0	330,215	44,484	2,698,086	2,765	481	$225,287	$6,392.74	$1,074.26
1998	3,026	588	23,282	377	587	5.9	352,114	44,087	2,715,958	2,834	483	$237,978	$6,525.68	$1,110.50
1999	3,012	587	23,871	381	605	5.8	370,784	44,172	2,746,453	2,862	473	$251,534	$6,607.51	$1,139.89
2000	3,003	583	24,452	382	618	5.7	393,168	43,655	2,833,615	2,919	472	$267,051	$6,717.48	$1,182.32
2001	2,998	585	24,983	385	628	5.6	404,901	43,640	2,829,691	2,971	473	$287,250	$7,051.76	$1,255.25
2002	3,025	582	25,425	391	646	5.6	416,910	43,241	2,820,159	3,039	471	$312,726	$7,457.84	$1,328.81
2003	2,984	575	25,668	389	647	5.5	424,215	42,965	2,854,764	3,059	473	$337,696	$7,904.93	$1,429.62
2004	2,967	568	25,757	388	655	5.5	430,262	41,968	2,844,617	3,077	470	$359,414	$8,266.64	$1,501.09
2005	2,958	561	25,881	388	667	5.5	441,653	41,585	2,876,677	3,155	473	$385,993	$8,670.83	$1,585.34
2006	2,919	559	25,798	385	671	5.4	453,501	40,888	2,905,275	3,207	478	$412,868	$9,189.58	$1,685.62

Table 1 (Continued)

CLASSIFICATION / YEAR	HOSPITALS	BEDS (in thousands)	ADMISSIONS (in thousands)	AVERAGE DAILY CENSUS (in thousands)	ADJUSTED AVERAGE DAILY CENSUS (in thousands)	AVERAGE LENGTH OF STAY (days)	OUTPATIENT VISITS (in thousands)	NEWBORNS Bassinets	NEWBORNS Births	FTE PERSONNEL Number (in thousands)	FTE PERSONNEL Per 100 Adjusted Census	EXPENSES Amount (in Millions of dollars)	EXPENSES Adjusted per Inpatient Stay	EXPENSES Adjusted per Inpatient Day (dollars)
Investor-owned (for-profit) community hospitals														
1975	775	73	2,646	48	53	6.6	7,713	4,062	141,392	139	263	$2,561	$876.48	$132.80
1976	752	76	2,734	50	54	6.6	8,048	4,044	144,751	147	272	$3,085	$1,031.91	$156.35
1979	727	83	2,963	53	59	6.6	9,289	4,110	174,843	174	300	$4,820	$1,476.42	$225.87
1980	730	87	3,165	57	62	6.5	9,696	4,439	199,722	189	304	$5,847	$1,675.85	$257.12
1981	729	88	3,239	58	63	6.5	9,961	4,523	207,405	203	322	$6,856	$1,952.56	$299.02
1982	748	91	3,316	60	66	6.6	13,193	4,736	219,675	212	320	$8,177	$2,224.75	$340.03
1983	757	94	3,299	59	66	6.5	10,389	5,039	228,883	213	323	$9,208	$2,517.53	$385.42
1984	786	100	3,314	57	64	6.3	11,090	5,807	242,088	214	335	$10,251	$2,748.51	$438.30
1985	805	104	3,242	54	63	6.1	12,378	6,117	266,839	221	350	$11,486	$3,033.06	$500.48
1986	834	107	3,231	54	65	6.1	14,896	6,305	291,112	229	354	$12,987	$3,341.79	$552.40
1987	828	106	3,157	54	66	6.2	16,566	6,391	306,492	242	367	$14,067	$3,617.19	$585.01
1988	790	104	3,090	53	66	6.2	17,926	6,254	308,828	249	379	$15,545	$4,022.77	$649.33
1989	769	102	3,071	53	67	6.3	19,341	6,354	325,711	261	390	$17,240	$4,406.20	$707.90
1990	749	101	3,066	54	69	6.4	20,110	6,261	340,555	273	396	$18,822	$4,727.27	$751.55
1991	738	100	3,016	52	69	6.3	21,174	6,358	359,115	281	409	$20,516	$5,133.53	$820.19
1992	723	99	2,969	51	69	6.3	22,900	6,519	357,776	285	412	$22,496	$5,548.24	$888.73
1993	717	99	2,946	51	69	6.2	24,936	6,395	363,358	289	417	$23,077	$5,643.21	$914.39
1994	719	101	3,035	50	70	6.1	26,443	6,329	354,477	302	434	$23,445	$5,528.91	$923.90
1995	752	106	3,428	55	77	5.8	31,940	7,164	408,339	343	443	$26,653	$5,425.20	$946.99
1996	759	109	3,684	56	82	5.6	37,347	7,441	444,697	359	437	$28,385	$5,207.44	$945.49
1997	797	115	3,953	60	89	5.5	40,919	8,026	465,919	385	433	$31,179	$5,218.69	$961.96
1998	771	113	3,971	58	90	5.5	42,072	7,895	466,025	383	425	$31,732	$5,262.44	$968.00
1999	747	107	3,905	58	86	5.5	39,896	7,486	467,585	362	422	$31,179	$5,350.07	$999.03
2000	749	110	4,141	61	90	5.4	43,378	7,792	503,497	378	418	$34,969	$5,642.18	$1,057.32
2001	754	109	4,197	63	92	5.4	44,706	7,413	494,669	379	413	$37,348	$5,971.81	$1,121.31
2002	766	108	4,365	64	93	5.3	45,215	7,467	496,988	380	407	$40,082	$6,161.44	$1,180.83
2003	790	110	4,481	65	95	5.3	44,246	7,491	515,693	391	411	$43,953	$6,589.91	$1,264.50
2004	835	113	4,599	68	100	5.4	44,962	7,763	534,503	406	406	$48,971	$7,139.13	$1,362.42
2005	868	114	4,618	68	101	5.3	46,016	7,714	546,307	421	418	$51,833	$7,351.96	$1,412.74
2006	890	115	4,735	68	103	5.2	44,237	8,012	574,113	423	413	$55,030	$7,422.08	$1,471.53
State and local government community hospitals														
1975	1,761	210	7,067	148	171	7.6	51,525	22,271	726,103	540	316	$8,463	$1,030.86	$135.64
1976	1,760	210	7,163	146	170	7.5	52,286	21,810	716,548	537	315	$9,391	$1,132.50	$151.00
1979	1,785	211	7,262	146	171	7.4	49,924	20,297	803,621	583	341	$13,247	$1,561.04	$211.89
1980	1,778	209	7,413	149	174	7.3	50,459	20,424	819,282	598	343	$15,204	$1,750.13	$238.63
1981	1,744	210	7,255	150	174	7.6	49,427	19,736	802,963	618	354	$17,449	$2,071.57	$274.25
1982	1,715	210	7,165	149	175	7.6	58,685	19,431	811,437	627	320	$19,893	$2,364.09	$311.56
1983	1,679	207	7,025	145	170	7.6	48,816	18,777	795,767	613	360	$21,593	$2,621.28	$347.56
1984	1,622	201	6,606	133	158	7.3	47,590	18,283	767,680	581	368	$22,271	$2,823.13	$385.17
1985	1,578	189	6,028	119	145	7.2	47,386	17,352	747,008	561	387	$22,863	$3,106.14	$432.84
1986	1,521	182	5,665	114	142	7.4	49,383	16,492	746,126	555	391	$24,143	$3,404.69	$466.17
1987	1,509	180	5,507	113	144	7.5	51,544	15,986	738,510	573	399	$26,192	$3,717.77	$499.33
1988	1,501	175	5,424	112	145	7.6	55,840	15,243	743,780	583	403	$28,474	$4,033.67	$538.63
1989	1,466	170	5,253	110	145	7.7	57,179	14,746	753,478	589	406	$30,769	$4,430.12	$582.15
1990	1,444	169	5,236	111	148	7.7	60,146	14,710	784,504	614	415	$34,198	$4,837.76	$634.45
1991	1,429	168	5,084	108	148	7.8	62,670	13,847	760,286	630	424	$37,701	$5,339.75	$695.89
1992	1,396	166	5,008	108	152	7.9	67,734	13,385	720,782	643	424	$41,806	$5,870.76	$753.92
1993	1,390	169	5,054	109	157	7.8	71,811	13,445	704,854	676	430	$45,825	$6,205.52	$799.73
1994	1,371	164	4,979	104	154	7.6	73,828	13,012	662,774	672	438	$48,115	$6,513.39	$858.62
1995	1,350	157	4,961	100	154	7.4	78,554	12,374	630,718	670	435	$49,322	$6,445.18	$877.85
1996	1,330	155	4,873	96	150	7.2	81,770	11,549	595,424	654	437	$49,420	$6,475.07	$903.41
1997	1,260	148	4,720	92	148	7.1	79,007	10,731	578,186	640	433	$49,298	$6,612.23	$913.62
1998	1,218	139	4,583	87	142	7.0	80,008	10,174	544,250	614	433	$49,123	$6,923.35	$949.36
1999	1,197	136	4,496	86	143	6.9	84,667	9,870	546,257	614	430	$52,534	$7,106.05	$1,006.91
2000	1,163	131	4,634	83	140	6.7	84,858	9,392	543,054	613	438	$54,544	$7,400.01	$1,063.75
2001	1,156	132	4,688	85	145	6.7	88,873	9,395	549,035	637	442	$59,137	$7,772.93	$1,113.79
2002	1,136	130	4,634	84	147	6.6	94,280	9,266	553,044	651	434	$63,783	$8,205.10	$1,188.12
2003	1,121	129	4,634	84	152	6.6	94,725	9,206	545,385	658	431	$68,475	$8,473.18	$1,237.64
2004	1,117	128	4,730	85	154	6.6	96,345	8,979	552,388	666	424	$72,861	$8,793.26	$1,291.06
2005	1,110	128	4,740	85	161	6.5	96,760	8,896	564,782	681	433	$77,914	$9,147.40	$1,329.64
2006	1,119	128	4,848	86	165	6.5	101,845	8,932	595,805	713	433	$83,974		$1,400.09

Table
2

2006 U.S. Registered Hospitals: Utilization, Personnel, and Finances

Excludes U.S.-Associated Areas, Puerto Rico, and nonregistered hospitals.

CLASSIFICATION	HOSPITALS	BEDS	ADMISSIONS	INPATIENT DAYS	ADJUSTED PATIENT DAYS	AVERAGE DAILY CENSUS	ADJUSTED AVERAGE DAILY CENSUS	AVERAGE STAY (days)	SURGICAL OPERATIONS	OUTPATIENT VISITS Emergency	OUTPATIENT VISITS Total	NEWBORNS Bassinets	NEWBORNS Births
UNITED STATES	5,747	947,412	37,188,775	238,203,381	—	653,136	—	—	28,112,193	122,628,450	690,425,395	58,670	4,126,598
6-24 Beds	421	7,188	209,870	908,846	—	2,504	—	—	262,222	1,511,299	9,976,504	505	13,534
25-49	1,171	37,976	1,274,475	6,743,355	—	18,634	—	—	1,261,884	7,809,121	43,309,225	3,048	116,708
50-99	1,227	88,341	2,722,781	20,105,210	—	55,243	—	—	2,336,303	12,144,702	69,279,626	5,806	266,896
100-199	1,306	186,904	7,113,924	44,482,688	—	122,007	—	—	5,771,266	28,025,133	142,409,621	13,204	814,996
200-299	699	171,001	7,314,537	43,078,712	—	118,075	—	—	5,415,552	24,344,525	121,444,563	11,769	819,706
300-399	402	138,092	5,852,121	35,488,902	—	97,235	—	—	4,033,213	17,351,012	90,408,489	8,523	682,838
400-499	205	91,039	3,953,048	24,424,839	—	66,918	—	—	2,876,508	10,569,145	65,617,888	5,176	450,952
500 or more	316	226,871	8,748,019	62,970,829	—	172,520	—	—	6,155,245	20,873,513	147,979,479	10,639	960,968
Psychiatric	462	84,322	723,906	26,098,172	—	71,518	—	—	19,847	153,708	8,241,833	0	0
Hospitals	454	80,329	723,328	25,212,172	—	69,090	—	—	19,847	153,708	8,237,097	0	0
Institutions for mentally retarded	8	3,993	578	886,000	—	2,428	—	—	0	0	4,736	0	0
General	4,771	815,947	35,594,789	199,829,412	—	547,948	—	—	27,431,696	121,496,288	663,824,771	57,769	4,052,307
Hospitals	4,749	813,506	35,571,147	199,162,759	—	546,124	—	—	27,430,207	121,462,721	663,546,848	57,769	4,052,307
Hospital units of institutions	22	2,441	23,642	666,653	—	1,824	—	—	1,489	33,567	277,923	0	0
TB and other respiratory diseases	2	97	141	19,454	—	54	—	—	0	0	1,499	6	0
Obstetrics and gynecology	17	2,238	124,571	564,950	—	1,550	—	—	86,015	164,448	1,160,714	804	68,926
Eye, ear, nose and throat	6	190	4,287	10,742	—	29	—	—	75,220	55,918	694,349	0	0
Rehabilitation	198	15,106	270,245	3,814,271	—	10,470	—	—	84,204	8,916	6,347,934	24	692
Orthopedic	25	1,427	56,861	263,930	—	723	—	—	96,566	61,607	894,026	0	0
Chronic Disease	8	743	6,209	227,515	—	624	—	—	2,296	6,627	119,541	0	0
Surgical	13	255	15,469	27,372	—	76	—	—	56,994	24,337	459,099	22	1,306
Cancer	11	1,776	75,697	527,963	—	1,446	—	—	64,712	25,741	2,999,222	0	0
Heart	8	708	54,174	205,961	—	564	—	—	36,721	40,203	167,128	0	0
Acute long-term care hospital	181	17,817	142,826	4,807,386	—	13,184	—	—	68,028	289,198	1,721,567	23	1,130
All other	45	6,786	119,600	1,806,253	—	4,950	—	—	89,894	301,459	3,793,712	22	2,237
Federal	221	46,691	1,008,486	11,324,376	—	31,025	—	—	756,031	3,867,623	83,973,864	814	51,371
Psychiatric	11	4,354	27,436	1,257,252	—	3,445	—	—	16,404	0	2,992,169	0	0
General and other special	210	42,337	981,050	10,067,124	—	27,580	—	—	739,627	3,867,623	80,981,695	814	51,371
Nonfederal	5,526	900,721	36,180,289	226,879,005	—	622,111	—	—	27,356,162	118,760,827	606,451,531	57,856	4,075,227
Psychiatric	451	79,968	696,470	24,840,920	—	68,073	—	—	3,443	153,708	5,249,664	0	0
Hospitals	443	75,975	695,892	23,954,920	—	65,645	—	—	3,443	153,708	5,244,928	0	0
Institutions for mentally retarded	8	3,993	578	886,000	—	2,428	—	—	0	0	4,736	0	0
TB and other respiratory diseases	2	97	141	19,454	—	54	—	—	0	0	1,499	6	0
Long-term general and other special	127	16,165	83,768	5,103,462	—	13,987	—	—	21,895	227,640	1,633,484	18	34
Short-term general and other special	4,946	804,491	35,399,910	196,915,169	—	539,997	—	—	27,330,824	118,379,479	599,566,884	57,832	4,075,193
Hospital units of institutions	19	1,833	22,251	548,657	—	1,501	—	—	0	5,450	13,859	0	0
Community Hospitals	4,927	802,658	35,377,659	196,366,512	342,281,133	538,496	938,580	5.6	27,330,824	118,374,029	599,553,025	57,832	4,075,193
6-24 Beds	375	6,446	191,951	772,553	2,939,621	2,122	8,062	4.0	250,147	1,269,428	7,802,940	458	12,310
25-49	1,066	34,217	1,187,667	5,837,190	16,552,272	16,149	45,580	4.9	1,212,190	7,198,343	37,053,602	2,857	108,279
50-99	969	69,408	2,300,638	14,534,929	32,354,104	39,970	88,962	6.3	2,180,211	11,175,926	52,974,785	5,488	249,458
100-199	1,117	160,426	6,661,921	36,835,335	70,991,261	101,054	194,707	5.5	5,629,729	27,389,126	124,426,326	13,092	806,893
200-299	607	148,541	7,007,798	36,681,087	61,096,942	100,555	167,456	5.2	5,237,059	23,583,282	103,431,461	11,599	803,495
300-399	354	121,747	5,720,821	30,853,206	49,178,882	84,533	134,729	5.4	3,980,191	17,144,271	82,916,312	8,523	682,838
400-499	180	79,732	3,871,574	20,851,846	32,931,013	57,128	90,216	5.4	2,837,465	10,442,303	60,439,877	5,176	450,952
500 or more	259	182,141	8,435,289	50,000,366	76,237,038	136,985	208,868	5.9	6,003,832	20,171,350	130,507,722	10,639	960,968
Nongovernment not-for-profit	2,919	559,216	25,797,616	140,275,730	244,934,607	384,522	671,387	5.4	20,038,250	83,394,426	453,501,060	40,888	2,905,275
Investor-owned (for profit)	889	115,337	4,731,773	24,658,958	37,369,075	67,680	102,582	5.2	3,689,801	15,703,033	44,207,427	8,012	574,113
State and Local Government	1,119	128,105	4,848,270	31,431,824	59,977,451	86,294	164,611	6.5	3,602,773	19,276,570	101,844,538	8,932	595,805

Table 2 (Continued)

CLASSIFICATION	FULL-TIME EQUIVALENT PERSONNEL					FULL-TIME EQUIVALENT TRAINEES			LABOR				EXPENSES TOTAL	TOTAL	
	Physicians and Dentists	Registered Nurses	Licensed Practical Nurses	Other Salaried Personnel	Total Personnel	Medical and Dental Residents	Other Trainees	Total Trainees	Payroll (in thousands)	Employee Benefits (in thousands)	Total (in thousands)	Percent of Total	Amount (in thousands)	Adjusted per Admission	Adjusted per Inpatient Day
UNITED STATES	113,870	1,227,951	139,009	3,426,541	4,907,371	97,234	13,679	110,913	$253,891,018	$65,669,628	$319,560,647	52.6	$607,355,354	—	—
6-24 Beds	1,228	8,668	2,954	32,425	45,275	161	46	207	$2,007,152	$702,015	$2,709,167	58.8	$4,608,752	—	—
25-49	4,943	43,989	11,814	159,547	220,293	275	468	743	$9,404,677	$2,324,331	$11,729,008	53.7	$21,840,922	—	—
50-99	8,873	83,608	18,185	283,604	394,270	1,216	876	2,092	$17,846,288	$4,520,571	$22,366,859	54.5	$41,060,250	—	—
100-199	18,180	214,272	31,121	614,413	877,986	6,452	717	7,169	$42,888,497	$11,006,856	$53,895,353	53.0	$101,707,669	—	—
200-299	18,389	225,801	23,458	612,396	880,044	10,563	1,621	12,184	$44,888,916	$11,709,092	$56,598,007	52.2	$108,347,048	—	—
300-399	14,081	182,704	17,396	486,049	700,230	11,417	2,096	13,513	$37,114,959	$9,480,590	$46,595,549	52.4	$88,993,552	—	—
400-499	10,141	138,493	10,926	358,446	518,006	14,467	1,518	15,985	$28,399,745	$7,378,017	$35,777,762	51.9	$68,994,776	—	—
500 or more	38,035	330,416	23,155	879,661	1,271,267	52,683	6,337	59,020	$71,340,784	$18,548,157	$89,888,941	52.3	$171,862,386	—	—
Psychiatric	5,047	25,437	8,298	154,503	193,285	522	318	840	$8,573,851	$2,674,852	$11,248,703	74.8	$15,043,142	—	—
Hospitals	5,009	25,177	7,958	147,011	185,155	522	318	840	$8,311,830	$2,598,089	$10,909,918	74.5	$14,646,830	—	—
Institutions for mentally retarded	38	260	340	7,492	8,130	0	0	0	$262,021	$76,763	$338,784	85.5	$396,312	—	—
General	103,293	1,162,054	122,416	3,123,255	4,511,018	94,193	12,149	106,342	$234,870,466	$60,453,576	$295,324,042	52.0	$568,114,301	—	—
Hospitals	103,002	1,161,388	121,832	3,119,888	4,506,110	94,176	12,144	106,320	$234,537,946	$60,333,652	$294,871,599	52.0	$567,551,192	—	—
Hospital units of institutions	291	666	584	3,367	4,908	17	5	22	$332,520	$119,924	$452,444	80.3	$563,109	—	—
TB and other respiratory diseases	0	22	17	131	170	0	0	0	$6,356	$2,102	$8,458	53.3	$15,861	—	—
Obstetrics and gynecology	142	4,144	213	7,975	12,474	43	4	47	$663,932	$156,290	$820,222	56.2	$1,459,347	—	—
Eye, ear, nose and throat	132	456	22	2,045	2,655	101	42	143	$129,044	$37,253	$166,297	47.5	$350,394	—	—
Rehabilitation	538	10,165	2,728	42,912	56,343	137	9	146	$2,413,853	$543,165	$2,957,018	56.6	$5,223,677	—	—
Orthopedic	378	2,102	162	7,454	10,096	76	9	85	$634,530	$164,987	$799,517	49.2	$1,625,902	—	—
Chronic Disease	41	380	147	1,842	2,410	0	7	7	$115,860	$27,199	$143,058	57.5	$248,835	—	—
Surgical	78	517	121	1,246	1,962	12	0	12	$106,174	$29,317	$135,492	47.1	$287,796	—	—
Cancer	2,366	6,146	139	28,391	37,042	1,218	804	2,022	$2,285,008	$592,652	$2,877,660	49.6	$5,803,782	—	—
Heart	38	1,491	28	2,728	4,285	0	0	0	$264,656	$66,273	$330,929	45.6	$725,017	—	—
Acute long-term care hospital	456	9,233	3,526	32,888	46,103	81	5	86	$2,222,049	$507,580	$2,729,629	55.9	$4,881,421	—	—
All other	1,361	5,804	1,192	21,171	29,528	851	332	1,183	$1,605,239	$414,382	$2,019,621	56.5	$3,575,880	—	—
Federal	26,390	58,189	15,442	238,540	338,561	11,384	5,944	17,328	$18,000,051	$4,882,281	$22,882,332	60.9	$37,553,880	—	—
Psychiatric	594	1,928	1,021	10,096	13,639	12	18	30	$864,442	$207,915	$1,072,357	70.4	$1,523,839	—	—
General and other special	25,796	56,261	14,421	228,444	324,922	11,372	5,926	17,298	$17,135,608	$4,674,366	$21,809,975	60.5	$36,030,041	—	—
Nonfederal	87,480	1,169,762	123,567	3,188,001	4,568,810	85,850	7,735	93,585	$235,890,968	$60,787,347	$296,678,315	52.1	$569,801,474	—	—
Psychiatric	4,453	23,509	7,277	144,407	179,646	510	300	810	$7,709,408	$2,466,937	$10,176,345	75.3	$13,519,303	—	—
Hospitals	4,415	23,249	6,937	136,915	171,516	510	300	810	$7,447,387	$2,390,174	$9,837,561	75.0	$13,122,991	—	—
Institutions for mentally retarded	38	260	340	7,492	8,130	0	0	0	$262,021	$76,763	$338,784	85.5	$396,312	—	—
Long-term general and other special	568	7,089	2,942	32,051	42,650	20	7	27	$2,041,085	$467,045	$2,508,130	62.3	$4,026,006	—	—
Short-term general and other special	82,459	1,139,142	113,331	3,011,412	4,346,344	85,320	7,428	92,748	$226,134,118	$57,851,263	$283,985,381	51.4	$552,240,305	—	—
Hospital units of institutions	210	509	434	1,711	2,864	0	0	0	$242,075	$69,736	$311,811	77.0	$404,976	—	—
Community Hospitals	82,249	1,138,633	112,897	3,009,701	4,343,480	85,320	7,428	92,748	$225,892,043	$57,781,527	$283,673,570	51.4	$551,835,328	$8,970.31	$1,612.23
6-24 Beds	590	7,436	2,023	26,253	36,302	24	5	29	$1,505,818	$366,730	$1,872,547	51.4	$3,644,293	$4,614.85	$1,239.72
25-49	3,375	40,434	10,446	140,784	195,039	231	219	450	$8,415,220	$2,110,511	$10,525,732	52.6	$20,009,399	$5,790.71	$1,208.86
50-99	4,011	70,534	14,017	218,787	307,349	253	118	371	$13,856,606	$3,592,532	$17,449,138	52.9	$32,959,605	$6,466.30	$1,018.71
100-199	12,543	195,902	25,707	536,811	770,963	4,500	429	4,929	$37,558,757	$9,591,230	$47,149,987	52.0	$90,741,588	$7,233.32	$1,278.21
200-299	10,626	207,784	19,322	530,235	767,967	8,128	944	9,072	$40,060,629	$10,290,043	$50,350,672	51.2	$98,273,431	$8,485.15	$1,608.48
300-399	11,536	174,446	14,711	448,812	649,505	10,330	636	10,966	$34,313,535	$8,722,030	$43,035,564	51.4	$83,742,334	$9,194.09	$1,702.81
400-499	8,334	133,513	9,090	332,341	483,278	14,046	1,434	15,480	$26,523,418	$6,787,814	$33,311,231	51.2	$65,100,973	$10,661.60	$1,976.89
500 or more	31,234	308,584	17,581	775,678	1,133,077	47,808	3,643	51,451	$63,658,061	$16,320,637	$79,978,697	50.8	$157,363,704	$12,260.94	$2,064.14
Nongovernment not-for-profit	65,018	835,540	69,265	2,237,635	3,207,458	60,366	5,618	65,984	$169,129,068	$43,715,293	$212,844,361	51.6	$412,867,575	$9,189.58	$1,685.62
Investor-owned (for profit)	1,777	129,573	19,133	272,704	423,187	2,426	251	2,677	$21,007,074	$4,568,674	$25,575,748	46.5	$54,994,199	$7,421.49	$1,471.65
State and Local Government	15,454	173,520	24,499	499,362	712,835	22,528	1,559	24,087	$35,755,902	$9,497,560	$45,253,462	53.9	$83,973,554	$9,147.40	$1,400.09

TABLE 4

BED SIZE CATEGORY 6-24

U.S. Registered Community Hospitals
(Nonfederal, short-term general and other special hospitals)

Utilization, Personnel, Revenue and Expenses 2002–2006

	2006	2005	2004	2003	2002
TOTAL FACILITY (Includes Hospital and Nursing Home Units)					
Utilization - Inpatient					
Beds	6,446	6,316	6,030	5,635	5,629
Admissions	191,951	185,689	181,662	162,231	161,716
Inpatient Days	772,553	772,972	745,115	658,374	666,858
Average Length of Stay.	4.0	4.2	4.1	4.1	4.1
Inpatient Surgeries.	37,527	36,766	36,110	33,263	26,172
Births.	12,310	12,004	10,695	9,347	10,297
Utilization - Outpatient					
Emergency Outpatient Visits	1,269,428	1,312,747	1,223,838	1,159,015	1,053,994
Other Outpatient Visits.	6,533,512	6,657,699	6,018,718	5,353,309	4,875,803
Total Outpatient Visits	7,802,940	7,970,446	7,242,556	6,512,324	5,929,797
Outpatient Surgeries	212,620	209,196	194,560	176,609	160,854
Personnel					
Full Time RNs	5,759	5,438	5,058	4,612	4,451
Full Time LPNs	1,632	1,633	1,794	1,710	1,677
Part Time RNs.	3,354	3,374	3,064	2,647	2,498
Part Time LPNs	800	782	783	779	709
Total Full Time.	29,489	28,924	26,579	24,113	23,058
Total Part Time	13,707	13,649	12,320	10,942	10,753
Revenue - Inpatient					
Gross Inpatient Revenue.	$1,828,399,829	$1,794,653,960	$1,722,861,214	$1,238,430,927	$1,187,061,180
Revenue - Outpatient					
Gross Outpatient Revenue	$4,642,506,692	$4,326,712,250	$3,677,188,569	$2,945,148,175	$2,471,688,778
Revenue and Expenses - Totals					
(Includes Inpatient and Outpatient)					
Total Gross Revenue.	$6,470,906,521	$6,121,366,210	$5,400,049,783	$4,183,579,102	$3,658,749,958
Deductions from Revenue.	3,001,843,000	2,937,005,012	2,539,972,888	1,799,934,162	1,513,681,706
Net Patient Revenue	3,469,063,521	3,184,361,198	2,860,076,895	2,383,644,940	2,145,068,252
Other Operating Revenue	323,188,226	299,545,114	192,978,846	198,380,153	162,911,063
Other Nonoperating Revenue	86,665,700	61,973,855	41,904,855	36,877,876	28,315,990
Total Net Revenue.	3,891,511,549	3,545,880,167	3,094,960,596	2,618,902,969	2,336,295,305
Total Expenses.	3,644,293,348	3,494,293,653	2,922,377,161	2,456,994,289	2,235,953,879
HOSPITAL UNIT (Excludes Separate Nursing Home Units)					
Utilization - Inpatient					
Beds	6,355	6,210	5,902	5,569	5,470
Admissions	191,730	185,287	181,141	162,101	161,090
Inpatient Days	740,244	741,578	710,462	639,363	619,452
Average Length of Stay.	3.9	4.0	3.9	3.9	3.8
Personnel					
Total Full Time.	29,285	28,752	26,475	23,964	22,960
Total Part Time	13,619	13,519	12,211	10,854	10,689
Revenue and Expenses - Totals					
(Includes Inpatient and Outpatient)					
Total Net Revenue.	$3,882,018,849	$3,535,620,933	$3,082,667,170	$2,612,681,706	$2,324,685,737
Total Expenses.	3,636,207,924	3,486,754,501	2,914,954,576	2,454,449,892	2,230,173,614

Bed Size Categories

TABLE 4

BED SIZE CATEGORY 25-49

U.S. Registered Community Hospitals
(Nonfederal, short-term general and other special hospitals)

Overview 2002–2006

	2006	2005	2004	2003	2002
Total Community Hospitals in Bed Size Category 25-49	**1,066**	**1,032**	**988**	**965**	**931**
Location					
Hospitals Urban	341	319	237	225	220
Hospitals Rural	725	713	751	740	711
Control					
State and Local Government	395	388	375	371	363
Not for Profit	506	492	479	475	461
Investor owned	165	152	134	119	107
Physician Models					
Independent Practice Association	134	120	132	130	128
Group Practice without Walls	32	35	27	28	27
Open Physician-Hospital Organization	95	96	88	88	87
Closed Physician-Hospital Organization . . .	32	28	24	32	33
Management Service Organization	54	48	54	55	56
Integrated Salary Model	292	257	250	252	212
Equity Model	13	6	6	7	6
Foundation	36	29	24	23	19
Insurance Products					
Health Maintenance Organization	84	87	94	86	78
Preferred Provider Organization	154	171	172	171	152
Indemnity Fee for Service	48	53	48	53	41
Managed Care Contracts					
Health Maintenance Organization	433	422	415	424	421
Preferred Provider Organization	633	618	597	591	578
Affiliations					
Hospitals in a System*	507	485	451	428	393
Hospitals in a Network	301	277	278	249	221
Hospitals in a Group Purchasing Organization	768	739	669	699	643

---

* Please note that system affiliate information for hospitals is derived from AHA membership. In years prior to 2003 the affiliation was derived from a question on the AHA Annual Survey of hospitals; therefore, non-responding hospitals were not included in the system affiliation counts. Years prior to 2003 have been updated to reflect this change, which now include affiliation for non-reporting hospitals.

14   AHA Hospital Statistics © 2008 Health Forum LLC, an affiliate of the American Hospital Association

TABLE 4

BED SIZE CATEGORY 200-299

U.S. Registered Community Hospitals
(Nonfederal, short-term general and other special hospitals)

Utilization, Personnel, Revenue and Expenses 2002–2006

	2006	2005	2004	2003	2002
TOTAL FACILITY (Includes Hospital and Nursing Home Units)					
Utilization - Inpatient					
Beds	148,541	151,290	151,197	152,487	152,682
Admissions	7,007,798	7,075,077	6,928,872	6,887,304	6,799,664
Inpatient Days	36,681,087	37,345,741	37,128,574	37,271,468	37,122,247
Average Length of Stay	5.2	5.3	5.4	5.4	5.5
Inpatient Surgeries	1,981,815	2,052,544	1,976,550	1,985,604	1,957,651
Births	803,495	807,357	783,857	764,095	753,559
Utilization - Outpatient					
Emergency Outpatient Visits	23,583,282	22,775,575	21,997,288	21,701,788	21,513,390
Other Outpatient Visits	79,848,179	84,556,147	77,828,723	78,393,455	80,910,560
Total Outpatient Visits	103,431,461	107,331,722	99,826,011	100,095,243	102,423,950
Outpatient Surgeries	3,255,244	3,456,049	3,507,669	3,435,799	3,394,622
Personnel					
Full Time RNs	161,572	159,272	150,192	146,013	141,467
Full Time LPNs	15,865	17,210	16,612	18,329	18,402
Part Time RNs	92,421	93,256	90,059	87,456	85,147
Part Time LPNs	6,919	7,525	8,246	8,691	8,442
Total Full Time	641,525	647,445	618,528	618,665	616,865
Total Part Time	271,052	276,003	268,734	271,315	260,312
Revenue - Inpatient					
Gross Inpatient Revenue	$180,028,152,728	$170,616,345,762	$155,294,785,296	$138,068,942,960	$119,690,492,836
Revenue - Outpatient					
Gross Outpatient Revenue	$103,386,338,141	$94,794,997,798	$82,164,264,391	$72,993,639,658	$64,425,216,711
Revenue and Expenses - Totals (Includes Inpatient and Outpatient)					
Total Gross Revenue	$283,414,490,869	$265,411,343,560	$237,459,049,687	$211,062,582,618	$184,115,709,547
Deductions from Revenue	186,023,673,013	172,106,934,465	151,887,190,782	130,733,370,398	108,902,937,426
Net Patient Revenue	97,390,817,856	93,304,409,095	85,571,858,905	80,329,212,220	75,212,772,121
Other Operating Revenue	5,003,781,859	4,083,925,703	3,962,288,724	3,686,516,113	3,204,222,444
Other Nonoperating Revenue	2,257,123,002	1,672,783,382	1,510,698,932	1,211,869,399	836,318,819
Total Net Revenue	104,622,047,660	99,061,118,180	91,044,846,561	85,227,597,732	79,253,313,384
Total Expenses	98,273,430,973	93,355,766,103	86,077,421,150	81,020,518,283	75,580,360,702
HOSPITAL UNIT (Excludes Separate Nursing Home Units)					
Utilization - Inpatient					
Beds	138,521	141,761	140,504	140,386	140,310
Admissions	6,933,995	7,003,676	6,857,430	6,798,001	6,706,901
Inpatient Days	33,409,499	34,317,326	33,667,207	33,411,165	33,216,134
Average Length of Stay	4.8	4.9	4.9	4.9	5.0
Personnel					
Total Full Time	633,780	640,026	602,684	609,113	608,134
Total Part Time	267,116	272,208	261,307	266,160	256,082
Revenue and Expenses - Totals (Includes Inpatient and Outpatient)					
Total Net Revenue	$103,386,452,224	$98,249,103,654	$90,313,938,352	$84,316,957,990	$78,446,952,108
Total Expenses	97,628,510,565	92,716,630,522	85,489,134,699	80,276,845,970	74,919,598,886

Bed Size Categories

TABLE 4

BED SIZE CATEGORY 300-399

U.S. Registered Community Hospitals
(Nonfederal, short-term general and other special hospitals)

Overview 2002–2006

	2006	2005	2004	2003	2002
Total Community Hospitals in Bed Size Category 300-399	354	368	351	349	358
Location					
Hospitals Urban......................	332	345	327	320	328
Hospitals Rural	22	23	24	29	30
Control					
State and Local Government	50	48	47	43	41
Not for Profit	259	277	258	263	270
Investor owned	45	43	46	43	47
Physician Models					
Independent Practice Association........	59	73	58	72	81
Group Practice without Walls...........	13	12	10	10	14
Open Physician-Hospital Organization....	65	71	76	78	89
Closed Physician-Hospital Organization...	21	33	34	38	38
Management Service Organization.......	53	58	55	59	65
Integrated Salary Model	132	131	118	119	108
Equity Model	3	5	4	4	6
Foundation.........................	23	33	25	22	20
Insurance Products					
Health Maintenance Organization........	78	76	82	79	80
Preferred Provider Organization.........	78	84	84	83	88
Indemnity Fee for Service..............	23	24	28	23	19
Managed Care Contracts					
Health Maintenance Organization........	254	262	253	255	257
Preferred Provider Organization.........	263	270	255	257	263
Affiliations					
Hospitals in a System*	220	233	218	221	224
Hospitals in a Network	129	120	117	113	122
Hospitals in a Group Purchasing Organization......................	283	291	274	285	270

* Please note that system affiliate information for hospitals is derived from AHA membership. In years prior to 2003 the affiliation was derived from a question on the AHA Annual Survey of hospitals; therefore, non-responding hospitals were not included in the system affiliation counts. Years prior to 2003 have been updated to reflect this change, which now include affiliation for non-reporting hospitals.

TABLE 4

BED SIZE CATEGORY 300-399

U.S. Registered Community Hospitals
(Nonfederal, short-term general and other special hospitals)

Utilization, Personnel, Revenue and Expenses 2002–2006

	2006	2005	2004	2003	2002
TOTAL FACILITY (Includes Hospital and Nursing Home Units)					
Utilization - Inpatient					
Beds	121,747	126,899	120,509	119,903	123,399
Admissions	5,720,821	6,025,261	5,764,742	5,589,833	5,606,593
Inpatient Days	30,853,206	32,448,452	30,711,591	29,998,416	30,625,907
Average Length of Stay	5.4	5.4	5.3	5.4	5.5
Inpatient Surgeries	1,634,694	1,725,447	1,659,042	1,596,627	1,670,246
Births	682,838	710,328	681,445	662,053	634,624
Utilization - Outpatient					
Emergency Outpatient Visits	17,144,271	17,521,842	16,519,917	15,897,067	16,337,980
Other Outpatient Visits	65,772,041	67,844,183	67,812,543	65,040,946	62,754,461
Total Outpatient Visits	82,916,312	85,366,025	84,332,460	80,938,013	79,092,441
Outpatient Surgeries	2,345,497	2,470,707	2,414,313	2,400,933	2,501,205
Personnel					
Full Time RNs	139,473	141,847	130,202	124,882	124,773
Full Time LPNs	12,244	13,443	14,178	14,381	15,634
Part Time RNs	69,952	74,727	70,366	71,225	66,826
Part Time LPNs	4,932	5,408	5,510	5,717	5,895
Total Full Time	554,388	568,290	536,011	534,706	546,123
Total Part Time	212,170	219,278	212,832	208,123	198,483
Revenue - Inpatient					
Gross Inpatient Revenue	$159,727,014,412	$159,263,214,837	$139,637,421,386	$122,641,223,447	$104,931,029,759
Revenue - Outpatient					
Gross Outpatient Revenue	$85,030,303,818	$82,354,123,219	$69,588,216,914	$59,808,208,882	$52,506,396,042
Revenue and Expenses - Totals **(Includes Inpatient and Outpatient)**					
Total Gross Revenue	$244,757,318,230	$241,617,338,056	$209,225,638,300	$182,449,432,329	$157,437,425,801
Deductions from Revenue	161,994,484,185	158,773,214,706	134,268,491,890	114,079,609,997	92,566,575,914
Net Patient Revenue	82,762,834,045	82,844,123,350	74,957,146,410	68,369,822,332	64,870,849,887
Other Operating Revenue	4,311,575,332	4,584,684,323	4,238,436,521	4,730,386,954	3,898,682,632
Other Nonoperating Revenue	1,820,794,415	1,454,600,821	1,504,494,878	1,184,335,242	518,357,079
Total Net Revenue	88,895,203,792	88,883,408,494	80,700,077,809	74,284,544,528	69,287,889,598
Total Expenses	83,742,334,417	83,960,197,153	76,000,965,751	70,380,924,713	66,128,522,671
HOSPITAL UNIT (Excludes Separate Nursing Home Units)					
Utilization - Inpatient					
Beds	114,872	120,190	114,080	113,798	116,100
Admissions	5,673,915	5,973,783	5,713,580	5,542,090	5,547,159
Inpatient Days	28,602,063	30,289,334	28,646,372	28,032,233	28,315,464
Average Length of Stay	5.0	5.1	5.0	5.1	5.1
Personnel					
Total Full Time	548,927	562,625	522,514	529,334	539,889
Total Part Time	209,541	216,580	207,159	205,408	195,895
Revenue and Expenses - Totals **(Includes Inpatient and Outpatient)**					
Total Net Revenue	$87,874,129,969	$88,248,210,144	$80,124,386,205	$73,673,285,779	$68,590,373,760
Total Expenses	83,178,661,808	83,379,302,567	75,569,639,844	69,826,896,240	65,561,221,517

TABLE 4

BED SIZE CATEGORY 400-499

U.S. Registered Community Hospitals
(Nonfederal, short-term general and other special hospitals)

Overview 2002–2006

	2006	2005	2004	2003	2002
Total Community Hospitals in Bed Size Category 400-499	180	173	185	172	174
Location					
Hospitals Urban	176	169	177	168	170
Hospitals Rural	4	4	8	4	4
Control					
State and Local Government	24	24	23	22	27
Not for Profit	141	138	150	141	139
Investor owned	15	11	12	9	8
Physician Models					
Independent Practice Association	27	22	31	40	34
Group Practice without Walls	8	8	9	10	6
Open Physician-Hospital Organization	45	35	47	41	37
Closed Physician-Hospital Organization...	21	17	14	15	19
Management Service Organization	31	25	36	38	34
Integrated Salary Model	81	72	73	58	63
Equity Model	2	4	4	3	5
Foundation	17	16	17	19	17
Insurance Products					
Health Maintenance Organization	42	36	43	46	54
Preferred Provider Organization	64	56	51	50	54
Indemnity Fee for Service	14	15	15	12	17
Managed Care Contracts					
Health Maintenance Organization	137	122	144	136	131
Preferred Provider Organization	147	127	145	136	135
Affiliations					
Hospitals in a System*	121	108	113	99	103
Hospitals in a Network	74	62	74	62	52
Hospitals in a Group Purchasing Organization	155	138	150	138	127

Bed Size Categories

Census Divisions

Census Division 1	**New England** Connecticut, Maine, Massachusetts, New Hampshire, Rhode Island, Vermont
Census Division 2	**Middle Atlantic** New Jersey, New York, Pennsylvania
Census Division 3	**South Atlantic** Delaware, District of Columbia, Florida, Georgia, Maryland, North Carolina, South Carolina, Virginia, West Virginia
Census Division 4	**East North Central** Illinois, Indiana, Michigan, Ohio, Wisconsin
Census Division 5	**East South Central** Alabama, Kentucky, Mississippi, Tennessee
Census Division 6	**West North Central** Iowa, Kansas, Minnesota, Missouri, Nebraska, North Dakota, South Dakota
Census Division 7	**West South Central** Arkansas, Louisiana, Oklahoma, Texas
Census Division 8	**Mountain** Arizona, Colorado, Idaho, Montana, Nevada, New Mexico, Utah, Wyoming
Census Division 9	**Pacific** Alaska, California, Hawaii, Oregon, Washington

U.S. Census Divisions

TABLE 5

U.S. CENSUS DIVISION 1: NEW ENGLAND

U.S. Registered Community Hospitals
(Nonfederal, short-term general and other special hospitals)

Overview 2002–2006

	2006	2005	2004	2003	2002
Total Community Hospitals in Census Division 1, New England	205	206	203	203	203
Bed Size Category					
6-24	9	8	4	6	8
25-49	38	42	43	36	32
50-99	44	44	43	46	46
100-199	56	54	56	61	58
200-299	26	29	25	28	30
300-399	16	13	16	12	15
400-499	3	3	2	2	1
500 + ...	13	13	14	12	13
Location					
Hospitals Urban..........................	147	148	126	126	126
Hospitals Rural	58	58	77	77	77
Control					
State and Local Government...............	6	6	6	6	7
Not for Profit.............................	183	184	182	183	185
Investor owned	16	16	15	14	11
Physician Models					
Independent Practice Association	50	56	54	58	58
Group Practice without Walls................	8	11	10	13	16
Open Physician-Hospital Organization	58	60	61	63	66
Closed Physician-Hospital Organization	17	14	12	15	18
Management Service Organization	21	23	25	26	33
Integrated Salary Model....................	101	96	90	82	73
Equity Model	5	5	3	6	6
Foundation................................	11	12	9	11	13
Insurance Products					
Health Maintenance Organization	20	21	25	22	23
Preferred Provider Organization..............	21	25	27	26	22
Indemnity Fee for Service	9	11	11	9	5
Managed Care Contracts					
Health Maintenance Organization	149	155	152	153	156
Preferred Provider Organization..............	142	151	147	150	143
Affiliations					
Hospitals in a System*.....................	79	74	71	71	71
Hospitals in a Network.....................	77	79	70	63	60
Hospitals in a Group Purchasing Organization..	174	168	160	171	161

* Please note that system affiliate information for hospitals is derived from AHA membership. In years prior to 2003 the affiliation was derived from a question on the AHA Annual Survey of hospitals; therefore, non-responding hospitals were not included in the system affiliation counts. Years prior to 2003 have been updated to reflect this change, which now include affiliation for non-reporting hospitals.

U.S. Census Divisions

TABLE 5

U.S. CENSUS DIVISION 1: NEW ENGLAND

U.S. Registered Community Hospitals
(Nonfederal, short-term general and other special hospitals)

Utilization, Personnel, Revenue and Expenses, Community Health Indicators 2002–2006

	2006	2005	2004	2003	2002
TOTAL FACILITY (Includes Hospital and Nursing Home Units)					
Utilization - Inpatient					
Beds	34,353	34,207	34,267	33,600	34,324
Admissions	1,688,920	1,651,462	1,637,291	1,598,123	1,580,396
Inpatient Days	9,240,145	9,213,139	9,158,050	8,854,347	9,120,976
Average Length of Stay	5.5	5.6	5.6	5.5	5.8
Inpatient Surgeries	444,881	463,184	455,130	454,152	459,541
Births	182,170	188,628	168,615	169,753	168,792
Utilization - Outpatient					
Emergency Outpatient Visits	6,691,531	6,379,473	6,262,078	6,275,074	6,233,520
Other Outpatient Visits	33,649,121	32,672,509	31,283,835	31,540,633	29,869,397
Total Outpatient Visits	40,340,652	39,051,982	37,545,913	37,815,707	36,102,917
Outpatient Surgeries	1,056,911	1,067,889	1,104,291	1,036,806	1,004,499
Personnel					
Full Time RNs	39,126	37,724	36,852	35,156	33,504
Full Time LPNs	2,069	2,067	2,185	2,189	2,408
Part Time RNs	37,918	35,874	35,790	34,385	33,457
Part Time LPNs	1,706	2,199	2,040	2,083	2,160
Total Full Time	198,629	192,138	187,759	186,008	186,629
Total Part Time	116,013	110,168	109,769	108,478	105,969
Revenue - Inpatient					
Gross Inpatient Revenue	$37,170,857,983	$33,302,111,863	$31,824,799,153	$28,271,467,530	$25,243,211,994
Revenue - Outpatient					
Gross Outpatient Revenue	$35,925,073,139	$31,378,420,843	$27,637,479,556	$24,060,068,236	$20,277,289,066
Revenue and Expenses - Totals					
(Includes Inpatient and Outpatient)					
Total Gross Revenue	$73,095,931,122	$64,680,532,706	$59,462,278,709	$52,331,535,766	$45,520,501,060
Deductions from Revenue	40,515,901,458	35,025,138,133	32,160,783,569	27,574,266,243	22,938,130,804
Net Patient Revenue	32,580,029,664	29,655,394,573	27,301,495,140	24,757,269,523	22,582,370,256
Other Operating Revenue	3,113,979,625	2,601,207,927	2,606,545,163	3,069,276,617	2,275,478,442
Other Nonoperating Revenue	748,697,662	523,042,046	473,318,177	210,317,295	69,173,336
Total Net Revenue	36,442,706,951	32,779,644,546	30,381,358,480	28,036,863,435	24,927,022,034
Total Expenses	34,779,690,838	31,439,056,968	29,161,999,714	26,783,737,017	24,762,701,274
HOSPITAL UNIT (Excludes Separate Nursing Home Units)					
Utilization - Inpatient					
Beds	32,825	32,330	32,598	31,720	32,069
Admissions	1,675,178	1,636,168	1,623,243	1,577,277	1,563,633
Inpatient Days	8,728,611	8,586,567	8,590,889	8,217,257	8,350,064
Average Length of Stay	5.2	5.2	5.3	5.2	5.3
Personnel					
Total Full Time	197,029	190,898	183,892	183,960	185,430
Total Part Time	114,872	108,937	106,988	106,700	104,927
Revenue and Expenses - Totals					
(Includes Inpatient and Outpatient)					
Total Net Revenue	$36,238,128,346	$32,614,381,638	$30,237,644,809	$27,883,105,011	$24,763,704,581
Total Expenses	34,618,507,186	31,303,107,618	29,026,346,841	26,640,736,159	24,599,025,809
COMMUNITY HEALTH INDICATORS PER 1000 POPULATION					
Total Population (in thousands)	14,270	14,255	14,241	14,208	14,145
Inpatient					
Beds	2.4	2.4	2.4	2.4	2.4
Admissions	118.4	115.9	115.0	112.5	111.7
Inpatient Days	647.5	646.3	643.1	623.2	644.8
Inpatient Surgeries	31.2	32.5	32.0	32.0	32.5
Births	12.8	13.2	11.8	11.9	11.9
Outpatient					
Emergency Outpatient Visits	468.9	447.5	439.7	441.6	440.7
Other Outpatient Visits	2,358.0	2,292.0	2,196.7	2,219.9	2,111.7
Total Outpatient Visits	2,827.0	2,739.5	2,636.4	2,661.5	2,552.4
Outpatient Surgeries	74.1	74.9	77.5	73.0	71.0
Expense per Capita (per person)	$2,437.3	$2,205.5	$2,047.7	$1,885.1	$1,750.7

U.S. Census Divisions

TABLE 5

U.S. CENSUS DIVISION 2: MIDDLE ATLANTIC

U.S. Registered Community Hospitals
(Nonfederal, short-term general and other special hospitals)

Overview 2002–2006

	2006	2005	2004	2003	2002
Total Community Hospitals					
in Census Division 2, Middle Atlantic.......	470	474	483	486	493
Bed Size Category					
6-24	8	8	9	9	8
25-49	30	26	23	22	21
50-99	59	64	65	61	64
100-199	130	131	137	144	148
200-299	96	98	107	107	103
300-399	58	61	49	51	55
400-499	32	35	41	39	40
500 + ...	57	51	52	53	54
Location					
Hospitals Urban....................	382	386	403	406	412
Hospitals Rural	88	88	80	80	81
Control					
State and Local Government................	26	26	25	29	30
Not for Profit	412	418	427	429	441
Investor owned	32	30	31	28	22
Physician Models					
Independent Practice Association	64	66	75	92	99
Group Practice without Walls................	19	19	23	22	21
Open Physician-Hospital Organization	55	55	63	70	76
Closed Physician-Hospital Organization	15	18	15	19	26
Management Service Organization	55	47	54	56	64
Integrated Salary Model....................	143	134	130	132	118
Equity Model	7	8	8	9	9
Foundation..........................	8	9	10	12	11
Insurance Products					
Health Maintenance Organization	74	70	79	87	82
Preferred Provider Organization..............	70	74	84	85	79
Indemnity Fee for Service	27	25	32	24	17
Managed Care Contracts					
Health Maintenance Organization	290	277	302	319	317
Preferred Provider Organization..............	276	265	286	304	300
Affiliations					
Hospitals in a System*....................	231	224	222	220	215
Hospitals in a Network....................	151	134	146	147	152
Hospitals in a Group Purchasing Organization..	324	303	314	351	350

* Please note that system affiliate information for hospitals is derived from AHA membership. In years prior to 2003 the affiliation was derived from a question on the AHA Annual Survey of hospitals; therefore, non-responding hospitals were not included in the system affiliation counts. Years prior to 2003 have been updated to reflect this change, which now include affiliation for non-reporting hospitals.

TABLE 5

U.S. CENSUS DIVISION 2: MIDDLE ATLANTIC

U.S. Registered Community Hospitals
(Nonfederal, short-term general and other special hospitals)

Utilization, Personnel, Revenue and Expenses, Community Health Indicators 2002–2006

	2006	2005	2004	2003	2002
TOTAL FACILITY (Includes Hospital and Nursing Home Units)					
Utilization - Inpatient					
Beds	125,252	124,760	126,236	128,420	130,198
Admissions	5,548,934	5,510,766	5,476,222	5,430,928	5,356,471
Inpatient Days	34,456,727	34,373,589	34,653,619	34,910,712	34,925,191
Average Length of Stay	6.2	6.2	6.3	6.4	6.5
Inpatient Surgeries	1,535,961	1,501,811	1,500,367	1,491,422	1,540,104
Births	500,614	499,733	493,349	504,382	503,700
Utilization - Outpatient					
Emergency Outpatient Visits	16,764,369	16,096,919	15,916,707	15,567,144	15,474,182
Other Outpatient Visits	89,966,865	87,179,404	84,948,606	80,640,481	79,593,390
Total Outpatient Visits	106,731,234	103,276,323	100,865,313	96,207,625	95,067,572
Outpatient Surgeries	2,759,965	2,677,026	2,704,979	2,717,736	2,779,831
Personnel					
Full Time RNs	145,453	139,183	134,422	128,214	124,834
Full Time LPNs	11,916	12,778	13,194	13,474	14,200
Part Time RNs	59,512	61,470	60,870	59,196	58,048
Part Time LPNs	4,433	4,916	5,143	5,444	5,567
Total Full Time	623,974	610,899	601,947	589,789	591,456
Total Part Time	186,861	188,090	187,381	185,751	182,720
Revenue - Inpatient					
Gross Inpatient Revenue	$177,688,048,241	$167,127,975,929	$151,115,513,963	$139,643,847,699	$114,499,007,759
Revenue - Outpatient					
Gross Outpatient Revenue	$90,009,081,885	$80,559,995,861	$72,056,564,602	$62,623,808,550	$53,178,962,709
Revenue and Expenses - Totals					
(Includes Inpatient and Outpatient)					
Total Gross Revenue	$267,697,130,126	$247,687,971,790	$223,172,078,565	$202,267,656,249	$167,677,970,468
Deductions from Revenue	181,556,755,763	166,798,862,867	147,628,349,961	131,171,564,551	101,832,776,300
Net Patient Revenue	86,140,374,363	80,889,108,923	75,543,728,604	71,096,091,698	65,845,194,168
Other Operating Revenue	6,577,538,742	5,939,476,131	5,615,764,568	5,043,277,779	4,945,663,508
Other Nonoperating Revenue	1,764,422,561	1,205,293,393	1,280,876,485	1,180,634,845	473,985,594
Total Net Revenue	94,482,335,756	88,033,878,447	82,440,369,657	77,320,004,322	71,264,843,270
Total Expenses	91,387,151,168	85,358,448,159	80,203,606,103	76,052,322,704	70,060,852,900
HOSPITAL UNIT (Excludes Separate Nursing Home Units)					
Utilization - Inpatient					
Beds	117,117	117,843	117,937	118,319	118,462
Admissions	5,508,450	5,472,172	5,433,347	5,382,414	5,305,173
Inpatient Days	31,721,535	32,104,839	31,812,952	31,572,094	30,977,155
Average Length of Stay	5.8	5.9	5.9	5.9	5.8
Personnel					
Total Full Time	617,422	605,638	574,772	581,806	582,279
Total Part Time	183,604	183,613	181,686	181,832	178,921
Revenue and Expenses - Totals					
(Includes Inpatient and Outpatient)					
Total Net Revenue	$93,800,512,716	$87,491,509,142	$81,836,025,189	$76,454,812,926	$70,357,276,445
Total Expenses	90,738,596,774	84,900,083,379	79,677,850,994	75,242,014,798	69,170,940,306
COMMUNITY HEALTH INDICATORS PER 1000 POPULATION					
Total Population (in thousands)	40,471	40,424	40,345	40,222	40,067
Inpatient					
Beds	3.1	3.1	3.1	3.2	3.2
Admissions	137.1	136.3	135.7	135.0	133.7
Inpatient Days	851.4	850.3	858.9	867.9	871.7
Inpatient Surgeries	38.0	37.2	37.2	37.1	38.4
Births	12.4	12.4	12.2	12.5	12.6
Outpatient					
Emergency Outpatient Visits	414.2	398.2	394.5	387.0	386.2
Other Outpatient Visits	2,223.0	2,156.6	2,105.6	2,004.9	1,986.5
Total Outpatient Visits	2,637.2	2,554.8	2,500.1	2,391.9	2,372.7
Outpatient Surgeries	68.2	66.2	67.0	67.6	69.4
Expense per Capita (per person)	$2,258.1	$2,111.6	$1,988.0	$1,890.8	$1,748.6

U.S. Census Divisions

TABLE 5

U.S. CENSUS DIVISION 3: SOUTH ATLANTIC

U.S. Registered Community Hospitals
(Nonfederal, short-term general and other special hospitals)

Overview 2002–2006

	2006	2005	2004	2003	2002
Total Community Hospitals					
in Census Division 3, South Atlantic	741	743	738	731	731
Bed Size Category					
6-24	17	20	21	23	21
25-49	111	106	99	94	97
50-99	128	127	141	137	135
100-199	203	207	205	207	200
200-299	118	126	113	111	116
300-399	72	66	64	70	73
400-499	33	34	38	30	30
500 + ...	59	57	57	59	59
Location					
Hospitals Urban.	496	495	447	442	442
Hospitals Rural	245	248	291	289	289
Control					
State and Local Government.	145	142	139	138	138
Not for Profit	396	402	405	403	407
Investor owned	200	199	194	190	186
Physician Models					
Independent Practice Association	57	62	65	66	54
Group Practice without Walls.	24	25	18	23	11
Open Physician-Hospital Organization	89	107	110	114	119
Closed Physician-Hospital Organization	40	45	34	41	39
Management Service Organization	53	47	49	58	64
Integrated Salary Model	228	193	196	187	175
Equity Model	17	14	17	17	15
Foundation.	18	14	13	17	20
Insurance Products					
Health Maintenance Organization	83	83	85	85	85
Preferred Provider Organization.	124	126	129	126	136
Indemnity Fee for Service	46	46	45	47	39
Managed Care Contracts					
Health Maintenance Organization	406	404	396	375	391
Preferred Provider Organization.	463	468	468	451	475
Affiliations					
Hospitals in a System*	451	449	443	425	432
Hospitals in a Network	219	215	225	225	228
Hospitals in a Group Purchasing Organization. .	497	488	465	502	471

* Please note that system affiliate information for hospitals is derived from AHA membership. In years prior to 2003 the affiliation was derived from a question on the AHA Annual Survey of hospitals; therefore, non-responding hospitals were not included in the system affiliation counts. Years prior to 2003 have been updated to reflect this change, which now include affiliation for non-reporting hospitals.

Utilization, Personnel, Revenue and Expenses, Community Health Indicators 2002–2006

	2006	2005	2004	2003	2002
TOTAL FACILITY (Includes Hospital and Nursing Home Units)					
Utilization - Inpatient					
Beds	153,115	152,564	151,039	151,754	152,236
Admissions	6,862,970	6,870,008	6,758,902	6,646,826	6,587,288
Inpatient Days	38,694,981	38,714,804	38,218,282	37,810,333	37,509,493
Average Length of Stay	5.6	5.6	5.7	5.7	5.7
Inpatient Surgeries	2,008,456	2,047,968	1,995,331	1,967,152	2,024,048
Births	754,948	734,589	717,018	695,242	695,805
Utilization - Outpatient					
Emergency Outpatient Visits	23,813,876	23,007,000	22,360,452	22,063,587	21,281,267
Other Outpatient Visits	66,355,974	65,404,860	64,181,107	61,832,573	61,195,587
Total Outpatient Visits	90,169,850	88,411,860	86,541,559	83,896,160	82,476,854
Outpatient Surgeries	3,294,862	3,440,867	3,392,029	3,348,605	3,403,716
Personnel					
Full Time RNs	182,267	173,865	165,119	158,536	154,257
Full Time LPNs	17,858	18,560	18,343	19,070	19,491
Part Time RNs	75,586	74,252	70,779	72,088	68,654
Part Time LPNs	5,540	5,857	6,154	7,195	6,084
Total Full Time	697,654	690,209	661,078	647,733	646,894
Total Part Time	211,258	209,300	201,834	206,568	196,385
Revenue - Inpatient					
Gross Inpatient Revenue	$165,578,390,457	$150,510,815,327	$134,169,078,228	$122,068,281,181	$109,659,179,223
Revenue - Outpatient					
Gross Outpatient Revenue	$97,769,350,198	$88,755,991,497	$75,463,034,619	$65,980,405,893	$59,025,023,880
Revenue and Expenses - Totals					
(Includes Inpatient and Outpatient)					
Total Gross Revenue	$263,347,740,655	$239,266,806,824	$209,632,112,847	$188,048,687,074	$168,684,203,103
Deductions from Revenue	165,215,098,511	147,502,610,445	124,405,790,632	109,766,909,281	95,540,558,726
Net Patient Revenue	98,132,642,144	91,764,196,379	85,226,322,215	78,281,777,793	73,143,644,377
Other Operating Revenue	4,785,098,906	4,231,278,257	4,044,693,679	3,910,102,561	3,729,711,113
Other Nonoperating Revenue	1,821,994,128	1,434,272,025	1,236,278,942	1,393,458,811	271,679,355
Total Net Revenue	104,739,735,178	97,429,746,661	90,507,294,836	83,585,339,165	77,145,034,845
Total Expenses	97,065,907,476	91,569,165,057	85,733,852,845	78,776,238,107	73,497,910,915
HOSPITAL UNIT (Excludes Separate Nursing Home Units)					
Utilization - Inpatient					
Beds	140,818	141,696	139,285	138,905	139,408
Admissions	6,814,310	6,825,392	6,710,353	6,592,950	6,530,617
Inpatient Days	34,675,520	35,145,534	34,248,832	33,500,043	33,321,870
Average Length of Stay	5.1	5.1	5.1	5.1	5.1
Personnel					
Total Full Time	686,079	680,932	646,868	636,985	636,583
Total Part Time	207,340	205,902	197,758	202,824	192,884
Revenue and Expenses - Totals					
(Includes Inpatient and Outpatient)					
Total Net Revenue	$101,638,027,688	$96,693,647,230	$89,524,617,669	$82,539,369,201	$76,360,437,261
Total Expenses	96,238,962,477	90,855,608,011	84,825,439,412	77,834,105,235	72,794,408,670
COMMUNITY HEALTH INDICATORS PER 1000 POPULATION					
Total Population (in thousands)	57,144	56,212	55,273	54,376	53,610
Inpatient					
Beds	2.7	2.7	2.7	2.8	2.8
Admissions	120.1	122.2	122.3	122.2	122.9
Inpatient Days	677.2	688.7	691.5	695.4	699.7
Inpatient Surgeries	35.1	36.4	36.1	36.2	37.8
Births	13.2	13.1	13.0	12.8	13.0
Outpatient					
Emergency Outpatient Visits	416.7	409.3	404.5	405.8	397.0
Other Outpatient Visits	1,161.2	1,163.5	1,161.2	1,137.1	1,141.5
Total Outpatient Visits	1,577.9	1,572.8	1,565.7	1,542.9	1,538.4
Outpatient Surgeries	57.7	61.2	61.4	61.6	63.5
Expense per Capita (per person)	$1,698.6	$1,629.0	$1,551.1	$1,448.7	$1,371.0

U.S. Census Divisions

TABLE 5

U.S. CENSUS DIVISION 4: EAST NORTH CENTRAL

U.S. Registered Community Hospitals
(Nonfederal, short-term general and other special hospitals)

Overview 2002–2006

	2006	2005	2004	2003	2002
Total Community Hospitals					
in Census Division 4, East North Central....	741	744	735	732	737
Bed Size Category					
6-24	33	36	32	25	28
25-49	161	147	134	128	121
50-99	148	160	165	170	173
100-199	178	177	178	184	189
200-299	100	95	94	99	101
300-399	51	63	63	60	59
400-499	30	29	29	28	26
500 + ...	40	37	40	38	40
Location					
Hospitals Urban.........................	468	469	446	442	444
Hospitals Rural	273	275	289	290	293
Control					
State and Local Government................	108	108	109	109	113
Not for Profit............................	580	591	587	588	592
Investor owned	53	45	39	35	32
Physician Models					
Independent Practice Association	90	81	85	107	102
Group Practice without Walls................	28	29	24	41	43
Open Physician-Hospital Organization	152	171	169	182	189
Closed Physician-Hospital Organization	69	62	67	80	72
Management Service Organization	94	105	102	109	106
Integrated Salary Model	257	249	242	256	235
Equity Model	16	13	9	6	12
Foundation................................	49	46	47	45	33
Insurance Products					
Health Maintenance Organization	157	138	142	149	142
Preferred Provider Organization..............	197	172	180	177	164
Indemnity Fee for Service	58	54	54	56	43
Managed Care Contracts					
Health Maintenance Organization	518	509	511	543	503
Preferred Provider Organization..............	564	572	563	596	554
Affiliations					
Hospitals in a System*.....................	405	405	393	378	370
Hospitals in a Network.....................	264	253	254	249	223
Hospitals in a Group Purchasing Organization..	634	631	603	635	592

---

* Please note that system affiliate information for hospitals is derived from AHA membership. In years prior to 2003 the affiliation was derived from a question on the AHA Annual Survey of hospitals; therefore, non-responding hospitals were not included in the system affiliation counts. Years prior to 2003 have been updated to reflect this change, which now include affiliation for non-reporting hospitals.

TABLE 5

U.S. CENSUS DIVISION 4: EAST NORTH CENTRAL

U.S. Registered Community Hospitals
(Nonfederal, short-term general and other special hospitals)

Utilization, Personnel, Revenue and Expenses, Community Health Indicators 2002–2006

	2006	2005	2004	2003	2002
TOTAL FACILITY (Includes Hospital and Nursing Home Units)					
Utilization - Inpatient					
Beds	125,144	126,170	127,568	127,610	129,716
Admissions	5,666,562	5,621,734	5,580,722	5,520,916	5,549,822
Inpatient Days	29,071,025	29,539,423	29,798,462	29,253,281	29,754,022
Average Length of Stay	5.1	5.3	5.3	5.3	5.4
Inpatient Surgeries	1,570,026	1,564,638	1,582,194	1,583,427	1,588,289
Births	596,871	591,825	601,542	600,200	594,899
Utilization - Outpatient					
Emergency Outpatient Visits	20,042,357	19,351,860	18,990,202	18,517,606	18,125,078
Other Outpatient Visits	99,366,389	96,055,128	94,959,549	92,718,085	88,307,662
Total Outpatient Visits	119,408,746	115,406,988	113,949,751	111,235,691	106,432,740
Outpatient Surgeries	3,160,980	3,243,949	3,136,209	3,170,597	3,101,230
Personnel					
Full Time RNs	141,688	136,639	129,203	126,117	120,224
Full Time LPNs	11,206	11,896	11,799	12,233	12,113
Part Time RNs	98,318	96,025	95,914	93,802	91,896
Part Time LPNs	7,058	7,595	7,806	7,637	7,846
Total Full Time	616,060	608,538	587,245	582,922	573,239
Total Part Time	307,330	299,308	296,832	289,862	288,607
Revenue - Inpatient					
Gross Inpatient Revenue	$128,438,375,170	$118,813,927,360	$108,311,909,673	$96,047,624,484	$87,407,038,737
Revenue - Outpatient					
Gross Outpatient Revenue	$101,789,022,674	$89,993,491,249	$78,870,661,671	$68,892,199,155	$59,494,801,802
Revenue and Expenses - Totals					
(Includes Inpatient and Outpatient)					
Total Gross Revenue	$230,227,397,844	$208,807,418,609	$187,182,571,344	$164,939,823,639	$146,901,840,539
Deductions from Revenue	137,355,334,545	121,595,959,764	106,120,808,063	90,427,903,676	77,136,739,719
Net Patient Revenue	92,872,063,299	87,211,458,845	81,061,763,281	74,511,919,963	69,765,100,820
Other Operating Revenue	5,159,399,104	4,846,875,073	4,398,960,733	4,093,763,516	3,815,440,330
Other Nonoperating Revenue	2,568,302,789	1,839,512,478	1,580,505,955	972,806,700	293,313,105
Total Net Revenue	100,599,765,192	93,897,846,396	87,041,229,969	79,578,490,179	73,873,854,255
Total Expenses	94,345,981,361	87,901,348,738	81,708,366,236	76,040,358,335	71,241,901,629
HOSPITAL UNIT (Excludes Separate Nursing Home Units)					
Utilization - Inpatient					
Beds	116,691	116,938	118,362	118,053	120,239
Admissions	5,612,044	5,565,439	5,524,664	5,458,596	5,486,852
Inpatient Days	26,473,334	26,735,473	27,024,447	26,320,238	26,833,806
Average Length of Stay	4.7	4.8	4.9	4.8	4.9
Personnel					
Total Full Time	610,220	602,139	569,647	576,932	567,494
Total Part Time	302,984	295,315	286,298	285,379	284,867
Revenue and Expenses - Totals					
(Includes Inpatient and Outpatient)					
Total Net Revenue	$99,932,380,489	$93,191,654,589	$86,457,086,696	$78,947,912,790	$73,267,139,602
Total Expenses	93,726,813,114	87,189,659,740	81,171,474,485	75,500,191,134	70,722,664,220
COMMUNITY HEALTH INDICATORS PER 1000 POPULATION					
Total Population (in thousands)	46,276	46,131	45,990	45,815	45,641
Inpatient					
Beds	2.7	2.7	2.8	2.8	2.8
Admissions	122.5	121.9	121.3	120.5	121.6
Inpatient Days	628.2	640.3	647.9	638.5	651.9
Inpatient Surgeries	33.9	33.9	34.4	34.6	34.8
Births	12.9	12.8	13.1	13.1	13.0
Outpatient					
Emergency Outpatient Visits	433.1	419.5	412.9	404.2	397.1
Other Outpatient Visits	2,147.3	2,082.2	2,064.8	2,023.8	1,934.8
Total Outpatient Visits	2,580.4	2,501.7	2,477.7	2,428.0	2,332.0
Outpatient Surgeries	68.3	70.3	68.2	69.2	67.9
Expense per Capita (per person)	$2,038.8	$1,905.5	$1,776.6	$1,659.7	$1,560.9

TABLE 5

U.S. CENSUS DIVISION 5: EAST SOUTH CENTRAL

U.S. Registered Community Hospitals
(Nonfederal, short-term general and other special hospitals)

Overview 2002–2006

	2006	2005	2004	2003	2002
Total Community Hospitals in Census Division 5, East South Central . . .	437	438	433	427	426
Bed Size Category					
6-24	15	14	13	14	15
25-49	109	108	101	96	83
50-99	107	111	111	108	118
100-199	112	109	110	112	113
200-299	36	39	44	41	41
300-399	26	26	21	22	23
400-499	14	13	14	12	12
500 + ...	18	18	19	22	21
Location					
Hospitals Urban.	201	202	173	169	168
Hospitals Rural	236	236	260	258	258
Control					
State and Local Government.	119	117	116	117	118
Not for Profit	186	194	196	197	197
Investor owned	132	127	121	113	111
Physician Models					
Independent Practice Association	34	35	37	44	50
Group Practice without Walls.	9	8	7	9	17
Open Physician-Hospital Organization	51	58	45	55	58
Closed Physician-Hospital Organization	10	9	5	15	15
Management Service Organization	37	38	32	46	53
Integrated Salary Model	76	74	59	81	81
Equity Model	1	2	—	1	2
Foundation.	16	22	12	23	28
Insurance Products					
Health Maintenance Organization	50	54	39	53	56
Preferred Provider Organization.	100	113	65	116	130
Indemnity Fee for Service	30	32	16	29	32
Managed Care Contracts					
Health Maintenance Organization	153	159	163	178	184
Preferred Provider Organization.	212	217	207	215	244
Affiliations					
Hospitals in a System*	276	276	264	262	254
Hospitals in a Network	109	108	111	103	99
Hospitals in a Group Purchasing Organization. .	244	254	241	252	222

---

* Please note that system affiliate information for hospitals is derived from AHA membership. In years prior to 2003 the affiliation was derived from a question on the AHA Annual Survey of hospitals; therefore, non-responding hospitals were not included in the system affiliation counts. Years prior to 2003 have been updated to reflect this change, which now include affiliation for non-reporting hospitals.

TABLE 5

U.S. CENSUS DIVISION 5: EAST SOUTH CENTRAL

U.S. Registered Community Hospitals
(Nonfederal, short-term general and other special hospitals)

Utilization, Personnel, Revenue and Expenses, Community Health Indicators 2002–2006

	2006	2005	2004	2003	2002
TOTAL FACILITY (Includes Hospital and Nursing Home Units)					
Utilization - Inpatient					
Beds	63,514	63,708	64,110	63,959	64,591
Admissions	2,565,449	2,568,031	2,574,086	2,538,273	2,492,114
Inpatient Days	14,300,824	14,461,395	14,494,590	14,171,337	13,856,950
Average Length of Stay	5.6	5.6	5.6	5.6	5.6
Inpatient Surgeries	755,751	757,883	731,898	736,740	727,890
Births	237,866	238,061	232,379	228,955	224,418
Utilization - Outpatient					
Emergency Outpatient Visits	8,840,824	9,051,997	8,843,497	8,827,897	8,643,710
Other Outpatient Visits	23,078,091	23,114,077	22,776,351	22,769,805	23,996,038
Total Outpatient Visits	31,918,915	32,166,074	31,619,848	31,597,702	32,639,748
Outpatient Surgeries	1,289,816	1,264,386	1,233,939	1,231,214	1,226,607
Personnel					
Full Time RNs	65,926	62,979	59,783	58,601	55,716
Full Time LPNs	9,818	10,148	10,484	11,555	10,859
Part Time RNs	24,318	23,762	23,045	23,463	23,303
Part Time LPNs	2,901	2,902	3,056	3,101	3,233
Total Full Time	260,548	248,959	244,738	242,696	237,483
Total Part Time	72,460	69,677	67,555	68,463	70,708
Revenue - Inpatient					
Gross Inpatient Revenue	$57,208,623,237	$51,625,768,080	$47,935,661,161	$42,807,554,660	$37,236,405,608
Revenue - Outpatient					
Gross Outpatient Revenue	$37,377,336,043	$32,822,416,403	$28,945,624,483	$24,877,139,678	$21,335,998,517
Revenue and Expenses - Totals					
(Includes Inpatient and Outpatient)					
Total Gross Revenue	$94,585,959,280	$84,448,184,483	$76,881,285,644	$67,684,694,338	$58,572,404,125
Deductions from Revenue	62,204,265,707	54,555,698,031	48,750,345,308	41,532,647,725	33,820,962,603
Net Patient Revenue	32,381,693,573	29,892,486,452	28,130,940,336	26,152,046,613	24,751,441,522
Other Operating Revenue	1,346,242,721	1,218,309,114	1,278,446,046	1,382,136,450	1,112,863,364
Other Nonoperating Revenue	658,282,487	520,488,052	480,174,247	392,950,942	246,155,552
Total Net Revenue	34,386,218,781	31,631,283,618	29,889,560,629	27,927,134,005	26,110,460,438
Total Expenses	32,228,480,833	29,947,795,643	27,999,718,544	26,377,671,189	24,262,441,941
HOSPITAL UNIT (Excludes Separate Nursing Home Units)					
Utilization - Inpatient					
Beds	58,500	58,491	58,988	58,436	59,825
Admissions	2,543,509	2,541,254	2,548,390	2,509,212	2,464,015
Inpatient Days	12,688,369	12,722,810	12,853,927	12,442,021	12,297,077
Average Length of Stay	5.0	5.0	5.0	5.0	5.0
Personnel					
Total Full Time	256,346	244,904	235,081	238,017	233,711
Total Part Time	71,329	68,430	65,522	67,226	69,573
Revenue and Expenses - Totals					
(Includes Inpatient and Outpatient)					
Total Net Revenue	$34,060,819,744	$31,310,742,372	$29,559,557,540	$27,597,631,434	$25,813,696,396
Total Expenses	31,986,666,215	29,673,466,971	27,745,269,836	26,092,562,236	24,024,754,092
COMMUNITY HEALTH INDICATORS PER 1000 POPULATION					
Total Population (in thousands)	17,754	17,585	17,436	17,318	17,218
Inpatient					
Beds	3.6	3.6	3.7	3.7	3.8
Admissions	144.5	146.0	147.6	146.6	144.7
Inpatient Days	805.5	822.4	831.3	818.3	804.8
Inpatient Surgeries	42.6	43.1	42.0	42.5	42.3
Births	13.4	13.5	13.3	13.2	13.0
Outpatient					
Emergency Outpatient Visits	497.9	514.8	507.2	509.7	502.0
Other Outpatient Visits	1,299.8	1,314.4	1,306.3	1,314.8	1,393.7
Total Outpatient Visits	1,797.8	1,829.2	1,813.5	1,824.5	1,895.7
Outpatient Surgeries	72.6	71.9	70.8	71.1	71.2
Expense per Capita (per person)	$1,815.2	$1,703.0	$1,605.8	$1,523.1	$1,409.1

TABLE 5

U.S. CENSUS DIVISION 6: WEST NORTH CENTRAL

U.S. Registered Community Hospitals
(Nonfederal, short-term general and other special hospitals)

Overview 2002–2006

	2006	2005	2004	2003	2002
Total Community Hospitals in Census Division 6, West North Central ...	674	678	676	675	679
Bed Size Category					
6-24	93	97	91	91	89
25-49	213	206	204	196	192
50-99	167	170	175	181	186
100-199	106	110	108	109	111
200-299	41	41	43	42	46
300-399	23	24	23	23	22
400-499	15	14	15	15	15
500 +	16	16	17	18	18
Location					
Hospitals Urban	209	211	179	179	180
Hospitals Rural	465	467	497	496	499
Control					
State and Local Government	241	242	242	243	247
Not for Profit	396	398	399	400	404
Investor owned	37	38	35	32	28
Physician Models					
Independent Practice Association	97	105	104	103	96
Group Practice without Walls	21	23	24	26	18
Open Physician-Hospital Organization	89	91	79	84	86
Closed Physician-Hospital Organization	32	36	36	44	45
Management Service Organization	31	30	29	30	33
Integrated Salary Model	306	284	272	269	240
Equity Model	6	5	6	4	8
Foundation	20	21	17	11	13
Insurance Products					
Health Maintenance Organization	69	73	81	80	84
Preferred Provider Organization	133	142	144	142	137
Indemnity Fee for Service	31	32	32	35	39
Managed Care Contracts					
Health Maintenance Organization	312	320	319	327	321
Preferred Provider Organization	488	483	494	500	485
Affiliations					
Hospitals in a System*	326	328	323	321	319
Hospitals in a Network	296	284	281	266	257
Hospitals in a Group Purchasing Organization	587	568	570	584	551

* Please note that system affiliate information for hospitals is derived from AHA membership. In years prior to 2003 the affiliation was derived from a question on the AHA Annual Survey of hospitals; therefore, non-responding hospitals were not included in the system affiliation counts. Years prior to 2003 have been updated to reflect this change, which now include affiliation for non-reporting hospitals.

TABLE 5

U.S. CENSUS DIVISION 8: MOUNTAIN

U.S. Registered Community Hospitals
(Nonfederal, short-term general and other special hospitals)

Utilization, Personnel, Revenue and Expenses, Community Health Indicators 2002–2006

	2006	2005	2004	2003	2002
TOTAL FACILITY (Includes Hospital and Nursing Home Units)					
Utilization - Inpatient					
Beds...........................	43,792	43,796	43,182	42,159	42,499
Admissions.....................	2,013,762	2,004,384	1,959,133	1,936,327	1,894,701
Inpatient Days	10,300,681	10,165,433	10,015,692	9,825,461	9,643,564
Average Length of Stay...........	5.1	5.1	5.1	5.1	5.1
Inpatient Surgeries..............	640,838	604,787	590,717	570,828	573,886
Births.........................	312,461	303,119	294,508	298,539	292,890
Utilization - Outpatient					
Emergency Outpatient Visits.......	6,901,098	6,851,313	6,243,490	6,191,190	6,124,812
Other Outpatient Visits...........	25,201,852	26,019,382	24,571,238	25,210,413	23,424,496
Total Outpatient Visits	32,102,950	32,870,695	30,814,728	31,401,603	29,549,308
Outpatient Surgeries	842,579	886,545	881,616	824,022	868,934
Personnel					
Full Time RNs	52,261	49,918	48,001	44,847	42,583
Full Time LPNs	4,308	4,502	4,521	4,688	4,955
Part Time RNs..................	23,766	23,173	21,260	22,105	20,935
Part Time LPNs.................	1,982	1,975	2,009	2,130	2,112
Total Full Time.................	204,327	201,681	190,186	186,346	179,836
Total Part Time	73,473	71,634	64,583	67,402	65,555
Revenue - Inpatient					
Gross Inpatient Revenue..........	$53,107,976,721	$48,458,007,228	$42,470,879,422	$37,659,338,009	$33,651,462,085
Revenue - Outpatient					
Gross Outpatient Revenue	$30,552,510,790	$27,312,023,316	$23,013,525,198	$20,005,569,335	$17,572,433,747
Revenue and Expenses - Totals					
(Includes Inpatient and Outpatient)					
Total Gross Revenue.............	$83,660,487,511	$75,770,030,544	$65,484,404,620	$57,664,907,344	$51,223,895,832
Deductions from Revenue.........	53,002,070,673	47,144,479,539	39,364,474,737	34,069,882,506	29,266,253,620
Net Patient Revenue	30,658,416,838	28,625,551,005	26,119,929,883	23,595,024,838	21,957,642,212
Other Operating Revenue	1,599,894,899	1,363,620,777	1,222,669,757	1,183,351,784	1,082,083,144
Other Nonoperating Revenue	481,150,834	357,911,606	358,187,063	279,791,570	247,116,847
Total Net Revenue..............	32,739,462,571	30,347,083,388	27,700,786,703	25,058,168,192	23,286,842,203
Total Expenses.................	29,827,199,413	27,941,395,174	25,258,325,366	23,296,281,246	21,439,442,983
HOSPITAL UNIT (Excludes Separate Nursing Home Units)					
Utilization - Inpatient					
Beds...........................	39,887	39,623	39,064	38,192	38,104
Admissions.....................	2,001,347	1,993,334	1,948,586	1,922,484	1,878,936
Inpatient Days	9,089,752	8,898,953	8,802,367	8,601,499	8,282,586
Average Length of Stay...........	4.5	4.5	4.5	4.5	4.4
Personnel					
Total Full Time.................	201,619	198,836	184,390	183,583	176,918
Total Part Time	72,021	69,885	62,492	65,741	63,778
Revenue and Expenses - Totals					
(Includes Inpatient and Outpatient)					
Total Net Revenue..............	$32,520,772,718	$30,134,818,660	$27,502,747,526	$24,854,081,925	$23,087,760,662
Total Expenses.................	29,635,161,921	27,747,618,911	25,083,681,922	23,103,787,089	21,258,843,110
COMMUNITY HEALTH INDICATORS PER 1000 POPULATION					
Total Population (in thousands)	20,846	20,318	19,825	19,389	19,050
Inpatient					
Beds...........................	2.1	2.2	2.2	2.2	2.2
Admissions.....................	96.6	98.7	98.8	99.9	99.5
Inpatient Days	494.1	500.3	505.2	506.8	506.2
Inpatient Surgeries..............	30.7	29.8	29.8	29.4	30.1
Births.........................	15.0	14.9	14.9	15.4	15.4
Outpatient					
Emergency Outpatient Visits.......	331.1	337.2	314.9	319.3	321.5
Other Outpatient Visits...........	1,209.0	1,280.6	1,239.4	1,300.3	1,229.7
Total Outpatient Visits	1,540.0	1,617.8	1,554.3	1,619.6	1,551.2
Outpatient Surgeries	40.4	43.6	44.5	42.5	45.6
Expense per Capita (per person)....	$1,430.8	$1,375.2	$1,274.1	$1,201.5	$1,125.5

U.S. Census Divisions

TABLE 5

U.S. CENSUS DIVISION 9: PACIFIC

U.S. Registered Community Hospitals
(Nonfederal, short-term general and other special hospitals)

Overview 2002–2006

	2006	2005	2004	2003	2002
Total Community Hospitals in Census Division 9, Pacific	549	548	547	556	573
Bed Size Category					
6-24	38	39	38	32	32
25-49	99	97	93	98	96
50-99	85	89	88	92	105
100-199	144	142	142	144	153
200-299	91	87	94	96	95
300-399	52	58	52	50	48
400-499	22	19	21	22	25
500 + ...	18	17	19	22	19
Location					
Hospitals Urban	424	422	409	418	433
Hospitals Rural	125	126	138	138	140
Control					
State and Local Government	144	136	137	135	140
Not for Profit	316	319	311	319	332
Investor owned	89	93	99	102	101
Physician Models					
Independent Practice Association	117	123	130	123	142
Group Practice without Walls	21	18	19	18	27
Open Physician-Hospital Organization	31	29	29	28	33
Closed Physician-Hospital Organization	9	16	16	18	17
Management Service Organization	51	46	53	47	56
Integrated Salary Model	113	117	90	87	100
Equity Model	3	3	1	—	1
Foundation	48	48	38	32	33
Insurance Products					
Health Maintenance Organization	70	75	76	71	76
Preferred Provider Organization	55	62	56	56	58
Indemnity Fee for Service	21	23	25	26	23
Managed Care Contracts					
Health Maintenance Organization	258	267	256	247	275
Preferred Provider Organization	285	289	281	271	300
Affiliations					
Hospitals in a System*	342	329	329	336	342
Hospitals in a Network	106	103	97	76	80
Hospitals in a Group Purchasing Organization . .	350	352	325	327	359

* Please note that system affiliate information for hospitals is derived from AHA membership. In years prior to 2003 the affiliation was derived from a question on the AHA Annual Survey of hospitals; therefore, non-responding hospitals were not included in the system affiliation counts. Years prior to 2003 have been updated to reflect this change, which now include affiliation for non-reporting hospitals.

TABLE 5

U.S. CENSUS DIVISION 9: PACIFIC

U.S. Registered Community Hospitals
(Nonfederal, short-term general and other special hospitals)

Utilization, Personnel, Revenue and Expenses, Community Health Indicators 2002–2006

	2006	2005	2004	2003	2002
TOTAL FACILITY (Includes Hospital and Nursing Home Units)					
Utilization - Inpatient					
Beds	92,077	91,864	93,975	96,854	97,048
Admissions	4,491,195	4,478,621	4,497,690	4,489,795	4,453,054
Inpatient Days	23,419,759	23,367,424	23,439,112	23,850,078	23,756,101
Average Length of Stay	5.2	5.2	5.2	5.3	5.3
Inpatient Surgeries	1,251,269	1,258,460	1,276,765	1,254,159	1,309,119
Births	670,591	644,267	645,833	630,788	616,819
Utilization - Outpatient					
Emergency Outpatient Visits	14,623,874	13,513,811	13,832,185	12,947,101	13,731,605
Other Outpatient Visits	61,615,935	57,116,950	54,773,146	56,929,025	60,828,353
Total Outpatient Visits	76,239,809	70,630,761	68,605,331	69,876,126	74,559,958
Outpatient Surgeries	1,783,808	1,817,189	1,825,002	1,808,400	1,902,778
Personnel					
Full Time RNs	109,551	102,846	100,389	97,331	96,461
Full Time LPNs	9,538	9,880	10,293	11,134	11,299
Part Time RNs	73,766	68,963	67,130	63,567	53,794
Part Time LPNs	5,058	4,669	5,036	5,204	4,211
Total Full Time	444,221	425,327	419,721	419,189	426,704
Total Part Time	202,571	191,425	185,090	176,116	154,518
Revenue - Inpatient					
Gross Inpatient Revenue	$162,753,461,850	$153,582,565,621	$142,652,359,980	$131,147,209,263	$104,936,331,959
Revenue - Outpatient					
Gross Outpatient Revenue	$78,665,367,009	$70,108,626,775	$61,627,750,175	$55,318,628,115	$46,066,247,391
Revenue and Expenses - Totals					
(Includes Inpatient and Outpatient)					
Total Gross Revenue	$241,418,828,859	$223,691,192,396	$204,280,110,155	$186,465,837,378	$151,002,579,350
Deductions from Revenue	167,168,229,819	154,243,546,060	139,866,102,129	125,667,694,248	95,502,859,945
Net Patient Revenue	74,250,599,040	69,447,646,336	64,414,008,026	60,798,143,130	55,499,719,405
Other Operating Revenue	4,361,003,114	3,540,496,528	3,375,512,005	3,547,025,742	3,077,494,277
Other Nonoperating Revenue	2,124,134,857	1,782,114,508	1,652,444,385	1,397,694,045	1,219,640,462
Total Net Revenue	80,706,061,954	74,770,257,372	69,441,964,416	65,742,862,917	59,796,854,144
Total Expenses	76,421,525,696	71,652,944,767	66,689,227,653	62,875,657,935	57,386,669,321
HOSPITAL UNIT (Excludes Separate Nursing Home Units)					
Utilization - Inpatient					
Beds	86,878	86,221	87,995	88,955	87,870
Admissions	4,456,404	4,441,580	4,455,935	4,437,867	4,385,440
Inpatient Days	21,889,072	21,675,035	21,541,278	21,468,884	21,145,589
Average Length of Stay	4.9	4.9	4.8	4.8	4.8
Personnel					
Total Full Time	438,331	420,531	411,223	413,600	420,265
Total Part Time	199,539	189,337	182,133	173,941	152,674
Revenue and Expenses - Totals					
(Includes Inpatient and Outpatient)					
Total Net Revenue	$79,957,542,841	$74,213,917,886	$68,863,776,071	$64,948,547,194	$59,059,246,409
Total Expenses	75,989,209,712	71,197,475,636	66,179,943,341	62,298,298,365	56,802,766,053
COMMUNITY HEALTH INDICATORS PER 1000 POPULATION					
Total Population (in thousands)	48,510	48,021	47,552	47,051	46,492
Inpatient					
Beds	1.9	1.9	2.0	2.1	2.1
Admissions	92.6	93.3	94.6	95.4	95.8
Inpatient Days	482.8	486.6	492.9	506.9	511.0
Inpatient Surgeries	25.8	26.2	26.8	26.7	28.2
Births	13.8	13.4	13.6	13.4	13.3
Outpatient					
Emergency Outpatient Visits	301.5	281.4	290.9	275.2	295.4
Other Outpatient Visits	1,270.2	1,189.4	1,151.9	1,209.9	1,308.4
Total Outpatient Visits	1,571.6	1,470.8	1,442.7	1,485.1	1,603.7
Outpatient Surgeries	36.8	37.8	38.4	38.4	40.9
Expense per Capita (per person)	$1,575.4	$1,492.1	$1,402.4	$1,336.3	$1,234.3

U.S. Census Divisions

TABLE 6

ALABAMA

U.S. Registered Community Hospitals
(Nonfederal, short-term general and other special hospitals)

Overview 2002–2006

	2006	2005	2004	2003	2002
Total Community Hospitals in Alabama	109	109	108	107	106
Bed Size Category					
6-24	6	7	7	7	6
25-49	22	23	20	19	15
50-99	24	24	25	24	30
100-199	34	31	33	34	30
200-299	11	13	13	11	13
300-399	7	6	5	6	7
400-499	1	1	1	2	1
500 + ...	4	4	4	4	4
Location					
Hospitals Urban..........................	60	60	57	57	57
Hospitals Rural	49	49	51	50	49
Control					
State and Local Government...............	41	39	37	37	36
Not for Profit	26	31	35	35	35
Investor owned	42	39	36	35	35
Physician Models					
Independent Practice Association	7	7	6	11	4
Group Practice without Walls...............	1	0	0	1	3
Open Physician-Hospital Organization	3	4	3	4	2
Closed Physician-Hospital Organization	1	3	1	0	0
Management Service Organization	7	9	7	8	8
Integrated Salary Model	12	11	12	13	9
Equity Model	0	0	0	0	0
Foundation...............................	2	5	3	8	6
Insurance Products					
Health Maintenance Organization	9	7	5	5	2
Preferred Provider Organization..............	8	12	11	16	13
Indemnity Fee for Service	2	3	2	3	3
Managed Care Contracts					
Health Maintenance Organization	27	35	36	41	33
Preferred Provider Organization..............	39	50	46	56	42
Affiliations					
Hospitals in a System*....................	65	68	63	70	66
Hospitals in a Network	10	12	13	12	8
Hospitals in a Group Purchasing Organization..	55	60	52	66	49

* Please note that system affiliate information for hospitals is derived from AHA membership. In years prior to 2003 the affiliation was derived from a question on the AHA Annual Survey of hospitals; therefore, non-responding hospitals were not included in the system affiliation counts. Years prior to 2003 have been updated to reflect this change, which now include affiliation for non-reporting hospitals.

TABLE 6

ALABAMA

U.S. Registered Community Hospitals
(Nonfederal, short-term general and other special hospitals)

Utilization, Personnel, Revenue and Expenses, Community Health Indicators 2002–2006

	2006	2005	2004	2003	2002
TOTAL FACILITY (Includes Hospital and Nursing Home Units)					
Utilization - Inpatient					
Beds	15,639	15,486	15,328	15,666	15,935
Admissions	683,726	706,442	715,709	708,995	676,337
Inpatient Days	3,556,939	3,628,012	3,664,493	3,547,203	3,244,123
Average Length of Stay	5.2	5.1	5.1	5.0	4.8
Inpatient Surgeries	223,876	210,076	204,461	210,149	198,225
Births	59,456	59,570	57,793	57,580	55,677
Utilization - Outpatient					
Emergency Outpatient Visits	2,192,221	2,085,573	2,026,709	2,145,885	2,162,011
Other Outpatient Visits	5,831,133	5,461,629	6,235,601	6,753,290	7,883,504
Total Outpatient Visits	8,023,354	7,547,202	8,262,310	8,899,175	10,045,515
Outpatient Surgeries	373,688	356,034	340,943	323,743	319,658
Personnel					
Full Time RNs	17,308	16,617	15,209	16,063	15,328
Full Time LPNs	2,225	2,356	2,488	2,975	2,680
Part Time RNs	6,677	6,097	5,804	5,543	5,382
Part Time LPNs	890	716	780	784	750
Total Full Time	65,120	65,221	62,248	64,944	63,011
Total Part Time	18,703	16,142	15,825	16,435	14,924
Revenue - Inpatient					
Gross Inpatient Revenue	$16,275,203,299	$15,022,125,418	$14,229,244,584	$13,225,879,008	$10,908,904,536
Revenue - Outpatient					
Gross Outpatient Revenue	$9,484,229,706	$8,417,319,841	$7,369,023,127	$6,504,097,756	$5,203,241,240
Revenue and Expenses - Totals					
(Includes Inpatient and Outpatient)					
Total Gross Revenue	$25,759,433,005	$23,439,445,259	$21,598,267,711	$19,729,976,764	$16,112,145,776
Deductions from Revenue	18,197,677,398	16,193,032,176	15,026,334,977	13,372,289,500	10,194,892,253
Net Patient Revenue	7,561,755,607	7,246,413,083	6,571,932,734	6,357,687,264	5,917,253,523
Other Operating Revenue	441,333,070	371,786,311	407,758,534	322,785,134	343,884,634
Other Nonoperating Revenue	203,736,118	149,232,438	139,283,436	165,592,463	66,577,418
Total Net Revenue	8,206,824,795	7,767,431,832	7,118,974,704	6,846,064,861	6,327,715,575
Total Expenses	7,550,751,275	7,180,554,012	6,733,585,986	6,507,392,947	5,767,179,494
HOSPITAL UNIT (Excludes Separate Nursing Home Units)					
Utilization - Inpatient					
Beds	14,917	14,692	14,615	14,823	15,678
Admissions	680,564	703,117	713,126	704,540	672,860
Inpatient Days	3,335,678	3,367,589	3,441,086	3,280,487	3,178,161
Average Length of Stay	4.9	4.8	4.8	4.7	4.7
Personnel					
Total Full Time	64,631	64,700	61,790	64,365	62,861
Total Part Time	18,617	16,035	15,768	16,309	14,895
Revenue and Expenses - Totals					
(Includes Inpatient and Outpatient)					
Total Net Revenue	$8,172,214,723	$7,734,917,420	$7,067,657,683	$6,778,019,599	$6,315,357,773
Total Expenses	7,526,811,142	7,153,872,718	6,691,220,104	6,441,833,027	5,754,090,214
COMMUNITY HEALTH INDICATORS PER 1000 POPULATION					
Total Population (in thousands)	4,599	4,548	4,517	4,495	4,478
Inpatient					
Beds	3.4	3.4	3.4	3.5	3.6
Admissions	148.7	155.3	158.4	157.7	151.0
Inpatient Days	773.4	797.7	811.2	789.1	724.5
Inpatient Surgeries	48.7	46.2	45.3	46.8	44.3
Births	12.9	13.1	12.8	12.8	12.4
Outpatient					
Emergency Outpatient Visits	476.7	458.5	448.6	477.4	482.9
Other Outpatient Visits	1,267.9	1,200.8	1,380.3	1,502.4	1,760.7
Total Outpatient Visits	1,744.6	1,659.3	1,829.0	1,979.8	2,243.5
Outpatient Surgeries	81.3	78.3	75.5	72.0	71.4
Expense per Capita (per person)	$1,641.8	$1,578.7	$1,490.6	$1,447.7	$1,288.0

States

TABLE 6

ALASKA

U.S. Registered Community Hospitals
(Nonfederal, short-term general and other special hospitals)

Overview 2002–2006

	2006	2005	2004	2003	2002
Total Community Hospitals in Alaska	22	22	19	19	19
Bed Size Category					
6-24	7	7	5	5	5
25-49	7	8	8	7	6
50-99	4	3	2	3	4
100-199	2	3	2	2	3
200-299	1	0	1	1	0
300-399	1	1	1	1	1
400-499	0	0	0	0	0
500 +	0	0	0	0	0
Location					
Hospitals Urban	5	5	3	3	3
Hospitals Rural	17	17	16	16	16
Control					
State and Local Government	7	7	7	7	7
Not for Profit	13	13	10	10	11
Investor owned	2	2	2	2	1
Physician Models					
Independent Practice Association	2	1	2	2	3
Group Practice without Walls	1	1	3	2	3
Open Physician-Hospital Organization	2	1	1	3	3
Closed Physician-Hospital Organization	0	1	0	0	0
Management Service Organization	0	0	0	0	0
Integrated Salary Model	6	6	2	6	5
Equity Model	0	0	0	0	0
Foundation	1	1	0	0	0
Insurance Products					
Health Maintenance Organization	0	0	0	0	0
Preferred Provider Organization	2	3	1	3	1
Indemnity Fee for Service	0	0	0	0	0
Managed Care Contracts					
Health Maintenance Organization	0	0	0	0	0
Preferred Provider Organization	8	6	4	7	6
Affiliations					
Hospitals in a System*	8	8	12	12	11
Hospitals in a Network	4	4	4	6	2
Hospitals in a Group Purchasing Organization	13	11	6	10	11

* Please note that system affiliate information for hospitals is derived from AHA membership. In years prior to 2003 the affiliation was derived from a question on the AHA Annual Survey of hospitals; therefore, non-responding hospitals were not included in the system affiliation counts. Years prior to 2003 have been updated to reflect this change, which now include affiliation for non-reporting hospitals.

TABLE 6

ALASKA

U.S. Registered Community Hospitals
(Nonfederal, short-term general and other special hospitals)

Utilization, Personnel, Revenue and Expenses, Community Health Indicators 2002–2006

	2006	2005	2004	2003	2002
TOTAL FACILITY (Includes Hospital and Nursing Home Units)					
Utilization - Inpatient					
Beds	1,551	1,393	1,427	1,456	1,378
Admissions	52,357	51,022	45,359	45,982	47,560
Inpatient Days	304,978	306,027	285,999	287,351	300,060
Average Length of Stay	5.8	6.0	6.3	6.2	6.3
Inpatient Surgeries	26,787	18,091	27,473	15,879	22,359
Births	9,128	8,554	7,366	7,608	7,596
Utilization - Outpatient					
Emergency Outpatient Visits	610,324	326,528	253,405	213,380	254,592
Other Outpatient Visits	1,165,596	1,340,089	1,077,327	1,230,029	1,083,024
Total Outpatient Visits	1,775,920	1,666,617	1,330,732	1,443,409	1,337,616
Outpatient Surgeries	34,522	41,155	44,071	35,682	35,136
Personnel					
Full Time RNs	2,071	2,135	1,583	1,749	1,734
Full Time LPNs	191	222	184	155	144
Part Time RNs	826	702	509	758	752
Part Time LPNs	56	55	58	55	58
Total Full Time	8,668	8,299	6,191	6,990	7,447
Total Part Time	2,304	2,031	1,532	2,266	2,221
Revenue - Inpatient					
Gross Inpatient Revenue	$1,619,128,443	$1,503,737,136	$1,338,181,466	$1,034,651,499	$960,861,590
Revenue - Outpatient					
Gross Outpatient Revenue	$1,283,765,424	$1,156,015,492	$971,620,399	$729,867,341	$665,750,510
Revenue and Expenses - Totals					
(Includes Inpatient and Outpatient)					
Total Gross Revenue	$2,902,893,867	$2,659,752,628	$2,309,801,865	$1,764,518,840	$1,626,612,100
Deductions from Revenue	1,529,429,013	1,433,497,046	1,302,835,817	864,446,975	755,063,643
Net Patient Revenue	1,373,464,854	1,226,255,582	1,006,966,048	900,071,865	871,548,457
Other Operating Revenue	73,602,633	53,752,321	43,170,801	45,996,074	40,119,994
Other Nonoperating Revenue	27,681,282	18,810,420	13,685,375	49,486,775	53,664,515
Total Net Revenue	1,474,748,769	1,298,818,323	1,063,822,224	995,554,714	965,332,966
Total Expenses	1,424,479,572	1,281,505,051	1,053,847,164	1,016,056,121	942,611,948
HOSPITAL UNIT (Excludes Separate Nursing Home Units)					
Utilization - Inpatient					
Beds	1,359	1,268	1,344	1,264	1,146
Admissions	51,957	50,773	45,140	45,690	47,038
Inpatient Days	242,591	270,302	261,976	229,735	228,355
Average Length of Stay	4.7	5.3	5.8	5.0	4.9
Personnel					
Total Full Time	8,483	8,182	6,115	6,896	7,261
Total Part Time	2,203	1,969	1,486	2,201	2,099
Revenue and Expenses - Totals					
(Includes Inpatient and Outpatient)					
Total Net Revenue	$1,446,879,893	$1,283,490,046	$1,055,506,617	$971,914,169	$938,542,659
Total Expenses	1,402,317,116	1,272,419,936	1,048,048,983	997,720,331	923,049,072
COMMUNITY HEALTH INDICATORS PER 1000 POPULATION					
Total Population (in thousands)	670	663	657	648	641
Inpatient					
Beds	2.3	2.1	2.2	2.2	2.2
Admissions	78.1	76.9	69.1	71.0	74.2
Inpatient Days	455.2	461.4	435.4	443.6	468.4
Inpatient Surgeries	40.0	27.3	41.8	24.5	34.9
Births	13.6	12.9	11.2	11.7	11.9
Outpatient					
Emergency Outpatient Visits	910.9	492.3	385.8	329.4	397.5
Other Outpatient Visits	1,739.6	2,020.5	1,640.2	1,898.9	1,690.8
Total Outpatient Visits	2,650.4	2,512.8	2,026.0	2,228.4	2,088.2
Outpatient Surgeries	51.5	62.1	67.1	55.1	54.9
Expense per Capita (per person)	$2,125.9	$1,932.2	$1,604.4	$1,568.6	$1,471.6

States

TABLE 6

ARIZONA

U.S. Registered Community Hospitals
(Nonfederal, short-term general and other special hospitals)

Overview 2002–2006

	2006	2005	2004	2003	2002
Total Community Hospitals in Arizona	66	67	62	61	61
Bed Size Category					
6-24	5	6	6	4	3
25-49	9	8	7	8	10
50-99	14	13	10	12	11
100-199	13	15	15	14	14
200-299	12	13	12	12	13
300-399	6	7	6	5	4
400-499	2	0	1	2	3
500 + ...	5	5	5	4	3
Location					
Hospitals Urban	50	51	47	46	46
Hospitals Rural	16	16	15	15	15
Control					
State and Local Government	5	5	5	5	5
Not for Profit	41	40	38	38	37
Investor owned	20	22	19	18	19
Physician Models					
Independent Practice Association	6	7	5	7	5
Group Practice without Walls	2	3	4	2	2
Open Physician-Hospital Organization	9	10	7	8	4
Closed Physician-Hospital Organization	5	5	2	2	3
Management Service Organization	2	3	2	3	1
Integrated Salary Model	11	10	12	13	7
Equity Model	1	1	1	1	0
Foundation	4	4	2	1	0
Insurance Products					
Health Maintenance Organization	10	10	9	7	7
Preferred Provider Organization	9	9	7	3	3
Indemnity Fee for Service	7	7	6	3	2
Managed Care Contracts					
Health Maintenance Organization	28	31	28	34	27
Preferred Provider Organization	32	36	32	36	29
Affiliations					
Hospitals in a System*	45	47	44	45	43
Hospitals in a Network	12	14	12	14	11
Hospitals in a Group Purchasing Organization . .	37	42	35	41	33

* Please note that system affiliate information for hospitals is derived from AHA membership. In years prior to 2003 the affiliation was derived from a question on the AHA Annual Survey of hospitals; therefore, non-responding hospitals were not included in the system affiliation counts. Years prior to 2003 have been updated to reflect this change, which now include affiliation for non-reporting hospitals.

TABLE 6

ARIZONA

U.S. Registered Community Hospitals
(Nonfederal, short-term general and other special hospitals)

Utilization, Personnel, Revenue and Expenses, Community Health Indicators 2002–2006

	2006	2005	2004	2003	2002
TOTAL FACILITY (Includes Hospital and Nursing Home Units)					
Utilization - Inpatient					
Beds	11,947	11,767	11,166	10,801	10,930
Admissions	664,773	664,595	624,583	603,310	591,094
Inpatient Days	3,023,329	2,936,640	2,781,888	2,669,152	2,544,370
Average Length of Stay	4.5	4.4	4.5	4.4	4.3
Inpatient Surgeries	218,604	186,097	179,548	172,178	150,482
Births	96,797	92,519	87,924	87,912	85,418
Utilization - Outpatient					
Emergency Outpatient Visits	2,073,320	2,050,938	1,747,614	1,781,590	1,559,078
Other Outpatient Visits	4,482,315	4,725,513	3,661,990	4,925,127	3,577,803
Total Outpatient Visits	6,555,635	6,776,451	5,409,604	6,706,717	5,136,881
Outpatient Surgeries	224,424	217,836	217,574	210,079	208,797
Personnel					
Full Time RNs	16,858	15,017	13,772	12,411	11,156
Full Time LPNs	1,041	1,042	964	1,015	1,115
Part Time RNs	5,535	5,982	5,195	5,489	5,226
Part Time LPNs	298	364	335	348	388
Total Full Time	61,165	58,488	52,349	47,524	45,502
Total Part Time	16,607	18,331	14,547	14,299	15,229
Revenue - Inpatient					
Gross Inpatient Revenue	$19,051,058,791	$17,448,393,885	$14,738,387,044	$13,150,302,688	$10,826,730,126
Revenue - Outpatient					
Gross Outpatient Revenue	$9,001,251,090	$8,162,904,498	$6,246,095,056	$5,741,277,192	$4,770,650,607
Revenue and Expenses - Totals					
(Includes Inpatient and Outpatient)					
Total Gross Revenue	$28,052,309,881	$25,611,298,383	$20,984,482,100	$18,891,579,880	$15,597,380,733
Deductions from Revenue	19,016,673,089	17,078,729,257	13,840,885,226	12,305,048,935	9,857,162,745
Net Patient Revenue	9,035,636,792	8,532,569,126	7,143,596,874	6,586,530,945	5,740,217,988
Other Operating Revenue	512,917,408	330,874,226	254,898,935	237,792,616	225,138,375
Other Nonoperating Revenue	103,114,887	83,188,540	61,100,042	41,239,855	34,008,928
Total Net Revenue	9,651,669,087	8,946,631,892	7,459,595,851	6,865,563,416	5,999,365,291
Total Expenses	8,959,776,857	8,025,631,963	6,861,149,144	6,256,631,400	5,647,682,344
HOSPITAL UNIT (Excludes Separate Nursing Home Units)					
Utilization - Inpatient					
Beds	11,739	11,630	11,093	10,584	10,653
Admissions	662,251	664,082	624,492	600,373	587,452
Inpatient Days	2,953,137	2,893,566	2,756,345	2,586,665	2,449,864
Average Length of Stay	4.5	4.4	4.4	4.3	4.2
Personnel					
Total Full Time	61,087	58,341	49,656	47,297	45,138
Total Part Time	16,567	18,288	14,076	14,247	15,130
Revenue and Expenses - Totals					
(Includes Inpatient and Outpatient)					
Total Net Revenue	$9,632,434,792	$8,939,787,932	$7,456,265,078	$6,835,799,648	$5,976,493,274
Total Expenses	8,946,668,918	8,012,166,227	6,856,080,845	6,226,275,219	5,623,701,779
COMMUNITY HEALTH INDICATORS PER 1000 POPULATION					
Total Population (in thousands)	6,166	5,953	5,746	5,582	5,445
Inpatient					
Beds	1.9	2.0	1.9	1.9	2.0
Admissions	107.8	111.6	108.7	108.1	108.6
Inpatient Days	490.3	493.3	484.2	478.1	467.3
Inpatient Surgeries	35.5	31.3	31.2	30.8	27.6
Births	15.7	15.5	15.3	15.7	15.7
Outpatient					
Emergency Outpatient Visits	336.2	344.5	304.2	319.2	286.3
Other Outpatient Visits	726.9	793.8	637.3	882.3	657.0
Total Outpatient Visits	1,063.1	1,138.3	941.5	1,201.4	943.4
Outpatient Surgeries	36.4	36.6	37.9	37.6	38.3
Expense per Capita (per person)	$1,453.0	$1,348.2	$1,194.1	$1,120.8	$1,037.2

States

TABLE 6

ARKANSAS

U.S. Registered Community Hospitals
(Nonfederal, short-term general and other special hospitals)

Overview 2002–2006

	2006	2005	2004	2003	2002
Total Community Hospitals in Arkansas.......	84	85	87	88	87
Bed Size Category					
6-24	5	6	5	5	6
25-49	29	29	28	26	20
50-99	20	19	21	24	28
100-199	16	18	20	20	21
200-299	7	6	7	6	5
300-399	5	5	4	5	5
400-499	0	0	0	0	0
500 + ...	2	2	2	2	2
Location					
Hospitals Urban..........................	35	35	32	32	31
Hospitals Rural	49	50	55	56	56
Control					
State and Local Government................	15	15	15	15	15
Not for Profit.............................	45	47	50	52	51
Investor owned	24	23	22	21	21
Physician Models					
Independent Practice Association	20	20	21	22	18
Group Practice without Walls................	5	8	5	6	6
Open Physician-Hospital Organization	32	32	30	32	29
Closed Physician-Hospital Organization	4	4	6	6	9
Management Service Organization	13	12	13	15	18
Integrated Salary Model....................	18	16	15	17	15
Equity Model.............................	2	2	2	2	2
Foundation...............................	8	7	8	9	10
Insurance Products					
Health Maintenance Organization	14	15	22	21	21
Preferred Provider Organization..............	11	17	23	31	30
Indemnity Fee for Service	4	5	7	6	8
Managed Care Contracts					
Health Maintenance Organization	45	45	47	48	48
Preferred Provider Organization..............	62	66	70	68	73
Affiliations					
Hospitals in a System*.....................	47	47	47	48	47
Hospitals in a Network.....................	28	29	29	27	28
Hospitals in a Group Purchasing Organization..	78	80	79	82	79

* Please note that system affiliate information for hospitals is derived from AHA membership. In years prior to 2003 the affiliation was derived from a question on the AHA Annual Survey of hospitals; therefore, non-responding hospitals were not included in the system affiliation counts. Years prior to 2003 have been updated to reflect this change, which now include affiliation for non-reporting hospitals.

TABLE 6

ARKANSAS

U.S. Registered Community Hospitals
(Nonfederal, short-term general and other special hospitals)

Utilization, Personnel, Revenue and Expenses, Community Health Indicators 2002–2006

	2006	2005	2004	2003	2002
TOTAL FACILITY (Includes Hospital and Nursing Home Units)					
Utilization - Inpatient					
Beds	9,309	9,389	9,580	9,909	9,942
Admissions	373,067	380,067	382,836	388,046	383,509
Inpatient Days	1,943,363	2,002,721	2,050,766	2,088,391	2,110,323
Average Length of Stay	5.2	5.3	5.4	5.4	5.5
Inpatient Surgeries	108,651	126,374	115,512	117,181	119,478
Births	39,232	37,939	36,734	38,892	38,191
Utilization - Outpatient					
Emergency Outpatient Visits	1,267,198	1,263,822	1,220,658	1,251,391	1,224,053
Other Outpatient Visits	3,818,276	3,707,485	3,621,645	3,330,961	3,614,451
Total Outpatient Visits	5,085,474	4,971,307	4,842,303	4,582,352	4,838,504
Outpatient Surgeries	144,619	141,104	146,074	151,653	159,314
Personnel					
Full Time RNs	9,699	9,578	8,903	9,019	8,417
Full Time LPNs	2,572	2,670	2,674	2,743	2,717
Part Time RNs	3,309	3,299	3,557	3,585	3,744
Part Time LPNs	859	884	1,015	1,045	969
Total Full Time	37,651	37,444	36,721	37,429	36,967
Total Part Time	10,845	10,766	11,816	12,127	11,843
Revenue - Inpatient					
Gross Inpatient Revenue	$7,346,539,305	$6,962,421,549	$6,513,778,911	$6,115,623,287	$5,484,336,913
Revenue - Outpatient					
Gross Outpatient Revenue	$4,655,737,561	$4,238,194,924	$3,861,410,128	$3,592,960,043	$3,139,609,992
Revenue and Expenses - Totals					
(Includes Inpatient and Outpatient)					
Total Gross Revenue	$12,002,276,866	$11,200,616,473	$10,375,189,039	$9,708,583,330	$8,623,946,905
Deductions from Revenue	7,572,665,742	6,945,017,078	6,360,783,014	5,790,602,643	4,920,059,934
Net Patient Revenue	4,429,611,124	4,255,599,395	4,014,406,025	3,917,980,687	3,703,886,971
Other Operating Revenue	154,744,439	153,253,789	134,780,857	127,642,206	134,834,877
Other Nonoperating Revenue	74,174,385	51,496,442	57,186,707	49,276,715	34,677,549
Total Net Revenue	4,658,529,948	4,460,349,626	4,206,373,589	4,094,899,608	3,873,399,397
Total Expenses	4,437,596,804	4,225,289,800	4,015,475,758	3,947,107,676	3,612,279,530
HOSPITAL UNIT (Excludes Separate Nursing Home Units)					
Utilization - Inpatient					
Beds	8,855	8,914	9,107	9,341	9,388
Admissions	371,143	377,594	380,311	384,978	380,945
Inpatient Days	1,799,422	1,852,272	1,903,513	1,921,041	1,935,371
Average Length of Stay	4.8	4.9	5.0	5.0	5.1
Personnel					
Total Full Time	37,231	37,086	36,344	37,063	36,629
Total Part Time	10,671	10,632	11,689	11,998	11,717
Revenue and Expenses - Totals					
(Includes Inpatient and Outpatient)					
Total Net Revenue	$4,637,882,611	$4,435,802,386	$4,184,016,644	$4,072,785,097	$3,850,828,585
Total Expenses	4,419,957,774	4,206,167,940	4,001,964,554	3,928,888,652	3,598,316,687
COMMUNITY HEALTH INDICATORS PER 1000 POPULATION					
Total Population (in thousands)	2,811	2,776	2,747	2,724	2,706
Inpatient					
Beds	3.3	3.4	3.5	3.6	3.7
Admissions	132.7	136.9	139.4	142.5	141.7
Inpatient Days	691.4	721.5	746.6	766.8	779.8
Inpatient Surgeries	38.7	45.5	42.1	43.0	44.1
Births	14.0	13.7	13.4	14.3	14.1
Outpatient					
Emergency Outpatient Visits	450.8	455.3	444.4	459.5	452.3
Other Outpatient Visits	1,358.4	1,335.7	1,318.5	1,223.0	1,335.6
Total Outpatient Visits	1,809.2	1,791.0	1,762.9	1,682.4	1,787.9
Outpatient Surgeries	51.4	50.8	53.2	55.7	58.9
Expense per Capita (per person)	$1,578.7	$1,522.2	$1,461.9	$1,449.2	$1,334.8

States

TABLE 6

CALIFORNIA

U.S. Registered Community Hospitals
(Nonfederal, short-term general and other special hospitals)

Overview 2002–2006

	2006	2005	2004	2003	2002
Total Community Hospitals in California	**357**	**357**	**361**	**370**	**383**
Bed Size Category					
6-24	11	11	14	9	10
25-49	39	39	37	42	47
50-99	53	54	59	63	63
100-199	109	107	102	105	114
200-299	71	70	74	74	74
300-399	43	49	44	41	38
400-499	16	12	14	16	20
500 + ...	15	15	17	20	17
Location					
Hospitals Urban........................	324	323	321	330	343
Hospitals Rural	33	34	40	40	40
Control					
State and Local Government...............	76	69	72	71	74
Not for Profit.........................	202	204	200	207	217
Investor owned	79	84	89	92	92
Physician Models					
Independent Practice Association	93	94	108	96	107
Group Practice without Walls..............	13	10	10	10	18
Open Physician-Hospital Organization	12	11	16	13	14
Closed Physician-Hospital Organization	3	6	9	9	11
Management Service Organization	38	32	41	37	43
Integrated Salary Model..................	36	35	30	24	35
Equity Model	2	2	1	0	1
Foundation............................	41	40	35	29	30
Insurance Products					
Health Maintenance Organization	52	54	58	51	50
Preferred Provider Organization.............	25	27	30	28	29
Indemnity Fee for Service	15	15	18	16	18
Managed Care Contracts					
Health Maintenance Organization	182	183	182	168	180
Preferred Provider Organization.............	184	186	189	174	184
Affiliations					
Hospitals in a System*...................	240	237	234	243	247
Hospitals in a Network...................	61	58	56	41	42
Hospitals in a Group Purchasing Organization..	212	211	217	203	219

* Please note that system affiliate information for hospitals is derived from AHA membership. In years prior to 2003 the affiliation was derived from a question on the AHA Annual Survey of hospitals; therefore, non-responding hospitals were not included in the system affiliation counts. Years prior to 2003 have been updated to reflect this change, which now include affiliation for non-reporting hospitals.

States

TABLE 6

DELAWARE

U.S. Registered Community Hospitals
(Nonfederal, short-term general and other special hospitals)

Utilization, Personnel, Revenue and Expenses, Community Health Indicators 2002–2006

	2006	2005	2004	2003	2002
TOTAL FACILITY (Includes Hospital and Nursing Home Units)					
Utilization - Inpatient					
Beds	2,138	1,909	1,955	2,051	2,014
Admissions	105,164	103,863	103,169	97,074	93,275
Inpatient Days	669,392	639,855	642,401	606,183	546,058
Average Length of Stay	6.4	6.2	6.2	6.2	5.9
Inpatient Surgeries	31,881	32,532	31,553	31,611	29,696
Births	12,361	12,014	11,974	11,837	11,350
Utilization - Outpatient					
Emergency Outpatient Visits	382,935	330,570	325,692	300,450	305,634
Other Outpatient Visits	1,456,973	1,537,157	1,540,257	1,721,410	1,642,184
Total Outpatient Visits	1,839,908	1,867,727	1,865,949	2,021,860	1,947,818
Outpatient Surgeries	62,593	60,754	62,461	62,989	66,987
Personnel					
Full Time RNs	2,995	2,918	2,605	2,170	2,609
Full Time LPNs	212	179	185	202	198
Part Time RNs	2,107	2,162	2,063	1,865	1,671
Part Time LPNs	126	109	108	145	86
Total Full Time	12,774	13,019	12,452	11,585	12,044
Total Part Time	5,541	5,809	5,704	5,771	4,759
Revenue - Inpatient					
Gross Inpatient Revenue	$2,060,178,931	$1,995,823,039	$1,753,513,945	$1,483,137,026	$1,257,109,446
Revenue - Outpatient					
Gross Outpatient Revenue	$1,315,656,776	$1,157,724,434	$990,566,571	$840,915,945	$697,074,088
Revenue and Expenses - Totals					
(Includes Inpatient and Outpatient)					
Total Gross Revenue	$3,375,835,707	$3,153,547,473	$2,744,080,516	$2,324,052,971	$1,954,183,534
Deductions from Revenue	1,626,506,667	1,461,877,504	1,219,630,928	984,738,879	821,168,346
Net Patient Revenue	1,749,329,040	1,691,669,969	1,524,449,588	1,339,314,092	1,133,015,188
Other Operating Revenue	144,361,451	133,359,882	119,498,615	109,287,307	81,264,100
Other Nonoperating Revenue	52,564,940	28,598,147	27,000,467	-21,627,318	-14,105,872
Total Net Revenue	1,946,255,431	1,853,627,998	1,670,948,670	1,426,974,081	1,200,173,416
Total Expenses	1,802,837,132	1,738,206,074	1,584,087,451	1,444,199,303	1,201,883,266
HOSPITAL UNIT (Excludes Separate Nursing Home Units)					
Utilization - Inpatient					
Beds	1,742	1,727	1,765	1,723	1,686
Admissions	104,253	103,078	102,359	95,493	91,880
Inpatient Days	532,566	578,748	580,519	493,165	440,860
Average Length of Stay	5.1	5.6	5.7	5.2	4.8
Personnel					
Total Full Time	12,551	12,851	12,292	11,300	11,753
Total Part Time	5,450	5,724	5,647	5,676	4,630
Revenue and Expenses - Totals					
(Includes Inpatient and Outpatient)					
Total Net Revenue	$1,913,476,298	$1,835,773,035	$1,654,004,709	$1,406,722,580	$1,174,652,121
Total Expenses	1,760,866,423	1,708,544,323	1,561,247,907	1,421,578,543	1,174,014,509
COMMUNITY HEALTH INDICATORS PER 1000 POPULATION					
Total Population (in thousands)	853	842	829	817	806
Inpatient					
Beds	2.5	2.3	2.4	2.5	2.5
Admissions	123.2	123.4	124.5	118.8	115.8
Inpatient Days	784.3	760.2	775.1	742.1	677.8
Inpatient Surgeries	37.4	38.6	38.1	38.7	36.9
Births	14.5	14.3	14.4	14.5	14.1
Outpatient					
Emergency Outpatient Visits	448.7	392.7	393.0	367.8	379.4
Other Outpatient Visits	1,707.1	1,826.2	1,858.5	2,107.3	2,038.5
Total Outpatient Visits	2,155.8	2,218.9	2,251.5	2,475.2	2,417.9
Outpatient Surgeries	73.3	72.2	75.4	77.1	83.2
Expense per Capita (per person)	$2,112.3	$2,065.0	$1,911.4	$1,768.0	$1,491.9

States

TABLE 6

DISTRICT OF COLUMBIA

U.S. Registered Community Hospitals
(Nonfederal, short-term general and other special hospitals)

Overview 2002–2006

	2006	2005	2004	2003	2002
Total Community Hospitals in					
District of Columbia	11	11	11	10	10
Bed Size Category					
6-24	0	0	0	0	0
25-49	0	0	0	0	0
50-99	1	0	0	0	0
100-199	2	4	4	3	3
200-299	2	2	3	2	1
300-399	4	3	2	3	4
400-499	0	0	0	0	0
500 + ...	2	2	2	2	2
Location					
Hospitals Urban	11	11	11	10	10
Hospitals Rural	0	0	0	0	0
Control					
State and Local Government	0	0	0	0	0
Not for Profit	7	7	7	7	7
Investor owned	4	4	4	3	3
Physician Models					
Independent Practice Association	0	1	1	1	1
Group Practice without Walls	1	0	0	0	0
Open Physician-Hospital Organization	1	1	1	1	1
Closed Physician-Hospital Organization	1	1	1	1	2
Management Service Organization	1	1	1	1	1
Integrated Salary Model	6	3	5	4	4
Equity Model	0	0	0	0	0
Foundation	1	1	0	0	0
Insurance Products					
Health Maintenance Organization	4	4	4	5	3
Preferred Provider Organization	1	1	1	2	1
Indemnity Fee for Service	1	1	1	2	0
Managed Care Contracts					
Health Maintenance Organization	8	7	6	7	8
Preferred Provider Organization	8	6	6	7	6
Affiliations					
Hospitals in a System*	8	6	5	4	7
Hospitals in a Network	0	0	1	0	0
Hospitals in a Group Purchasing Organization . .	8	7	7	8	7

* Please note that system affiliate information for hospitals is derived from AHA membership. In years prior to 2003 the affiliation was derived from a question on the AHA Annual Survey of hospitals; therefore, non-responding hospitals were not included in the system affiliation counts. Years prior to 2003 have been updated to reflect this change, which now include affiliation for non-reporting hospitals.

States

TABLE 6

GEORGIA

U.S. Registered Community Hospitals
(Nonfederal, short-term general and other special hospitals)

Utilization, Personnel, Revenue and Expenses, Community Health Indicators 2002–2006

	2006	2005	2004	2003	2002
TOTAL FACILITY (Includes Hospital and Nursing Home Units)					
Utilization - Inpatient					
Beds	24,772	25,015	24,709	24,624	24,500
Admissions	956,395	961,195	943,837	925,681	885,142
Inpatient Days	6,221,330	6,191,628	6,093,697	6,024,083	5,774,911
Average Length of Stay	6.5	6.4	6.5	6.5	6.5
Inpatient Surgeries	273,420	300,754	286,215	276,917	288,573
Births	140,741	139,577	136,501	133,692	128,981
Utilization - Outpatient					
Emergency Outpatient Visits	3,629,453	3,683,883	3,492,747	3,542,261	3,227,698
Other Outpatient Visits	10,153,274	10,119,196	9,905,204	9,307,084	9,256,245
Total Outpatient Visits	13,782,727	13,803,079	13,397,951	12,849,345	12,483,943
Outpatient Surgeries	504,293	556,126	513,356	507,592	511,906
Personnel					
Full Time RNs	25,671	25,269	23,256	23,431	22,730
Full Time LPNs	3,965	4,217	4,043	4,053	4,063
Part Time RNs	12,286	12,174	11,800	11,974	12,269
Part Time LPNs	1,230	1,285	1,361	1,277	1,189
Total Full Time	104,111	104,406	99,205	100,288	98,246
Total Part Time	32,617	32,953	33,537	31,452	32,518
Revenue - Inpatient					
Gross Inpatient Revenue	$22,163,780,319	$20,093,353,401	$18,156,528,430	$16,113,698,381	$14,445,750,952
Revenue - Outpatient					
Gross Outpatient Revenue	$14,777,650,188	$13,622,377,234	$11,618,489,833	$10,259,708,558	$9,240,551,617
Revenue and Expenses - Totals					
(Includes Inpatient and Outpatient)					
Total Gross Revenue	$36,941,430,507	$33,715,730,635	$29,775,018,263	$26,373,406,939	$23,686,302,569
Deductions from Revenue	23,269,007,568	20,520,952,593	17,743,170,185	15,113,531,785	13,112,710,432
Net Patient Revenue	13,672,422,939	13,194,778,042	12,031,848,078	11,259,875,154	10,573,592,137
Other Operating Revenue	830,795,303	613,617,105	609,415,034	634,628,403	553,755,731
Other Nonoperating Revenue	257,847,975	179,448,150	163,439,074	227,288,500	29,263,979
Total Net Revenue	14,761,066,217	13,987,843,297	12,804,702,186	12,121,792,057	11,156,611,847
Total Expenses	13,846,913,245	13,345,809,666	12,162,763,316	11,386,865,460	10,576,054,877
HOSPITAL UNIT (Excludes Separate Nursing Home Units)					
Utilization - Inpatient					
Beds	21,036	21,121	21,291	19,969	20,655
Admissions	950,054	954,725	936,806	918,417	880,499
Inpatient Days	4,942,793	4,864,313	4,945,631	4,426,838	4,466,878
Average Length of Stay	5.2	5.1	5.3	4.8	5.1
Personnel					
Total Full Time	101,590	101,435	95,311	96,825	95,471
Total Part Time	31,890	32,052	32,682	30,446	31,711
Revenue and Expenses - Totals					
(Includes Inpatient and Outpatient)					
Total Net Revenue	$14,592,684,941	$13,807,327,170	$12,641,676,379	$11,896,757,187	$11,012,776,470
Total Expenses	13,687,516,954	13,178,754,987	12,012,826,005	11,201,806,143	10,446,159,150
COMMUNITY HEALTH INDICATORS PER 1000 POPULATION					
Total Population (in thousands)	9,364	9,133	8,935	8,750	8,598
Inpatient					
Beds	2.6	2.7	2.8	2.8	2.8
Admissions	102.1	105.2	105.6	105.8	102.9
Inpatient Days	664.4	678.0	682.0	688.4	671.7
Inpatient Surgeries	29.2	32.9	32.0	31.6	33.6
Births	15.0	15.3	15.3	15.3	15.0
Outpatient					
Emergency Outpatient Visits	387.6	403.4	390.9	404.8	375.4
Other Outpatient Visits	1,084.3	1,108.0	1,108.6	1,063.6	1,076.6
Total Outpatient Visits	1,471.9	1,511.4	1,499.5	1,468.5	1,452.0
Outpatient Surgeries	53.9	60.9	57.5	58.0	59.5
Expense per Capita (per person)	$1,478.7	$1,461.3	$1,361.2	$1,301.3	$1,230.1

States

TABLE 6

HAWAII

U.S. Registered Community Hospitals
(Nonfederal, short-term general and other special hospitals)

Overview 2002–2006

	2006	2005	2004	2003	2002
Total Community Hospitals in Hawaii	24	25	24	24	25
Bed Size Category					
6-24	4	4	2	3	3
25-49	4	4	5	5	5
50-99	3	5	3	2	3
100-199	7	7	9	9	9
200-299	5	4	4	4	4
300-399	0	0	0	0	0
400-499	1	1	1	1	1
500 + ...	0	0	0	0	0
Location					
Hospitals Urban	13	13	13	13	13
Hospitals Rural	11	12	11	11	12
Control					
State and Local Government	7	8	7	6	7
Not for Profit	17	17	17	18	18
Investor owned	0	0	0	0	0
Physician Models					
Independent Practice Association	1	2	1	4	3
Group Practice without Walls	0	0	0	0	0
Open Physician-Hospital Organization	2	3	4	1	1
Closed Physician-Hospital Organization	1	1	0	1	1
Management Service Organization	0	0	0	0	0
Integrated Salary Model	5	5	3	3	3
Equity Model	0	0	0	0	0
Foundation	1	1	1	1	1
Insurance Products					
Health Maintenance Organization	1	1	2	3	3
Preferred Provider Organization	1	1	2	2	1
Indemnity Fee for Service	0	0	2	1	0
Managed Care Contracts					
Health Maintenance Organization	11	11	9	9	13
Preferred Provider Organization	9	11	10	6	9
Affiliations					
Hospitals in a System*	20	21	20	19	21
Hospitals in a Network	4	4	4	1	1
Hospitals in a Group Purchasing Organization ..	14	15	15	11	14

* Please note that system affiliate information for hospitals is derived from AHA membership. In years prior to 2003 the affiliation was derived from a question on the AHA Annual Survey of hospitals; therefore, non-responding hospitals were not included in the system affiliation counts. Years prior to 2003 have been updated to reflect this change, which now include affiliation for non-reporting hospitals.

States

TABLE 6

ILLINOIS

U.S. Registered Community Hospitals
(Nonfederal, short-term general and other special hospitals)

Utilization, Personnel, Revenue and Expenses, Community Health Indicators 2002–2006

	2006	2005	2004	2003	2002
TOTAL FACILITY (Includes Hospital and Nursing Home Units)					
Utilization - Inpatient					
Beds	34,178	34,498	34,844	35,048	36,309
Admissions	1,583,620	1,583,328	1,586,401	1,594,007	1,615,269
Inpatient Days	8,072,145	8,258,893	8,405,800	8,174,779	8,326,561
Average Length of Stay	5.1	5.2	5.3	5.1	5.2
Inpatient Surgeries	407,498	398,425	418,369	419,711	429,366
Births	170,858	169,531	173,700	177,192	172,338
Utilization - Outpatient					
Emergency Outpatient Visits	5,079,148	5,021,453	4,947,646	4,867,066	4,699,328
Other Outpatient Visits	24,485,471	23,707,111	23,387,196	22,358,135	21,811,988
Total Outpatient Visits	29,564,619	28,728,564	28,334,842	27,225,201	26,511,316
Outpatient Surgeries	729,602	715,216	715,470	710,827	745,579
Personnel					
Full Time RNs	36,521	35,229	33,613	34,297	32,720
Full Time LPNs	2,271	2,297	2,542	2,590	2,608
Part Time RNs	24,837	24,748	25,332	25,372	25,875
Part Time LPNs	1,220	1,222	1,365	1,376	1,361
Total Full Time	158,757	156,434	153,720	157,106	156,627
Total Part Time	79,025	77,647	77,912	76,983	80,497
Revenue - Inpatient					
Gross Inpatient Revenue	$38,493,305,193	$36,286,660,043	$33,428,553,596	$30,474,701,629	$27,722,800,143
Revenue - Outpatient					
Gross Outpatient Revenue	$26,754,990,338	$23,617,488,823	$20,355,331,327	$18,096,235,944	$15,980,470,692
Revenue and Expenses - Totals					
(Includes Inpatient and Outpatient)					
Total Gross Revenue	$65,248,295,531	$59,904,148,866	$53,783,884,923	$48,570,937,573	$43,703,270,835
Deductions from Revenue	42,114,856,257	37,220,464,082	32,823,525,854	28,856,859,436	25,017,360,640
Net Patient Revenue	23,133,439,274	22,683,684,784	20,960,359,069	19,714,078,137	18,685,910,195
Other Operating Revenue	1,399,916,299	1,368,531,305	1,314,989,573	1,137,597,475	1,174,384,266
Other Nonoperating Revenue	713,723,481	606,480,110	369,884,276	320,997,567	56,898,594
Total Net Revenue	25,247,079,054	24,658,696,199	22,645,232,918	21,172,673,179	19,917,193,055
Total Expenses	24,077,972,512	23,329,645,752	21,729,619,998	20,458,310,850	19,597,944,423
HOSPITAL UNIT (Excludes Separate Nursing Home Units)					
Utilization - Inpatient					
Beds	31,932	32,006	32,180	32,267	33,876
Admissions	1,565,855	1,562,755	1,563,815	1,568,413	1,588,707
Inpatient Days	7,450,541	7,577,711	7,637,905	7,382,487	7,652,143
Average Length of Stay	4.8	4.8	4.9	4.7	4.8
Personnel					
Total Full Time	157,039	154,165	150,603	155,219	154,973
Total Part Time	77,948	76,823	76,889	75,920	79,653
Revenue and Expenses - Totals					
(Includes Inpatient and Outpatient)					
Total Net Revenue	$25,089,859,015	$24,503,316,065	$22,478,149,114	$21,024,338,670	$19,771,409,995
Total Expenses	23,875,608,006	23,137,091,202	21,520,879,222	20,332,186,270	19,476,432,848
COMMUNITY HEALTH INDICATORS PER 1000 POPULATION					
Total Population (in thousands)	12,832	12,765	12,714	12,650	12,595
Inpatient					
Beds	2.7	2.7	2.7	2.8	2.9
Admissions	123.4	124.0	124.8	126.0	128.2
Inpatient Days	629.1	647.0	661.2	646.2	661.1
Inpatient Surgeries	31.8	31.2	32.9	33.2	34.1
Births	13.3	13.3	13.7	14.0	13.7
Outpatient					
Emergency Outpatient Visits	395.8	393.4	389.2	384.8	373.1
Other Outpatient Visits	1,908.2	1,857.1	1,839.5	1,767.5	1,731.8
Total Outpatient Visits	2,304.0	2,250.5	2,228.7	2,152.2	2,104.9
Outpatient Surgeries	56.9	56.0	56.3	56.2	59.2
Expense per Capita (per person)	$1,876.4	$1,827.6	$1,709.2	$1,617.3	$1,556.0

States

TABLE 6

INDIANA

U.S. Registered Community Hospitals
(Nonfederal, short-term general and other special hospitals)

Overview 2002–2006

	2006	2005	2004	2003	2002
Total Community Hospitals in Indiana	114	113	113	112	112
Bed Size Category					
6-24	5	5	5	4	5
25-49	35	32	27	28	23
50-99	20	26	31	28	33
100-199	22	20	18	20	21
200-299	17	14	15	15	13
300-399	3	6	6	6	6
400-499	5	3	3	2	3
500 + ...	7	7	8	9	8
Location					
Hospitals Urban	74	72	68	67	67
Hospitals Rural	40	41	45	45	45
Control					
State and Local Government	39	36	37	38	40
Not for Profit	56	58	60	59	58
Investor owned	19	19	16	15	14
Physician Models					
Independent Practice Association	8	7	11	11	14
Group Practice without Walls	4	5	2	5	4
Open Physician-Hospital Organization	26	29	26	27	29
Closed Physician-Hospital Organization	9	8	10	11	13
Management Service Organization	12	12	16	15	16
Integrated Salary Model	41	40	38	33	37
Equity Model	1	0	0	0	0
Foundation	6	3	2	3	3
Insurance Products					
Health Maintenance Organization	29	31	26	25	17
Preferred Provider Organization	42	45	40	35	31
Indemnity Fee for Service	9	11	9	10	6
Managed Care Contracts					
Health Maintenance Organization	60	58	64	66	65
Preferred Provider Organization	75	80	79	82	78
Affiliations					
Hospitals in a System*	68	66	65	56	57
Hospitals in a Network	41	39	37	37	41
Hospitals in a Group Purchasing Organization..	94	91	87	87	87

* Please note that system affiliate information for hospitals is derived from AHA membership. In years prior to 2003 the affiliation was derived from a question on the AHA Annual Survey of hospitals; therefore, non-responding hospitals were not included in the system affiliation counts. Years prior to 2003 have been updated to reflect this change, which now include affiliation for non-reporting hospitals.

States

TABLE 6

INDIANA

U.S. Registered Community Hospitals
(Nonfederal, short-term general and other special hospitals)

Utilization, Personnel, Revenue and Expenses, Community Health Indicators 2002–2006

	2006	2005	2004	2003	2002
TOTAL FACILITY (Includes Hospital and Nursing Home Units)					
Utilization - Inpatient					
Beds	18,076	17,750	18,796	18,932	18,961
Admissions	726,020	717,490	730,610	712,151	715,936
Inpatient Days	3,801,325	3,763,741	4,059,031	3,997,353	4,077,032
Average Length of Stay	5.2	5.2	5.6	5.6	5.7
Inpatient Surgeries	201,896	212,497	210,455	201,344	199,279
Births	85,960	83,336	85,670	81,200	78,921
Utilization - Outpatient					
Emergency Outpatient Visits	2,704,727	2,594,196	2,624,977	2,492,597	2,437,268
Other Outpatient Visits	13,815,730	13,857,787	12,887,708	12,505,299	11,650,167
Total Outpatient Visits	16,520,457	16,451,983	15,512,685	14,997,896	14,087,435
Outpatient Surgeries	443,997	415,756	430,099	452,206	416,641
Personnel					
Full Time RNs	18,592	17,532	17,385	16,836	17,176
Full Time LPNs	2,197	2,259	2,217	2,292	2,408
Part Time RNs	14,729	14,843	14,650	12,701	11,544
Part Time LPNs	1,381	1,523	1,507	1,456	1,399
Total Full Time	81,503	78,337	78,178	76,985	79,408
Total Part Time	43,210	42,031	41,619	37,643	35,876
Revenue - Inpatient					
Gross Inpatient Revenue	$15,861,935,722	$14,091,962,851	$13,296,387,383	$11,665,904,141	$10,700,904,487
Revenue - Outpatient					
Gross Outpatient Revenue	$13,095,278,016	$11,464,712,812	$10,362,964,783	$8,771,505,233	$7,508,632,761
Revenue and Expenses - Totals					
(Includes Inpatient and Outpatient)					
Total Gross Revenue	$28,957,213,738	$25,556,675,663	$23,659,352,166	$20,437,409,374	$18,209,537,248
Deductions from Revenue	16,266,448,623	13,874,036,226	12,303,799,992	10,322,060,345	8,632,745,626
Net Patient Revenue	12,690,765,115	11,682,639,437	11,355,552,174	10,115,349,029	9,576,791,622
Other Operating Revenue	729,382,635	660,605,999	495,987,318	584,230,112	433,611,706
Other Nonoperating Revenue	394,167,657	224,037,175	252,320,225	196,893,476	63,204,269
Total Net Revenue	13,814,315,407	12,567,282,611	12,103,859,717	10,896,472,617	10,073,607,597
Total Expenses	12,642,920,543	11,413,287,976	10,916,451,392	9,985,287,171	9,272,854,799
HOSPITAL UNIT (Excludes Separate Nursing Home Units)					
Utilization - Inpatient					
Beds	17,194	16,841	17,907	17,907	17,867
Admissions	716,630	707,682	720,545	701,648	704,094
Inpatient Days	3,532,765	3,484,986	3,812,707	3,690,772	3,751,265
Average Length of Stay	4.9	4.9	5.3	5.3	5.3
Personnel					
Total Full Time	80,597	77,768	77,283	76,249	78,630
Total Part Time	42,664	41,496	40,858	36,759	35,272
Revenue and Expenses - Totals					
(Includes Inpatient and Outpatient)					
Total Net Revenue	$13,752,934,410	$12,495,533,140	$12,051,572,873	$10,836,544,994	$9,996,393,418
Total Expenses	12,580,110,810	11,352,451,392	10,871,754,546	9,927,768,129	9,204,932,252
COMMUNITY HEALTH INDICATORS PER 1000 POPULATION					
Total Population (in thousands)	6,314	6,266	6,223	6,192	6,155
Inpatient					
Beds	2.9	2.8	3.0	3.1	3.1
Admissions	115.0	114.5	117.4	115.0	116.3
Inpatient Days	602.1	600.7	652.2	645.6	662.4
Inpatient Surgeries	32.0	33.9	33.8	32.5	32.4
Births	13.6	13.3	13.8	13.1	12.8
Outpatient					
Emergency Outpatient Visits	428.4	414.0	421.8	402.6	396.0
Other Outpatient Visits	2,188.3	2,211.6	2,070.9	2,019.7	1,892.9
Total Outpatient Visits	2,616.7	2,625.6	2,492.7	2,422.3	2,288.9
Outpatient Surgeries	70.3	66.4	69.1	73.0	67.7
Expense per Capita (per person)	$2,002.5	$1,821.5	$1,754.1	$1,612.7	$1,506.6

TABLE 6

IOWA

U.S. Registered Community Hospitals
(Nonfederal, short-term general and other special hospitals)

Overview 2002–2006

	2006	2005	2004	2003	2002
Total Community Hospitals in Iowa...........	117	116	115	116	116
Bed Size Category					
6-24.....................................	13	13	10	11	12
25-49....................................	51	50	49	47	45
50-99....................................	26	25	28	30	29
100-199..................................	12	13	13	13	14
200-299..................................	7	6	6	6	7
300-399..................................	4	5	4	5	5
400-499..................................	2	2	3	2	2
500 +....................................	2	2	2	2	2
Location					
Hospitals Urban.........................	33	32	20	21	21
Hospitals Rural.........................	84	84	95	95	95
Control					
State and Local Government................	59	59	59	59	59
Not for Profit...........................	58	57	56	57	57
Investor owned..........................	0	0	0	0	0
Physician Models					
Independent Practice Association............	17	20	19	18	21
Group Practice without Walls...............	3	3	4	4	3
Open Physician-Hospital Organization........	26	24	21	19	18
Closed Physician-Hospital Organization.......	11	11	12	16	17
Management Service Organization...........	12	13	13	13	12
Integrated Salary Model....................	62	59	56	58	51
Equity Model............................	1	1	2	2	3
Foundation..............................	6	6	5	3	3
Insurance Products					
Health Maintenance Organization............	13	13	17	16	18
Preferred Provider Organization.............	29	31	37	37	35
Indemnity Fee for Service	7	7	8	9	8
Managed Care Contracts					
Health Maintenance Organization............	66	65	65	66	66
Preferred Provider Organization.............	99	93	94	97	96
Affiliations					
Hospitals in a System*....................	64	62	61	59	61
Hospitals in a Network....................	73	70	65	59	59
Hospitals in a Group Purchasing Organization..	110	108	105	105	105

* Please note that system affiliate information for hospitals is derived from AHA membership. In years prior to 2003 the affiliation was derived from a question on the AHA Annual Survey of hospitals; therefore, non-responding hospitals were not included in the system affiliation counts. Years prior to 2003 have been updated to reflect this change, which now include affiliation for non-reporting hospitals.

TABLE 6

IOWA

U.S. Registered Community Hospitals
(Nonfederal, short-term general and other special hospitals)

Utilization, Personnel, Revenue and Expenses, Community Health Indicators 2002–2006

	2006	2005	2004	2003	2002
TOTAL FACILITY (Includes Hospital and Nursing Home Units)					
Utilization - Inpatient					
Beds	10,500	10,753	10,943	11,002	11,267
Admissions	363,077	362,541	359,611	363,008	370,968
Inpatient Days	2,267,449	2,323,346	2,358,165	2,369,769	2,447,672
Average Length of Stay	6.2	6.4	6.6	6.5	6.6
Inpatient Surgeries	99,335	102,520	108,042	100,020	106,987
Births	39,560	38,899	38,419	37,936	37,342
Utilization - Outpatient					
Emergency Outpatient Visits	1,122,636	1,118,233	1,065,819	1,066,268	1,072,319
Other Outpatient Visits	9,172,457	8,979,828	8,619,047	8,669,111	8,258,357
Total Outpatient Visits	10,295,093	10,098,061	9,684,866	9,735,379	9,330,676
Outpatient Surgeries	335,367	348,557	334,652	273,026	302,995
Personnel					
Full Time RNs	10,218	9,842	9,268	8,926	8,967
Full Time LPNs	904	978	901	922	996
Part Time RNs	7,211	6,683	7,207	7,045	7,391
Part Time LPNs	759	737	836	832	836
Total Full Time	43,563	43,891	41,397	40,849	41,179
Total Part Time	25,228	23,884	25,233	24,861	25,648
Revenue - Inpatient					
Gross Inpatient Revenue	$6,041,189,863	$5,691,952,810	$5,138,048,080	$4,676,641,630	$4,245,474,792
Revenue - Outpatient					
Gross Outpatient Revenue	$5,765,745,834	$5,140,873,851	$4,509,250,053	$3,946,331,686	$3,390,410,867
Revenue and Expenses - Totals					
(Includes Inpatient and Outpatient)					
Total Gross Revenue	$11,806,935,697	$10,832,826,661	$9,647,298,133	$8,622,973,316	$7,635,885,659
Deductions from Revenue	6,158,463,230	5,563,253,766	4,779,712,534	3,993,879,715	3,333,435,082
Net Patient Revenue	5,648,472,467	5,269,572,895	4,867,585,599	4,629,093,601	4,302,450,577
Other Operating Revenue	423,197,979	422,215,028	397,098,611	352,052,586	328,828,491
Other Nonoperating Revenue	141,353,867	122,389,633	74,842,671	52,808,563	51,699,288
Total Net Revenue	6,213,024,313	5,814,177,556	5,339,526,881	5,033,954,750	4,682,978,356
Total Expenses	5,830,164,533	5,446,874,403	5,081,276,194	4,779,866,027	4,483,595,177
HOSPITAL UNIT (Excludes Separate Nursing Home Units)					
Utilization - Inpatient					
Beds	8,491	8,664	8,829	8,777	9,038
Admissions	354,676	353,704	351,217	352,526	360,065
Inpatient Days	1,605,060	1,653,640	1,685,270	1,643,007	1,723,431
Average Length of Stay	4.5	4.7	4.8	4.7	4.8
Personnel					
Total Full Time	42,578	42,873	39,785	39,856	40,108
Total Part Time	24,254	22,882	23,980	23,844	24,625
Revenue and Expenses - Totals					
(Includes Inpatient and Outpatient)					
Total Net Revenue	$6,108,192,223	$5,707,539,421	$5,244,048,673	$4,927,832,564	$4,581,452,200
Total Expenses	5,746,268,857	5,359,185,888	5,006,432,721	4,695,594,251	4,406,423,753
COMMUNITY HEALTH INDICATORS PER 1000 POPULATION					
Total Population (in thousands)	2,982	2,966	2,954	2,942	2,935
Inpatient					
Beds	3.5	3.6	3.7	3.7	3.8
Admissions	121.8	122.3	121.8	123.4	126.4
Inpatient Days	760.4	783.5	798.4	805.5	833.9
Inpatient Surgeries	33.3	34.6	36.6	34.0	36.4
Births	13.3	13.1	13.0	12.9	12.7
Outpatient					
Emergency Outpatient Visits	376.5	377.1	360.8	362.4	365.3
Other Outpatient Visits	3,075.9	3,028.1	2,918.1	2,946.6	2,813.5
Total Outpatient Visits	3,452.3	3,405.2	3,278.9	3,309.0	3,178.8
Outpatient Surgeries	112.5	117.5	113.3	92.8	103.2
Expense per Capita (per person)	$1,955.1	$1,836.7	$1,720.3	$1,624.7	$1,527.5

States

TABLE 6

KANSAS

U.S. Registered Community Hospitals
(Nonfederal, short-term general and other special hospitals)

Overview 2002–2006

	2006	2005	2004	2003	2002
Total Community Hospitals in Kansas	129	131	134	134	132
Bed Size Category					
6-24	15	16	15	17	15
25-49	52	50	50	45	42
50-99	38	42	47	48	50
100-199	13	13	12	14	14
200-299	6	6	5	5	6
300-399	2	1	2	2	2
400-499	1	1	1	1	2
500 + ...	2	2	2	2	1
Location					
Hospitals Urban..............................	29	30	27	27	25
Hospitals Rural	100	101	107	107	107
Control					
State and Local Government................	61	61	61	61	61
Not for Profit	57	58	60	60	62
Investor owned	11	12	13	13	9
Physician Models					
Independent Practice Association	17	19	20	18	16
Group Practice without Walls................	5	4	5	6	5
Open Physician-Hospital Organization	14	16	14	16	18
Closed Physician-Hospital Organization	2	1	1	2	4
Management Service Organization	6	3	3	2	5
Integrated Salary Model....................	66	58	51	52	45
Equity Model	1	0	0	0	0
Foundation..................................	5	4	3	2	3
Insurance Products					
Health Maintenance Organization	5	6	8	8	7
Preferred Provider Organization..............	31	35	36	34	22
Indemnity Fee for Service	4	4	6	6	6
Managed Care Contracts					
Health Maintenance Organization	44	45	43	42	41
Preferred Provider Organization..............	113	111	111	103	105
Affiliations					
Hospitals in a System*.....................	48	50	51	54	52
Hospitals in a Network.....................	81	83	83	78	73
Hospitals in a Group Purchasing Organization..	124	125	127	124	121

* Please note that system affiliate information for hospitals is derived from AHA membership. In years prior to 2003 the affiliation was derived from a question on the AHA Annual Survey of hospitals; therefore, non-responding hospitals were not included in the system affiliation counts. Years prior to 2003 have been updated to reflect this change, which now include affiliation for non-reporting hospitals.

TABLE 6

KANSAS

U.S. Registered Community Hospitals
(Nonfederal, short-term general and other special hospitals)

Utilization, Personnel, Revenue and Expenses, Community Health Indicators 2002–2006

	2006	2005	2004	2003	2002
TOTAL FACILITY (Includes Hospital and Nursing Home Units)					
Utilization - Inpatient					
Beds	10,019	10,075	10,362	10,554	10,850
Admissions	332,524	330,429	330,712	331,244	328,987
Inpatient Days	2,024,257	2,070,956	2,115,015	2,148,111	2,165,195
Average Length of Stay	6.1	6.3	6.4	6.5	6.6
Inpatient Surgeries	82,929	95,685	96,928	89,889	88,704
Births	40,729	40,039	39,489	39,341	38,591
Utilization - Outpatient					
Emergency Outpatient Visits	972,761	959,699	933,816	945,208	940,408
Other Outpatient Visits	5,173,496	4,985,081	4,926,831	5,004,830	4,734,607
Total Outpatient Visits	6,146,257	5,944,780	5,860,647	5,950,038	5,675,015
Outpatient Surgeries	160,808	169,295	168,004	162,583	155,965
Personnel					
Full Time RNs	8,599	8,396	8,081	7,839	7,600
Full Time LPNs	1,055	1,066	1,085	1,169	1,138
Part Time RNs	4,671	4,756	4,046	4,217	4,088
Part Time LPNs	484	485	530	490	558
Total Full Time	35,113	34,326	33,963	34,022	33,790
Total Part Time	14,162	14,570	13,957	14,736	14,290
Revenue - Inpatient					
Gross Inpatient Revenue	$7,121,171,892	$6,492,436,141	$6,041,564,302	$5,466,344,640	$4,837,931,215
Revenue - Outpatient					
Gross Outpatient Revenue	$5,152,612,930	$4,575,808,221	$4,008,314,363	$3,554,053,357	$3,020,822,797
Revenue and Expenses - Totals					
(Includes Inpatient and Outpatient)					
Total Gross Revenue	$12,273,784,822	$11,068,244,362	$10,049,878,665	$9,020,397,997	$7,858,754,012
Deductions from Revenue	7,575,131,231	6,722,580,237	5,989,750,259	5,192,082,605	4,306,839,200
Net Patient Revenue	4,698,653,591	4,345,664,125	4,060,128,406	3,828,315,392	3,551,914,812
Other Operating Revenue	183,451,488	160,393,655	167,277,373	145,873,173	150,197,636
Other Nonoperating Revenue	92,775,123	65,308,485	68,121,241	27,634,261	18,174,135
Total Net Revenue	4,974,880,202	4,571,366,265	4,295,527,020	4,001,822,826	3,720,286,583
Total Expenses	4,612,906,605	4,292,972,936	4,062,879,679	3,816,798,953	3,576,366,207
HOSPITAL UNIT (Excludes Separate Nursing Home Units)					
Utilization - Inpatient					
Beds	8,313	8,376	8,699	8,785	9,004
Admissions	329,818	327,686	327,208	326,144	322,983
Inpatient Days	1,498,214	1,547,593	1,588,632	1,600,483	1,630,230
Average Length of Stay	4.5	4.7	4.9	4.9	5.0
Personnel					
Total Full Time	34,042	33,277	32,568	32,915	32,669
Total Part Time	13,650	14,042	13,263	14,149	13,618
Revenue and Expenses - Totals					
(Includes Inpatient and Outpatient)					
Total Net Revenue	$4,908,181,882	$4,509,750,464	$4,236,126,636	$3,940,784,536	$3,656,845,788
Total Expenses	4,558,169,540	4,243,480,226	4,010,808,623	3,760,914,701	3,520,829,715
COMMUNITY HEALTH INDICATORS PER 1000 POPULATION					
Total Population (in thousands)	2,764	2,748	2,738	2,727	2,715
Inpatient					
Beds	3.6	3.7	3.8	3.9	4.0
Admissions	120.3	120.2	120.8	121.5	121.2
Inpatient Days	732.3	753.6	772.4	787.7	797.6
Inpatient Surgeries	30.0	34.8	35.4	33.0	32.7
Births	14.7	14.6	14.4	14.4	14.2
Outpatient					
Emergency Outpatient Visits	351.9	349.2	341.0	346.6	346.4
Other Outpatient Visits	1,871.7	1,814.0	1,799.2	1,835.3	1,744.0
Total Outpatient Visits	2,223.6	2,163.2	2,140.2	2,181.9	2,090.4
Outpatient Surgeries	58.2	61.6	61.4	59.6	57.5
Expense per Capita (per person)	$1,668.9	$1,562.1	$1,483.7	$1,399.6	$1,317.4

States

TABLE 6

KENTUCKY

U.S. Registered Community Hospitals
(Nonfederal, short-term general and other special hospitals)

Overview 2002–2006

	2006	2005	2004	2003	2002
Total Community Hospitals in Kentucky.......	104	105	105	103	104
Bed Size Category					
6-24	2	2	1	1	2
25-49	31	29	28	27	21
50-99	24	27	27	26	33
100-199	19	20	20	21	21
200-299	13	12	15	13	13
300-399	8	7	6	7	6
400-499	5	6	6	5	5
500 + ...	2	2	2	3	3
Location					
Hospitals Urban......................	40	41	35	32	32
Hospitals Rural	64	64	70	71	72
Control					
State and Local Government..............	13	13	13	13	14
Not for Profit........................	71	72	72	73	73
Investor owned	20	20	20	17	17
Physician Models					
Independent Practice Association	7	8	3	9	8
Group Practice without Walls..............	2	2	1	2	2
Open Physician-Hospital Organization	11	11	12	14	11
Closed Physician-Hospital Organization	4	3	2	1	1
Management Service Organization	3	2	2	4	3
Integrated Salary Model	34	30	27	29	31
Equity Model	0	0	0	0	0
Foundation............................	3	2	3	2	9
Insurance Products					
Health Maintenance Organization	17	20	21	25	23
Preferred Provider Organization.............	23	31	23	20	23
Indemnity Fee for Service	3	4	3	3	1
Managed Care Contracts					
Health Maintenance Organization	45	46	51	61	59
Preferred Provider Organization.............	67	66	64	73	70
Affiliations					
Hospitals in a System*...................	74	69	69	64	63
Hospitals in a Network....................	26	25	23	18	15
Hospitals in a Group Purchasing Organization..	83	80	77	91	82

* Please note that system affiliate information for hospitals is derived from AHA membership. In years prior to 2003 the affiliation was derived from a question on the AHA Annual Survey of hospitals; therefore, non-responding hospitals were not included in the system affiliation counts. Years prior to 2003 have been updated to reflect this change, which now include affiliation for non-reporting hospitals.

TABLE **6**

KENTUCKY

U.S. Registered Community Hospitals
(Nonfederal, short-term general and other special hospitals)

Utilization, Personnel, Revenue and Expenses, Community Health Indicators 2002–2006

	2006	2005	2004	2003	2002
TOTAL FACILITY (Includes Hospital and Nursing Home Units)					
Utilization - Inpatient					
Beds	14,574	14,891	15,276	14,940	15,066
Admissions	612,842	617,969	605,707	600,454	601,644
Inpatient Days	3,239,168	3,385,604	3,384,932	3,394,239	3,393,525
Average Length of Stay.	5.3	5.5	5.6	5.7	5.6
Inpatient Surgeries.	178,264	178,250	169,692	169,619	180,073
Births.	54,614	53,835	53,067	52,813	52,098
Utilization - Outpatient					
Emergency Outpatient Visits	2,191,969	2,238,194	2,257,276	2,137,500	2,109,556
Other Outpatient Visits.	6,623,337	6,620,883	6,622,870	6,405,609	6,536,556
Total Outpatient Visits	8,815,306	8,859,077	8,880,146	8,543,109	8,646,112
Outpatient Surgeries	373,174	375,953	365,854	370,684	363,052
Personnel					
Full Time RNs	15,106	14,515	14,319	13,620	13,224
Full Time LPNs	2,146	2,178	2,163	2,749	2,361
Part Time RNs	6,400	6,668	6,436	6,706	6,354
Part Time LPNs	547	665	614	655	714
Total Full Time.	59,725	57,617	56,989	56,016	56,104
Total Part Time	18,967	21,061	19,236	19,332	20,611
Revenue - Inpatient					
Gross Inpatient Revenue.	$12,527,888,281	$11,140,011,986	$10,211,530,486	$9,477,812,427	$8,677,558,625
Revenue - Outpatient					
Gross Outpatient Revenue	$9,475,429,030	$8,208,360,194	$7,156,929,150	$6,435,990,027	$5,544,182,284
Revenue and Expenses - Totals					
(Includes Inpatient and Outpatient)					
Total Gross Revenue.	$22,003,317,311	$19,348,372,180	$17,368,459,636	$15,913,802,454	$14,221,740,909
Deductions from Revenue	13,658,377,781	11,792,754,141	10,353,176,805	9,289,949,832	7,943,529,393
Net Patient Revenue.	8,344,939,530	7,555,618,039	7,015,282,831	6,623,852,622	6,278,211,516
Other Operating Revenue	257,873,549	292,730,942	314,482,516	286,235,427	264,424,862
Other Nonoperating Revenue	190,808,469	84,227,172	80,671,058	38,680,240	55,509,283
Total Net Revenue.	8,793,621,548	7,932,576,153	7,410,436,405	6,948,768,289	6,598,145,661
Total Expenses.	7,943,139,511	7,397,991,998	6,893,069,255	6,606,931,221	6,201,408,483
HOSPITAL UNIT (Excludes Separate Nursing Home Units)					
Utilization - Inpatient					
Beds	13,581	13,794	13,980	13,408	13,640
Admissions	606,435	609,253	597,247	590,914	591,970
Inpatient Days	2,928,444	3,010,129	2,992,615	2,932,767	2,999,495
Average Length of Stay.	4.8	4.9	5.0	5.0	5.1
Personnel					
Total Full Time.	58,711	56,719	54,461	54,630	54,958
Total Part Time	18,596	20,725	18,269	18,897	20,115
Revenue and Expenses - Totals					
(Includes Inpatient and Outpatient)					
Total Net Revenue.	$8,703,572,762	$7,815,800,206	$7,312,879,356	$6,840,739,073	$6,505,926,611
Total Expenses.	7,869,950,752	7,301,705,467	6,825,631,885	6,523,073,019	6,126,969,102
COMMUNITY HEALTH INDICATORS PER 1000 POPULATION					
Total Population (in thousands)	4,206	4,173	4,140	4,114	4,089
Inpatient					
Beds	3.5	3.6	3.7	3.6	3.7
Admissions	145.7	148.1	146.3	145.9	147.1
Inpatient Days	770.1	811.4	817.5	824.9	829.9
Inpatient Surgeries.	42.4	42.7	41.0	41.2	44.0
Births.	13.0	12.9	12.8	12.8	12.7
Outpatient					
Emergency Outpatient Visits	521.1	536.4	545.2	519.5	515.9
Other Outpatient Visits.	1,574.7	1,586.7	1,599.6	1,556.8	1,598.6
Total Outpatient Visits	2,095.9	2,123.2	2,144.7	2,076.3	2,114.5
Outpatient Surgeries	88.7	90.1	88.4	90.1	88.8
Expense per Capita (per person). . . .	$1,888.5	$1,773.0	$1,664.8	$1,605.8	$1,516.6

States

TABLE 6

LOUISIANA

U.S. Registered Community Hospitals
(Nonfederal, short-term general and other special hospitals)

Overview 2002–2006

	2006	2005	2004	2003	2002
Total Community Hospitals in Louisiana	132	128	131	127	128
Bed Size Category					
6-24	16	16	15	11	10
25-49	40	35	33	32	33
50-99	27	27	30	29	30
100-199	27	26	27	25	28
200-299	10	13	10	12	8
300-399	4	4	6	8	9
400-499	4	4	6	5	5
500 + ...	4	3	4	5	5
Location					
Hospitals Urban.........................	81	78	82	78	77
Hospitals Rural	51	50	49	49	51
Control					
State and Local Government...............	51	51	53	50	52
Not for Profit	38	32	34	34	35
Investor owned	43	45	44	43	41
Physician Models					
Independent Practice Association	14	8	12	13	13
Group Practice without Walls...............	4	4	5	4	5
Open Physician-Hospital Organization	14	11	13	14	17
Closed Physician-Hospital Organization	6	3	4	4	8
Management Service Organization	7	6	7	7	8
Integrated Salary Model...................	18	13	19	18	19
Equity Model.........................	1	1	1	1	1
Foundation.........................	4	2	1	1	3
Insurance Products					
Health Maintenance Organization	7	8	12	8	8
Preferred Provider Organization.............	12	10	12	10	14
Indemnity Fee for Service	6	2	2	1	3
Managed Care Contracts					
Health Maintenance Organization	41	45	50	55	51
Preferred Provider Organization.............	54	52	60	65	62
Affiliations					
Hospitals in a System*....................	72	65	67	68	68
Hospitals in a Network....................	19	17	22	20	18
Hospitals in a Group Purchasing Organization..	64	60	60	70	64

* Please note that system affiliate information for hospitals is derived from AHA membership. In years prior to 2003 the affiliation was derived from a question on the AHA Annual Survey of hospitals; therefore, non-responding hospitals were not included in the system affiliation counts. Years prior to 2003 have been updated to reflect this change, which now include affiliation for non-reporting hospitals.

States

TABLE 6

LOUISIANA

U.S. Registered Community Hospitals
(Nonfederal, short-term general and other special hospitals)

Utilization, Personnel, Revenue and Expenses, Community Health Indicators 2002–2006

	2006	2005	2004	2003	2002
TOTAL FACILITY (Includes Hospital and Nursing Home Units)					
Utilization - Inpatient					
Beds	15,864	15,534	17,199	17,829	17,867
Admissions	623,144	619,500	696,154	690,246	692,011
Inpatient Days	3,556,169	3,404,395	3,856,768	3,872,912	3,873,634
Average Length of Stay	5.7	5.5	5.5	5.6	5.6
Inpatient Surgeries	176,644	150,594	170,141	171,599	179,986
Births	69,455	56,499	56,218	63,923	57,564
Utilization - Outpatient					
Emergency Outpatient Visits	2,096,962	2,147,600	2,468,882	2,498,935	2,468,832
Other Outpatient Visits	7,764,689	7,659,204	7,911,215	8,325,075	8,262,795
Total Outpatient Visits	9,861,651	9,806,804	10,380,097	10,824,010	10,731,627
Outpatient Surgeries	281,956	239,027	269,918	254,242	287,954
Personnel					
Full Time RNs	15,502	15,017	16,231	15,350	15,320
Full Time LPNs	2,761	2,898	3,394	3,296	3,186
Part Time RNs	5,545	5,358	5,552	5,413	5,973
Part Time LPNs	778	786	936	853	921
Total Full Time	65,516	62,785	69,516	69,524	69,541
Total Part Time	17,124	16,770	18,508	17,344	19,700
Revenue - Inpatient					
Gross Inpatient Revenue	$12,833,233,745	$12,486,431,054	$12,631,245,465	$12,094,846,990	$10,679,535,909
Revenue - Outpatient					
Gross Outpatient Revenue	$7,529,943,140	$7,056,479,417	$7,060,262,549	$6,409,128,381	$5,523,762,540
Revenue and Expenses - Totals					
(Includes Inpatient and Outpatient)					
Total Gross Revenue	$20,363,176,885	$19,542,910,471	$19,691,508,014	$18,503,975,371	$16,203,298,449
Deductions from Revenue	13,060,049,470	12,631,005,388	12,335,668,769	11,323,461,934	9,401,154,343
Net Patient Revenue	7,303,127,415	6,911,905,083	7,355,839,245	7,180,513,437	6,802,144,106
Other Operating Revenue	495,512,730	394,178,196	383,145,135	342,156,916	271,896,066
Other Nonoperating Revenue	168,610,943	99,333,406	115,137,849	124,878,279	49,925,463
Total Net Revenue	7,979,845,190	7,405,416,685	7,854,122,229	7,647,548,632	7,123,965,635
Total Expenses	7,552,791,081	7,158,276,605	7,419,160,281	7,170,688,383	6,751,804,011
HOSPITAL UNIT (Excludes Separate Nursing Home Units)					
Utilization - Inpatient					
Beds	14,964	14,881	16,826	17,430	17,026
Admissions	621,068	617,435	693,562	687,450	687,478
Inpatient Days	3,276,461	3,212,644	3,737,214	3,747,426	3,657,799
Average Length of Stay	5.3	5.2	5.4	5.5	5.3
Personnel					
Total Full Time	64,629	62,136	68,744	68,913	68,904
Total Part Time	16,905	16,612	18,142	17,029	19,388
Revenue and Expenses - Totals					
(Includes Inpatient and Outpatient)					
Total Net Revenue	$7,947,920,310	$7,375,447,859	$7,829,455,901	$7,623,909,158	$7,079,640,911
Total Expenses	7,514,898,181	7,124,471,067	7,393,898,853	7,147,825,517	6,714,901,922
COMMUNITY HEALTH INDICATORS PER 1000 POPULATION					
Total Population (in thousands)	4,288	4,507	4,496	4,481	4,471
Inpatient					
Beds	3.7	3.4	3.8	4.0	4.0
Admissions	145.3	137.4	154.8	154.0	154.8
Inpatient Days	829.4	755.3	857.9	864.3	866.5
Inpatient Surgeries	41.2	33.4	37.8	38.3	40.3
Births	16.2	12.5	12.5	14.3	12.9
Outpatient					
Emergency Outpatient Visits	489.1	476.5	549.2	557.7	552.2
Other Outpatient Visits	1,810.9	1,699.3	1,759.7	1,857.9	1,848.3
Total Outpatient Visits	2,299.9	2,175.7	2,308.9	2,415.6	2,400.5
Outpatient Surgeries	65.8	53.0	60.0	56.7	64.4
Expense per Capita (per person)	$1,761.5	$1,588.1	$1,650.3	$1,600.3	$1,510.3

States

TABLE **6**

MAINE

U.S. Registered Community Hospitals
(Nonfederal, short-term general and other special hospitals)

Overview 2002–2006

	2006	2005	2004	2003	2002
Total Community Hospitals in Maine..........	37	37	37	37	37
Bed Size Category					
6-24	2	2	1	2	3
25-49	15	14	15	12	11
50-99	10	11	11	12	12
100-199	7	7	7	8	8
200-299	1	1	1	0	0
300-399	1	1	1	2	2
400-499	0	0	0	0	0
500 + ...	1	1	1	1	1
Location					
Hospitals Urban..........................	15	15	8	8	8
Hospitals Rural	22	22	29	29	29
Control					
State and Local Government...............	2	2	2	2	2
Not for Profit	34	34	34	34	34
Investor owned	1	1	1	1	1
Physician Models					
Independent Practice Association	4	4	4	5	4
Group Practice without Walls...............	2	1	1	2	2
Open Physician-Hospital Organization	14	15	14	14	15
Closed Physician-Hospital Organization	0	1	1	0	0
Management Service Organization	3	4	4	3	4
Integrated Salary Model...................	21	21	18	15	14
Equity Model	1	1	1	1	2
Foundation..............................	0	0	1	1	2
Insurance Products					
Health Maintenance Organization	3	2	2	2	3
Preferred Provider Organization.............	5	6	5	5	4
Indemnity Fee for Service	3	2	2	1	2
Managed Care Contracts					
Health Maintenance Organization	21	22	22	22	24
Preferred Provider Organization.............	20	22	20	19	21
Affiliations					
Hospitals in a System*....................	15	14	13	14	15
Hospitals in a Network	20	20	18	18	18
Hospitals in a Group Purchasing Organization..	33	32	30	33	34

States

* Please note that system affiliate information for hospitals is derived from AHA membership. In years prior to 2003 the affiliation was derived from a question on the AHA Annual Survey of hospitals; therefore, non-responding hospitals were not included in the system affiliation counts. Years prior to 2003 have been updated to reflect this change, which now include affiliation for non-reporting hospitals.

TABLE 6

MAINE

U.S. Registered Community Hospitals
(Nonfederal, short-term general and other special hospitals)

Utilization, Personnel, Revenue and Expenses, Community Health Indicators 2002–2006

	2006	2005	2004	2003	2002
TOTAL FACILITY (Includes Hospital and Nursing Home Units)					
Utilization - Inpatient					
Beds	3,489	3,526	3,549	3,702	3,694
Admissions	150,990	151,303	151,135	148,517	145,917
Inpatient Days	851,520	848,195	820,114	816,332	889,005
Average Length of Stay.	5.6	5.6	5.4	5.5	6.1
Inpatient Surgeries.	44,380	42,857	43,761	45,340	60,022
Births.	13,736	13,667	13,504	13,263	13,072
Utilization - Outpatient					
Emergency Outpatient Visits	757,685	728,701	711,570	710,201	709,091
Other Outpatient Visits.	3,447,664	3,570,798	3,406,226	3,215,263	3,022,170
Total Outpatient Visits	4,205,349	4,299,499	4,117,796	3,925,464	3,731,261
Outpatient Surgeries	125,183	118,469	118,131	115,386	97,665
Personnel					
Full Time RNs	4,337	4,369	4,132	4,035	3,754
Full Time LPNs	270	256	291	283	241
Part Time RNs	3,596	3,349	3,437	3,428	3,449
Part Time LPNs	150	169	171	185	193
Total Full Time	21,285	20,969	19,205	17,983	17,038
Total Part Time	11,494	10,914	10,723	10,496	10,681
Revenue - Inpatient					
Gross Inpatient Revenue.	$2,679,113,113	$2,540,202,810	$2,467,189,637	$2,191,849,628	$2,019,706,879
Revenue - Outpatient					
Gross Outpatient Revenue	$2,828,799,712	$2,491,229,223	$2,211,215,695	$1,869,295,933	$1,567,817,352
Revenue and Expenses - Totals					
(Includes Inpatient and Outpatient)					
Total Gross Revenue.	$5,507,912,825	$5,031,432,033	$4,678,405,332	$4,061,145,561	$3,587,524,231
Deductions from Revenue	2,428,063,405	2,169,148,932	2,111,297,150	1,774,902,165	1,488,086,115
Net Patient Revenue	3,079,849,420	2,862,283,101	2,567,108,182	2,286,243,396	2,099,438,116
Other Operating Revenue	90,802,554	86,008,208	80,994,871	76,610,152	72,149,218
Other Nonoperating Revenue	61,676,959	54,877,774	52,626,519	29,473,853	19,653,975
Total Net Revenue.	3,232,328,933	3,003,169,083	2,700,729,572	2,392,327,401	2,191,241,309
Total Expenses.	3,060,867,876	2,762,713,712	2,549,574,659	2,291,786,577	2,105,062,300
HOSPITAL UNIT (Excludes Separate Nursing Home Units)					
Utilization - Inpatient					
Beds	3,099	3,112	3,310	3,351	3,151
Admissions	149,665	150,031	150,073	146,917	144,016
Inpatient Days	721,622	714,678	745,357	704,903	714,141
Average Length of Stay.	4.8	4.8	5.0	4.8	5.0
Personnel					
Total Full Time	20,709	20,647	18,517	17,502	16,584
Total Part Time	11,123	10,639	10,225	9,843	10,351
Revenue and Expenses - Totals					
(Includes Inpatient and Outpatient)					
Total Net Revenue.	$3,203,268,060	$2,976,406,866	$2,684,324,134	$2,369,627,414	$2,161,952,361
Total Expenses.	3,034,440,927	2,736,792,556	2,533,017,594	2,269,425,051	2,081,511,605
COMMUNITY HEALTH INDICATORS PER 1000 POPULATION					
Total Population (in thousands)	1,322	1,318	1,314	1,307	1,297
Inpatient					
Beds	2.6	2.7	2.7	2.8	2.8
Admissions	114.3	114.8	115.0	113.6	112.5
Inpatient Days	644.3	643.4	624.2	624.5	685.5
Inpatient Surgeries.	33.6	32.5	33.3	34.7	46.3
Births.	10.4	10.4	10.3	10.1	10.1
Outpatient					
Emergency Outpatient Visits	573.3	552.8	541.6	543.3	546.8
Other Outpatient Visits.	2,608.8	2,708.8	2,592.4	2,459.7	2,330.5
Total Outpatient Visits	3,182.1	3,261.6	3,134.0	3,003.1	2,877.2
Outpatient Surgeries	94.7	89.9	89.9	88.3	75.3
Expense per Capita (per person). . . .	$2,316.1	$2,095.8	$1,940.4	$1,753.3	$1,623.3

TABLE 6

MARYLAND

U.S. Registered Community Hospitals
(Nonfederal, short-term general and other special hospitals)

Overview 2002–2006

	2006	2005	2004	2003	2002
Total Community Hospitals in Maryland	50	50	50	51	49
Bed Size Category					
6-24	0	0	0	0	0
25-49	3	3	2	3	4
50-99	7	5	6	7	5
100-199	13	16	17	16	15
200-299	16	15	11	12	11
300-399	6	6	8	8	9
400-499	2	2	3	2	2
500 +	3	3	3	3	3
Location					
Hospitals Urban	44	44	41	41	40
Hospitals Rural	6	6	9	10	9
Control					
State and Local Government	0	0	0	1	0
Not for Profit	48	48	48	47	46
Investor owned	2	2	2	3	3
Physician Models					
Independent Practice Association	4	3	6	7	5
Group Practice without Walls	2	1	2	2	2
Open Physician-Hospital Organization	7	8	10	8	7
Closed Physician-Hospital Organization	4	4	1	2	3
Management Service Organization	6	5	4	3	2
Integrated Salary Model	26	23	26	25	23
Equity Model	2	2	4	3	3
Foundation	2	1	1	2	2
Insurance Products					
Health Maintenance Organization	8	8	9	12	10
Preferred Provider Organization	4	4	5	7	4
Indemnity Fee for Service	2	1	3	3	1
Managed Care Contracts					
Health Maintenance Organization	36	33	36	39	36
Preferred Provider Organization	32	33	35	36	32
Affiliations					
Hospitals in a System*	32	30	30	30	26
Hospitals in a Network	10	9	13	11	9
Hospitals in a Group Purchasing Organization	46	45	46	48	41

* Please note that system affiliate information for hospitals is derived from AHA membership. In years prior to 2003 the affiliation was derived from a question on the AHA Annual Survey of hospitals; therefore, non-responding hospitals were not included in the system affiliation counts. Years prior to 2003 have been updated to reflect this change, which now include affiliation for non-reporting hospitals.

States

TABLE 6

MARYLAND

U.S. Registered Community Hospitals
(Nonfederal, short-term general and other special hospitals)

Utilization, Personnel, Revenue and Expenses, Community Health Indicators 2002–2006

	2006	2005	2004	2003	2002
TOTAL FACILITY (Includes Hospital and Nursing Home Units)					
Utilization - Inpatient					
Beds	11,479	11,404	11,489	11,613	11,417
Admissions	690,371	679,838	661,449	645,158	634,914
Inpatient Days	3,167,502	3,187,739	3,189,302	3,167,111	3,049,647
Average Length of Stay	4.6	4.7	4.8	4.9	4.8
Inpatient Surgeries	192,341	188,592	189,945	185,674	186,084
Births	69,138	67,813	68,201	65,861	63,744
Utilization - Outpatient					
Emergency Outpatient Visits	2,299,181	2,160,010	2,162,198	2,079,674	1,943,614
Other Outpatient Visits	4,708,636	4,590,267	4,769,543	4,442,692	4,520,569
Total Outpatient Visits	7,007,817	6,750,277	6,931,741	6,522,366	6,464,183
Outpatient Surgeries	349,370	357,194	361,757	347,734	347,715
Personnel					
Full Time RNs	14,709	13,933	13,664	13,209	11,975
Full Time LPNs	578	579	589	583	705
Part Time RNs	8,972	8,096	8,348	8,825	8,418
Part Time LPNs	264	252	326	300	357
Total Full Time	62,875	61,492	58,981	58,458	56,379
Total Part Time	25,458	23,583	25,011	25,552	24,293
Revenue - Inpatient					
Gross Inpatient Revenue	$7,817,701,056	$7,328,324,384	$6,825,359,796	$6,419,579,015	$6,314,536,604
Revenue - Outpatient					
Gross Outpatient Revenue	$4,043,062,566	$3,806,641,962	$3,472,795,225	$3,161,027,418	$3,110,642,148
Revenue and Expenses - Totals					
(Includes Inpatient and Outpatient)					
Total Gross Revenue	$11,860,763,622	$11,134,966,346	$10,298,155,021	$9,580,606,433	$9,425,178,752
Deductions from Revenue	2,108,964,137	2,153,177,051	1,940,994,076	2,111,602,747	2,597,808,764
Net Patient Revenue	9,751,799,485	8,981,789,295	8,357,160,945	7,469,003,686	6,827,369,988
Other Operating Revenue	395,195,238	326,183,274	322,420,713	293,576,216	303,127,043
Other Nonoperating Revenue	132,820,364	121,915,311	53,498,715	58,685,721	25,174,124
Total Net Revenue	10,279,815,087	9,429,887,880	8,733,080,373	7,821,265,623	7,155,671,155
Total Expenses	9,794,446,454	8,998,802,051	8,424,555,436	7,601,418,187	6,971,693,586
HOSPITAL UNIT (Excludes Separate Nursing Home Units)					
Utilization - Inpatient					
Beds	10,733	10,706	10,675	10,796	10,726
Admissions	682,097	671,054	652,166	634,981	624,477
Inpatient Days	2,948,727	2,965,422	2,928,619	2,899,226	2,832,577
Average Length of Stay	4.3	4.4	4.5	4.6	4.5
Personnel					
Total Full Time	62,242	60,750	58,217	57,729	55,681
Total Part Time	25,092	23,194	24,621	25,201	23,927
Revenue and Expenses - Totals					
(Includes Inpatient and Outpatient)					
Total Net Revenue	$10,172,144,312	$9,330,092,287	$8,631,033,566	$7,736,373,266	$7,070,224,974
Total Expenses	9,685,250,847	8,900,701,029	8,316,968,289	7,516,936,241	6,892,430,543
COMMUNITY HEALTH INDICATORS PER 1000 POPULATION					
Total Population (in thousands)	5,616	5,590	5,553	5,507	5,441
Inpatient					
Beds	2.0	2.0	2.1	2.1	2.1
Admissions	122.9	121.6	119.1	117.2	116.7
Inpatient Days	564.0	570.3	574.3	575.1	560.5
Inpatient Surgeries	34.3	33.7	34.2	33.7	34.2
Births	12.3	12.1	12.3	12.0	11.7
Outpatient					
Emergency Outpatient Visits	409.4	386.4	389.4	377.7	357.2
Other Outpatient Visits	838.5	821.2	858.9	806.8	830.8
Total Outpatient Visits	1,247.9	1,207.6	1,248.2	1,184.4	1,188.0
Outpatient Surgeries	62.2	63.9	65.1	63.1	63.9
Expense per Capita (per person)	$1,744.1	$1,609.9	$1,517.0	$1,380.4	$1,281.2

States

TABLE 6

MASSACHUSETTS

U.S. Registered Community Hospitals
(Nonfederal, short-term general and other special hospitals)

Overview 2002–2006

	2006	2005	2004	2003	2002
Total Community Hospitals in Massachusetts...	80	80	78	79	78
Bed Size Category					
6-24	6	5	2	3	4
25-49	7	11	13	10	9
50-99	12	10	8	9	7
100-199	25	23	25	28	27
200-299	14	17	13	17	18
300-399	8	6	9	5	6
400-499	1	1	1	1	1
500 + ...	7	7	7	6	6
Location					
Hospitals Urban...........................	78	78	67	68	67
Hospitals Rural	2	2	11	11	11
Control					
State and Local Government................	3	3	3	3	4
Not for Profit	67	67	66	68	68
Investor owned	10	10	9	8	6
Physician Models					
Independent Practice Association	30	33	30	33	34
Group Practice without Walls...............	6	8	7	7	8
Open Physician-Hospital Organization	15	15	18	15	17
Closed Physician-Hospital Organization	11	9	6	10	11
Management Service Organization	10	11	12	12	14
Integrated Salary Model....................	37	36	37	35	30
Equity Model	4	3	2	4	3
Foundation...............................	7	7	4	5	6
Insurance Products					
Health Maintenance Organization	11	11	10	10	9
Preferred Provider Organization.............	8	8	7	6	6
Indemnity Fee for Service	4	4	3	4	1
Managed Care Contracts					
Health Maintenance Organization	64	65	61	62	62
Preferred Provider Organization.............	59	61	58	61	58
Affiliations					
Hospitals in a System*....................	42	38	37	39	38
Hospitals in a Network	25	27	25	20	21
Hospitals in a Group Purchasing Organization..	62	56	52	62	54

* Please note that system affiliate information for hospitals is derived from AHA membership. In years prior to 2003 the affiliation was derived from a question on the AHA Annual Survey of hospitals; therefore, non-responding hospitals were not included in the system affiliation counts. Years prior to 2003 have been updated to reflect this change, which now include affiliation for non-reporting hospitals.

States

TABLE 6

MASSACHUSETTS

U.S. Registered Community Hospitals
(Nonfederal, short-term general and other special hospitals)

Utilization, Personnel, Revenue and Expenses, Community Health Indicators 2002–2006

	2006	2005	2004	2003	2002
TOTAL FACILITY (Includes Hospital and Nursing Home Units)					
Utilization - Inpatient					
Beds	16,344	16,213	16,215	16,001	16,033
Admissions	834,895	799,653	801,137	784,618	765,820
Inpatient Days	4,432,313	4,386,690	4,428,800	4,372,515	4,348,099
Average Length of Stay	5.3	5.5	5.5	5.6	5.7
Inpatient Surgeries	201,727	222,012	209,418	211,618	205,077
Births	94,228	99,215	79,299	80,016	80,034
Utilization - Outpatient					
Emergency Outpatient Visits	3,139,255	2,866,187	2,874,936	2,929,681	2,882,602
Other Outpatient Visits	16,404,673	15,998,978	16,161,749	16,703,465	16,141,885
Total Outpatient Visits	19,543,928	18,865,165	19,036,685	19,633,146	19,024,487
Outpatient Surgeries	515,027	507,335	543,250	484,786	486,143
Personnel					
Full Time RNs	17,773	17,644	17,751	16,736	16,799
Full Time LPNs	873	907	1,101	974	1,206
Part Time RNs	20,521	19,190	18,435	17,473	15,846
Part Time LPNs	827	1,280	971	984	961
Total Full Time	95,358	91,708	94,873	96,845	99,089
Total Part Time	61,747	56,704	54,831	55,781	51,096
Revenue - Inpatient					
Gross Inpatient Revenue	$18,131,480,820	$16,062,562,936	$16,030,894,805	$14,495,247,329	$12,947,175,259
Revenue - Outpatient					
Gross Outpatient Revenue	$18,765,595,188	$16,256,621,729	$14,502,126,803	$12,932,344,645	$10,988,975,820
Revenue and Expenses - Totals					
(Includes Inpatient and Outpatient)					
Total Gross Revenue	$36,897,076,008	$32,319,184,665	$30,533,021,608	$27,427,591,974	$23,936,151,079
Deductions from Revenue	20,747,996,172	17,830,536,310	17,030,539,095	15,140,167,010	12,756,840,606
Net Patient Revenue	16,149,079,836	14,488,648,355	13,502,482,513	12,287,424,964	11,179,310,473
Other Operating Revenue	2,378,723,094	1,919,801,409	1,999,130,082	2,515,283,376	1,822,811,119
Other Nonoperating Revenue	410,670,072	246,123,264	257,876,135	122,250,355	-20,027,456
Total Net Revenue	18,938,473,002	16,654,573,028	15,759,488,730	14,924,958,695	12,982,094,136
Total Expenses	18,075,916,295	16,079,248,699	15,124,176,850	14,000,779,782	12,979,804,604
HOSPITAL UNIT (Excludes Separate Nursing Home Units)					
Utilization - Inpatient					
Beds	15,959	15,552	15,565	15,255	15,301
Admissions	824,881	788,780	790,876	768,485	754,165
Inpatient Days	4,316,301	4,176,350	4,220,730	4,130,356	4,118,738
Average Length of Stay	5.2	5.3	5.3	5.4	5.5
Personnel					
Total Full Time	95,080	91,414	93,735	96,223	98,795
Total Part Time	61,339	56,275	53,268	55,245	50,699
Revenue and Expenses - Totals					
(Includes Inpatient and Outpatient)					
Total Net Revenue	$18,830,494,898	$16,584,625,538	$15,695,985,452	$14,864,520,506	$12,931,336,845
Total Expenses	18,007,708,627	16,036,372,144	15,066,414,424	13,946,133,825	12,931,961,619
COMMUNITY HEALTH INDICATORS PER 1000 POPULATION					
Total Population (in thousands)	6,437	6,433	6,436	6,440	6,431
Inpatient					
Beds	2.5	2.5	2.5	2.5	2.5
Admissions	129.7	124.3	124.5	121.8	119.1
Inpatient Days	688.5	681.9	688.1	679.0	676.1
Inpatient Surgeries	31.3	34.5	32.5	32.9	31.9
Births	14.6	15.4	12.3	12.4	12.4
Outpatient					
Emergency Outpatient Visits	487.7	445.5	446.7	454.9	448.2
Other Outpatient Visits	2,548.4	2,486.9	2,511.2	2,593.9	2,509.9
Total Outpatient Visits	3,036.1	2,932.4	2,957.8	3,048.8	2,958.1
Outpatient Surgeries	80.0	78.9	84.4	75.3	75.6
Expense per Capita (per person)	$2,808.0	$2,499.4	$2,349.9	$2,174.2	$2,018.2

States

TABLE 6

MICHIGAN

U.S. Registered Community Hospitals
(Nonfederal, short-term general and other special hospitals)

Overview 2002–2006

	2006	2005	2004	2003	2002
Total Community Hospitals in Michigan.......	**142**	**146**	**144**	**144**	**145**
Bed Size Category					
6-24.....................................	10	11	11	8	7
25-49....................................	25	25	21	22	24
50-99....................................	41	45	47	47	47
100-199..................................	21	20	20	20	19
200-299..................................	16	14	14	16	16
300-399..................................	12	16	16	16	16
400-499..................................	6	5	4	6	7
500 +....................................	11	10	11	9	9
Location					
Hospitals Urban..........................	84	87	85	85	86
Hospitals Rural..........................	58	59	59	59	59
Control					
State and Local Government................	17	18	18	18	19
Not for Profit...........................	120	124	122	122	122
Investor owned...........................	5	4	4	4	4
Physician Models					
Independent Practice Association..........	12	16	15	24	23
Group Practice without Walls..............	6	5	8	11	12
Open Physician-Hospital Organization......	36	39	46	53	55
Closed Physician-Hospital Organization....	19	17	15	19	17
Management Service Organization...........	16	23	19	24	22
Integrated Salary Model..................	70	69	66	65	60
Equity Model.............................	2	2	2	0	0
Foundation...............................	8	8	9	8	5
Insurance Products					
Health Maintenance Organization..........	49	51	49	50	44
Preferred Provider Organization..........	61	61	60	57	52
Indemnity Fee for Service................	17	21	17	16	13
Managed Care Contracts					
Health Maintenance Organization..........	111	106	110	117	111
Preferred Provider Organization..........	113	113	116	121	116
Affiliations					
Hospitals in a System*...................	74	77	76	77	73
Hospitals in a Network...................	64	66	63	57	50
Hospitals in a Group Purchasing Organization..	128	128	122	129	124

* Please note that system affiliate information for hospitals is derived from AHA membership. In years prior to 2003 the affiliation was derived from a question on the AHA Annual Survey of hospitals; therefore, non-responding hospitals were not included in the system affiliation counts. Years prior to 2003 have been updated to reflect this change, which now include affiliation for non-reporting hospitals.

States

TABLE 6

MICHIGAN

U.S. Registered Community Hospitals
(Nonfederal, short-term general and other special hospitals)

Utilization, Personnel, Revenue and Expenses, Community Health Indicators 2002–2006

	2006	2005	2004	2003	2002
TOTAL FACILITY (Includes Hospital and Nursing Home Units)					
Utilization - Inpatient					
Beds	25,945	26,214	25,953	25,820	26,130
Admissions	1,205,481	1,198,076	1,190,293	1,168,359	1,163,157
Inpatient Days	6,245,033	6,412,561	6,279,987	6,223,908	6,296,654
Average Length of Stay...........	5.2	5.4	5.3	5.3	5.4
Inpatient Surgeries..............	349,826	349,441	354,425	355,235	346,641
Births........................	123,600	124,808	127,666	128,886	127,754
Utilization - Outpatient					
Emergency Outpatient Visits.......	4,326,912	4,177,255	4,155,147	3,990,117	4,029,309
Other Outpatient Visits...........	23,798,191	21,972,261	23,580,862	23,184,923	21,837,056
Total Outpatient Visits	28,125,103	26,149,516	27,736,009	27,175,040	25,866,365
Outpatient Surgeries	755,353	769,424	780,943	792,887	739,878
Personnel					
Full Time RNs	30,490	29,501	27,994	25,864	25,067
Full Time LPNs	1,770	2,006	1,990	2,190	2,292
Part Time RNs..................	19,793	18,959	18,418	18,604	19,095
Part Time LPNs	1,241	1,420	1,518	1,568	1,750
Total Full Time..................	135,402	132,063	127,386	125,290	122,075
Total Part Time	65,321	63,532	62,069	61,194	63,009
Revenue - Inpatient					
Gross Inpatient Revenue..........	$26,450,363,373	$24,395,111,754	$22,587,070,811	$19,821,173,066	$18,067,876,124
Revenue - Outpatient					
Gross Outpatient Revenue	$22,637,487,899	$19,689,965,942	$17,786,301,382	$15,428,984,110	$13,502,108,253
Revenue and Expenses - Totals					
(Includes Inpatient and Outpatient)					
Total Gross Revenue.............	$49,087,851,272	$44,085,077,696	$40,373,372,193	$35,250,157,176	$31,569,984,377
Deductions from Revenue.........	28,905,181,590	25,570,765,697	23,170,867,760	19,419,489,941	16,694,090,957
Net Patient Revenue	20,182,669,682	18,514,311,999	17,202,504,433	15,830,667,235	14,875,893,420
Other Operating Revenue	1,018,637,486	888,745,004	811,237,389	784,324,482	700,959,929
Other Nonoperating Revenue	566,746,298	441,671,050	400,368,184	113,029,604	19,519,553
Total Net Revenue..............	21,768,053,466	19,844,728,053	18,414,110,006	16,728,021,321	15,596,372,902
Total Expenses.................	20,701,788,855	18,818,318,860	17,506,296,112	16,333,925,475	15,321,064,736
HOSPITAL UNIT (Excludes Separate Nursing Home Units)					
Utilization - Inpatient					
Beds	24,542	24,282	24,243	23,985	24,354
Admissions	1,201,976	1,192,956	1,186,198	1,163,656	1,159,116
Inpatient Days	5,766,423	5,811,312	5,779,770	5,641,185	5,724,932
Average Length of Stay...........	4.8	4.9	4.9	4.8	4.9
Personnel					
Total Full Time..................	134,441	130,712	125,902	124,127	120,860
Total Part Time	64,532	62,686	61,210	60,504	62,308
Revenue and Expenses - Totals					
(Includes Inpatient and Outpatient)					
Total Net Revenue..............	$21,641,889,153	$19,696,234,106	$18,292,566,711	$16,618,881,265	$15,477,617,658
Total Expenses.................	20,619,312,307	18,683,610,130	17,436,971,373	16,267,781,536	15,232,840,934
COMMUNITY HEALTH INDICATORS PER 1000 POPULATION					
Total Population (in thousands)	10,096	10,101	10,093	10,068	10,038
Inpatient					
Beds	2.6	2.6	2.6	2.6	2.6
Admissions	119.4	118.6	117.9	116.0	115.9
Inpatient Days	618.6	634.9	622.2	618.2	627.3
Inpatient Surgeries..............	34.7	34.6	35.1	35.3	34.5
Births........................	12.2	12.4	12.6	12.8	12.7
Outpatient					
Emergency Outpatient Visits.......	428.6	413.6	411.7	396.3	401.4
Other Outpatient Visits...........	2,357.3	2,175.3	2,336.3	2,302.8	2,175.4
Total Outpatient Visits	2,785.9	2,588.8	2,747.9	2,699.1	2,576.8
Outpatient Surgeries	74.8	76.2	77.4	78.8	73.7
Expense per Capita (per person)....	$2,050.6	$1,863.0	$1,734.4	$1,622.3	$1,526.3

States

TABLE 6

MINNESOTA

U.S. Registered Community Hospitals
(Nonfederal, short-term general and other special hospitals)

Overview 2002–2006

	2006	2005	2004	2003	2002
Total Community Hospitals in Minnesota......	131	133	132	131	133
Bed Size Category					
6-24	17	18	17	15	18
25-49	23	23	23	25	20
50-99	40	38	36	36	38
100-199	35	38	40	38	41
200-299	4	4	4	5	4
300-399	4	5	5	5	3
400-499	5	4	4	3	5
500 + ...	3	3	3	4	4
Location					
Hospitals Urban..........................	49	50	46	45	46
Hospitals Rural	82	83	86	86	87
Control					
State and Local Government................	40	41	41	42	44
Not for Profit............................	91	91	91	89	89
Investor owned	0	1	0	0	0
Physician Models					
Independent Practice Association	28	27	30	29	24
Group Practice without Walls................	5	4	5	6	2
Open Physician-Hospital Organization	9	10	9	13	8
Closed Physician-Hospital Organization	5	8	7	7	7
Management Service Organization	3	4	4	5	3
Integrated Salary Model....................	42	38	41	46	40
Equity Model.............................	1	1	2	1	1
Foundation...............................	1	2	3	2	2
Insurance Products					
Health Maintenance Organization	11	13	13	16	13
Preferred Provider Organization..............	16	17	15	16	16
Indemnity Fee for Service	3	4	4	5	5
Managed Care Contracts					
Health Maintenance Organization	53	55	63	65	64
Preferred Provider Organization..............	59	61	70	76	72
Affiliations					
Hospitals in a System*.....................	70	71	68	64	64
Hospitals in a Network	28	24	25	24	22
Hospitals in a Group Purchasing Organization..	95	85	92	103	95

* Please note that system affiliate information for hospitals is derived from AHA membership. In years prior to 2003 the affiliation was derived from a question on the AHA Annual Survey of hospitals; therefore, non-responding hospitals were not included in the system affiliation counts. Years prior to 2003 have been updated to reflect this change, which now include affiliation for non-reporting hospitals.

TABLE 6

MINNESOTA

U.S. Registered Community Hospitals
(Nonfederal, short-term general and other special hospitals)

Utilization, Personnel, Revenue and Expenses, Community Health Indicators 2002–2006

	2006	2005	2004	2003	2002
TOTAL FACILITY (Includes Hospital and Nursing Home Units)					
Utilization - Inpatient					
Beds	15,843	15,993	16,101	16,439	16,659
Admissions	633,225	635,162	626,693	614,867	598,852
Inpatient Days	3,955,503	4,020,255	4,004,183	4,113,264	4,162,994
Average Length of Stay	6.2	6.3	6.4	6.7	7.0
Inpatient Surgeries	182,856	204,762	190,791	175,001	178,443
Births	71,999	70,784	69,799	68,492	68,220
Utilization - Outpatient					
Emergency Outpatient Visits	1,711,528	1,717,155	1,558,720	1,581,734	1,605,237
Other Outpatient Visits	8,397,658	7,725,310	7,971,965	7,602,634	7,296,661
Total Outpatient Visits	10,109,186	9,442,465	9,530,685	9,184,368	8,901,898
Outpatient Surgeries	300,661	300,667	298,323	288,902	279,781
Personnel					
Full Time RNs	8,980	8,609	8,440	8,322	7,750
Full Time LPNs	1,481	1,477	1,436	1,525	1,383
Part Time RNs	20,193	21,070	17,218	19,140	18,637
Part Time LPNs	2,300	2,354	2,293	2,605	2,452
Total Full Time	48,647	47,471	46,782	45,873	45,546
Total Part Time	59,057	61,469	51,444	56,699	56,063
Revenue - Inpatient					
Gross Inpatient Revenue	$14,591,084,241	$13,866,748,412	$12,319,629,780	$11,089,213,807	$10,100,747,850
Revenue - Outpatient					
Gross Outpatient Revenue	$10,131,993,797	$9,152,203,023	$7,932,681,220	$6,771,151,253	$6,116,730,184
Revenue and Expenses - Totals					
(Includes Inpatient and Outpatient)					
Total Gross Revenue	$24,723,078,038	$23,018,951,435	$20,252,311,000	$17,860,365,060	$16,217,478,034
Deductions from Revenue	13,936,215,046	12,923,611,920	11,069,414,757	9,421,711,537	8,364,782,672
Net Patient Revenue	10,786,862,992	10,095,339,515	9,182,896,243	8,438,653,523	7,852,695,362
Other Operating Revenue	579,265,096	513,674,553	483,299,164	454,629,698	448,432,311
Other Nonoperating Revenue	241,843,240	131,543,838	125,102,720	96,685,979	42,923,367
Total Net Revenue	11,607,971,328	10,740,557,906	9,791,298,127	8,989,969,200	8,344,051,040
Total Expenses	10,886,427,005	10,169,803,966	9,202,353,673	8,522,793,912	7,883,926,731
HOSPITAL UNIT (Excludes Separate Nursing Home Units)					
Utilization - Inpatient					
Beds	12,729	12,969	12,881	12,304	13,078
Admissions	629,069	630,577	621,925	608,772	594,971
Inpatient Days	2,901,267	2,987,706	2,888,972	2,674,779	2,918,600
Average Length of Stay	4.6	4.7	4.6	4.4	4.9
Personnel					
Total Full Time	47,079	45,979	44,919	43,727	43,905
Total Part Time	56,638	59,124	48,693	53,056	53,701
Revenue and Expenses - Totals					
(Includes Inpatient and Outpatient)					
Total Net Revenue	$11,431,135,431	$10,568,197,592	$9,614,263,388	$8,766,867,394	$8,180,139,592
Total Expenses	10,704,577,635	9,999,347,164	9,023,305,159	8,297,651,895	7,729,649,102
COMMUNITY HEALTH INDICATORS PER 1000 POPULATION					
Total Population (in thousands)	5,167	5,127	5,094	5,059	5,025
Inpatient					
Beds	3.1	3.1	3.2	3.2	3.3
Admissions	122.5	123.9	123.0	121.5	119.2
Inpatient Days	765.5	784.2	786.0	813.1	828.5
Inpatient Surgeries	35.4	39.9	37.5	34.6	35.5
Births	13.9	13.8	13.7	13.5	13.6
Outpatient					
Emergency Outpatient Visits	331.2	334.9	306.0	312.7	319.5
Other Outpatient Visits	1,625.2	1,506.9	1,564.9	1,502.8	1,452.2
Total Outpatient Visits	1,956.5	1,841.8	1,870.9	1,815.4	1,771.7
Outpatient Surgeries	58.2	58.6	58.6	57.1	55.7
Expense per Capita (per person)	$2,106.9	$1,983.7	$1,806.4	$1,684.7	$1,569.1

States

TABLE 6

MISSISSIPPI

U.S. Registered Community Hospitals
(Nonfederal, short-term general and other special hospitals)

Overview 2002–2006

	2006	2005	2004	2003	2002
Total Community Hospitals in Mississippi	94	94	93	92	91
Bed Size Category					
6-24	1	1	1	2	2
25-49	28	26	25	22	19
50-99	26	25	23	25	26
100-199	24	27	29	28	29
200-299	4	3	4	4	4
300-399	3	7	4	4	4
400-499	3	1	2	2	2
500 + ...	5	4	5	5	5
Location					
Hospitals Urban	27	27	19	19	18
Hospitals Rural	67	67	74	73	73
Control					
State and Local Government	41	41	42	42	42
Not for Profit	29	29	25	26	25
Investor owned	24	24	26	24	24
Physician Models					
Independent Practice Association	7	6	9	8	11
Group Practice without Walls	4	4	3	4	10
Open Physician-Hospital Organization	18	21	8	20	21
Closed Physician-Hospital Organization	2	1	0	5	5
Management Service Organization	9	10	1	8	10
Integrated Salary Model	19	19	7	20	19
Equity Model	1	2	0	1	0
Foundation	7	8	2	8	11
Insurance Products					
Health Maintenance Organization	7	8	1	9	12
Preferred Provider Organization	43	39	7	45	50
Indemnity Fee for Service	10	11	2	13	15
Managed Care Contracts					
Health Maintenance Organization	6	1	6	2	10
Preferred Provider Organization	28	20	20	5	39
Affiliations					
Hospitals in a System*	39	41	38	35	36
Hospitals in a Network	32	31	35	34	35
Hospitals in a Group Purchasing Organization . .	24	31	31	7	8

* Please note that system affiliate information for hospitals is derived from AHA membership. In years prior to 2003 the affiliation was derived from a question on the AHA Annual Survey of hospitals; therefore, non-responding hospitals were not included in the system affiliation counts. Years prior to 2003 have been updated to reflect this change, which now include affiliation for non-reporting hospitals.

TABLE 6

MISSISSIPPI

U.S. Registered Community Hospitals
(Nonfederal, short-term general and other special hospitals)

Utilization, Personnel, Revenue and Expenses, Community Health Indicators 2002–2006

	2006	2005	2004	2003	2002
TOTAL FACILITY (Includes Hospital and Nursing Home Units)					
Utilization - Inpatient					
Beds	12,973	12,753	13,143	13,040	13,144
Admissions	415,577	414,373	427,401	415,909	416,815
Inpatient Days	2,697,952	2,679,961	2,771,304	2,696,522	2,745,516
Average Length of Stay	6.5	6.5	6.5	6.5	6.6
Inpatient Surgeries	122,509	116,048	122,339	123,033	121,710
Births	42,729	43,202	40,431	39,540	39,553
Utilization - Outpatient					
Emergency Outpatient Visits	1,650,523	1,665,894	1,602,016	1,597,509	1,556,488
Other Outpatient Visits	2,567,848	2,427,582	2,613,026	2,401,457	2,439,892
Total Outpatient Visits	4,218,371	4,093,476	4,215,042	3,998,966	3,996,380
Outpatient Surgeries	162,127	146,338	150,301	142,791	152,172
Personnel					
Full Time RNs	10,092	10,552	9,881	9,529	9,091
Full Time LPNs	1,803	1,742	1,929	1,951	1,923
Part Time RNs	3,583	3,493	3,757	3,763	3,906
Part Time LPNs	475	525	629	611	615
Total Full Time	43,338	42,140	42,182	41,081	40,107
Total Part Time	11,648	11,124	12,109	11,821	11,478
Revenue - Inpatient					
Gross Inpatient Revenue	$8,470,744,247	$7,660,349,400	$7,255,099,763	$6,235,537,687	$5,702,037,800
Revenue - Outpatient					
Gross Outpatient Revenue	$5,402,234,688	$4,830,456,007	$4,286,884,357	$3,630,142,778	$3,320,188,769
Revenue and Expenses - Totals					
(Includes Inpatient and Outpatient)					
Total Gross Revenue	$13,872,978,935	$12,490,805,407	$11,541,984,120	$9,865,680,465	$9,022,226,569
Deductions from Revenue	8,822,388,239	7,955,298,330	6,899,022,514	5,715,365,284	4,977,500,289
Net Patient Revenue	5,050,590,696	4,535,507,077	4,642,961,606	4,150,315,181	4,044,726,280
Other Operating Revenue	231,893,393	193,477,120	163,436,087	167,113,664	164,171,241
Other Nonoperating Revenue	62,006,706	71,401,765	63,508,641	66,551,838	60,542,992
Total Net Revenue	5,344,490,795	4,800,385,962	4,869,906,334	4,383,980,683	4,269,440,513
Total Expenses	5,237,172,195	4,738,973,161	4,470,158,941	4,056,824,801	3,907,203,934
HOSPITAL UNIT (Excludes Separate Nursing Home Units)					
Utilization - Inpatient					
Beds	11,247	11,190	11,695	11,510	11,579
Admissions	414,554	413,368	426,552	414,762	415,182
Inpatient Days	2,123,492	2,153,451	2,297,184	2,206,104	2,217,217
Average Length of Stay	5.1	5.2	5.4	5.3	5.3
Personnel					
Total Full Time	41,925	40,919	36,915	39,851	39,009
Total Part Time	11,290	10,802	11,523	11,510	11,212
Revenue and Expenses - Totals					
(Includes Inpatient and Outpatient)					
Total Net Revenue	$5,251,964,574	$4,752,934,290	$4,815,226,678	$4,326,841,865	$4,211,247,202
Total Expenses	5,189,913,198	4,700,533,201	4,429,693,154	4,010,876,381	3,866,957,946
COMMUNITY HEALTH INDICATORS PER 1000 POPULATION					
Total Population (in thousands)	2,911	2,908	2,893	2,874	2,863
Inpatient					
Beds	4.5	4.4	4.5	4.5	4.6
Admissions	142.8	142.5	147.8	144.7	145.6
Inpatient Days	927.0	921.4	958.0	938.2	958.9
Inpatient Surgeries	42.1	39.9	42.3	42.8	42.5
Births	14.7	14.9	14.0	13.8	13.8
Outpatient					
Emergency Outpatient Visits	567.1	572.8	553.8	555.8	543.6
Other Outpatient Visits	882.3	834.7	903.3	835.5	852.2
Total Outpatient Visits	1,449.3	1,407.4	1,457.1	1,391.3	1,395.8
Outpatient Surgeries	55.7	50.3	52.0	49.7	53.1
Expense per Capita (per person)	$1,799.4	$1,629.4	$1,545.3	$1,411.5	$1,364.7

TABLE 6

MISSOURI

U.S. Registered Community Hospitals
(Nonfederal, short-term general and other special hospitals)

Overview 2002–2006

	2006	2005	2004	2003	2002
Total Community Hospitals in Missouri	119	119	119	119	119
Bed Size Category					
6-24	5	7	6	6	6
25-49	36	32	33	31	31
50-99	18	19	21	25	25
100-199	28	28	23	22	22
200-299	13	14	17	15	17
300-399	9	9	8	8	9
400-499	4	4	5	6	4
500 + ...	6	6	6	6	5
Location					
Hospitals Urban	66	66	61	61	61
Hospitals Rural	53	53	58	58	58
Control					
State and Local Government	36	36	36	36	36
Not for Profit	62	63	64	67	68
Investor owned	21	20	19	16	15
Physician Models					
Independent Practice Association	13	17	15	18	17
Group Practice without Walls	1	2	3	5	2
Open Physician-Hospital Organization	19	21	18	19	21
Closed Physician-Hospital Organization	9	10	13	14	13
Management Service Organization	5	5	4	7	10
Integrated Salary Model	59	59	60	52	52
Equity Model	0	0	0	0	2
Foundation	2	2	3	1	1
Insurance Products					
Health Maintenance Organization	19	20	21	21	28
Preferred Provider Organization	14	15	15	13	22
Indemnity Fee for Service	7	7	6	6	11
Managed Care Contracts					
Health Maintenance Organization	99	104	102	102	100
Preferred Provider Organization	107	111	111	109	108
Affiliations					
Hospitals in a System*	68	69	67	67	66
Hospitals in a Network	40	34	35	33	39
Hospitals in a Group Purchasing Organization . .	114	114	113	110	107

---

* Please note that system affiliate information for hospitals is derived from AHA membership. In years prior to 2003 the affiliation was derived from a question on the AHA Annual Survey of hospitals; therefore, non-responding hospitals were not included in the system affiliation counts. Years prior to 2003 have been updated to reflect this change, which now include affiliation for non-reporting hospitals.

TABLE 6

MISSOURI

U.S. Registered Community Hospitals
(Nonfederal, short-term general and other special hospitals)

Utilization, Personnel, Revenue and Expenses, Community Health Indicators 2002–2006

	2006	2005	2004	2003	2002
TOTAL FACILITY (Includes Hospital and Nursing Home Units)					
Utilization - Inpatient					
Beds..........................	18,888	19,146	19,131	19,346	18,891
Admissions....................	830,882	836,179	831,892	831,210	809,355
Inpatient Days	4,331,742	4,421,138	4,407,818	4,342,987	4,235,298
Average Length of Stay...........	5.2	5.3	5.3	5.2	5.2
Inpatient Surgeries..............	219,027	210,112	216,568	205,270	209,739
Births.........................	79,240	77,542	77,638	78,564	74,815
Utilization - Outpatient					
Emergency Outpatient Visits.......	2,641,586	2,617,778	2,561,625	2,624,926	2,476,194
Other Outpatient Visits...........	13,696,600	14,595,386	13,624,807	13,043,778	12,427,894
Total Outpatient Visits	16,338,186	17,213,164	16,186,432	15,668,704	14,904,088
Outpatient Surgeries	384,189	398,992	397,142	393,167	393,761
Personnel					
Full Time RNs	21,839	20,275	19,212	19,034	19,236
Full Time LPNs	2,811	2,849	2,950	2,860	3,039
Part Time RNs	11,942	11,598	11,774	12,255	11,417
Part Time LPNs	1,001	1,069	1,133	1,192	1,174
Total Full Time.................	92,126	90,985	88,747	87,529	85,983
Total Part Time	35,565	36,195	36,403	37,338	35,177
Revenue - Inpatient					
Gross Inpatient Revenue..........	$19,488,280,323	$18,091,147,295	$16,624,521,378	$15,395,529,429	$13,686,358,547
Revenue - Outpatient					
Gross Outpatient Revenue	$13,820,205,178	$12,666,683,321	$11,220,642,518	$10,090,913,418	$8,390,580,917
Revenue and Expenses - Totals					
(Includes Inpatient and Outpatient)					
Total Gross Revenue.............	$33,308,485,501	$30,757,830,616	$27,845,163,896	$25,486,442,847	$22,076,939,464
Deductions from Revenue.........	20,127,195,935	18,464,345,424	16,534,751,958	14,843,065,456	12,532,916,322
Net Patient Revenue	13,181,289,566	12,293,485,192	11,310,411,938	10,643,377,391	9,544,023,142
Other Operating Revenue	882,120,238	646,016,294	745,387,376	720,949,265	570,212,535
Other Nonoperating Revenue	414,857,246	245,980,140	314,383,075	266,984,711	89,622,933
Total Net Revenue...............	14,478,267,050	13,185,481,626	12,370,182,389	11,631,311,367	10,203,858,610
Total Expenses..................	13,503,914,459	12,612,917,341	11,559,349,647	10,852,258,947	9,747,670,518
HOSPITAL UNIT (Excludes Separate Nursing Home Units)					
Utilization - Inpatient					
Beds..........................	17,664	17,767	17,735	17,898	17,396
Admissions....................	820,375	825,255	819,702	816,595	791,849
Inpatient Days	3,966,608	4,022,789	4,040,112	3,934,255	3,844,365
Average Length of Stay...........	4.8	4.9	4.9	4.8	4.9
Personnel					
Total Full Time.................	91,235	89,670	87,147	86,094	85,531
Total Part Time	35,082	35,617	35,705	36,831	34,767
Revenue and Expenses - Totals					
(Includes Inpatient and Outpatient)					
Total Net Revenue...............	$14,267,051,695	$13,071,840,233	$12,222,272,066	$11,480,749,638	$10,043,647,885
Total Expenses..................	13,315,304,412	12,505,733,147	11,428,018,346	10,738,245,530	9,620,134,560
COMMUNITY HEALTH INDICATORS PER 1000 POPULATION					
Total Population (in thousands)	5,843	5,798	5,753	5,712	5,680
Inpatient					
Beds..........................	3.2	3.3	3.3	3.4	3.3
Admissions....................	142.2	144.2	144.6	145.5	142.5
Inpatient Days	741.4	762.6	766.2	760.3	745.6
Inpatient Surgeries..............	37.5	36.2	37.6	35.9	36.9
Births.........................	13.6	13.4	13.5	13.8	13.2
Outpatient					
Emergency Outpatient Visits.......	452.1	451.5	445.3	459.5	435.9
Other Outpatient Visits...........	2,344.2	2,517.4	2,368.4	2,283.4	2,187.9
Total Outpatient Visits	2,796.3	2,969.0	2,813.6	2,742.9	2,623.8
Outpatient Surgeries	65.8	68.8	69.0	68.8	69.3
Expense per Capita (per person)....	$2,311.2	$2,175.5	$2,009.3	$1,899.8	$1,716.1

TABLE 6

MONTANA

U.S. Registered Community Hospitals
(Nonfederal, short-term general and other special hospitals)

Overview 2002–2006

	2006	2005	2004	2003	2002
Total Community Hospitals in Montana	52	54	54	53	53
Bed Size Category					
6-24	10	9	10	8	8
25-49	15	16	15	16	15
50-99	14	16	17	17	18
100-199	10	10	8	8	9
200-299	1	1	2	2	1
300-399	1	1	1	1	2
400-499	1	1	1	1	0
500 + ...	0	0	0	0	0
Location					
Hospitals Urban.........................	6	6	3	5	5
Hospitals Rural	46	48	51	48	48
Control					
State and Local Government	9	10	10	10	10
Not for Profit	42	44	44	43	43
Investor owned	1	0	0	0	0
Physician Models					
Independent Practice Association	9	10	9	10	6
Group Practice without Walls...............	2	2	3	3	3
Open Physician-Hospital Organization	8	8	8	7	7
Closed Physician-Hospital Organization	1	1	0	0	1
Management Service Organization	8	8	6	6	6
Integrated Salary Model....................	28	31	27	24	22
Equity Model	0	1	2	0	1
Foundation.............................	3	5	0	0	2
Insurance Products					
Health Maintenance Organization	7	6	5	4	4
Preferred Provider Organization.............	9	17	13	9	6
Indemnity Fee for Service	7	9	8	7	3
Managed Care Contracts					
Health Maintenance Organization	15	15	16	12	13
Preferred Provider Organization.............	29	32	31	28	23
Affiliations					
Hospitals in a System*	12	15	14	14	16
Hospitals in a Network....................	24	25	27	22	25
Hospitals in a Group Purchasing Organization..	48	50	48	47	47

* Please note that system affiliate information for hospitals is derived from AHA membership. In years prior to 2003 the affiliation was derived from a question on the AHA Annual Survey of hospitals; therefore, non-responding hospitals were not included in the system affiliation counts. Years prior to 2003 have been updated to reflect this change, which now include affiliation for non-reporting hospitals.

TABLE 6

MONTANA

U.S. Registered Community Hospitals
(Nonfederal, short-term general and other special hospitals)

Utilization, Personnel, Revenue and Expenses, Community Health Indicators 2002–2006

	2006	2005	2004	2003	2002
TOTAL FACILITY (Includes Hospital and Nursing Home Units)					
Utilization - Inpatient					
Beds	4,089	4,283	4,337	4,326	4,263
Admissions	106,826	106,457	106,619	107,024	106,758
Inpatient Days	975,390	1,023,301	1,042,530	1,049,607	1,071,834
Average Length of Stay	9.1	9.6	9.8	9.8	10.0
Inpatient Surgeries	32,099	32,081	32,550	34,689	32,343
Births	10,681	10,426	10,418	10,301	9,963
Utilization - Outpatient					
Emergency Outpatient Visits	333,504	311,144	294,359	301,772	276,829
Other Outpatient Visits	2,568,374	2,548,342	2,600,951	2,435,962	2,381,906
Total Outpatient Visits	2,901,878	2,859,486	2,895,310	2,737,734	2,658,735
Outpatient Surgeries	44,129	37,910	38,428	39,301	38,792
Personnel					
Full Time RNs	2,508	2,333	2,304	2,200	2,233
Full Time LPNs	490	502	501	489	487
Part Time RNs	1,882	1,979	1,736	1,798	1,819
Part Time LPNs	315	351	335	344	322
Total Full Time	13,081	12,773	12,372	11,912	11,834
Total Part Time	7,059	7,325	6,612	6,757	6,893
Revenue - Inpatient					
Gross Inpatient Revenue	$1,669,626,014	$1,566,799,646	$1,442,716,805	$1,311,517,596	$1,196,591,796
Revenue - Outpatient					
Gross Outpatient Revenue	$1,490,075,406	$1,315,545,776	$1,159,001,092	$1,029,438,041	$928,260,803
Revenue and Expenses - Totals					
(Includes Inpatient and Outpatient)					
Total Gross Revenue	$3,159,701,420	$2,882,345,422	$2,601,717,897	$2,340,955,637	$2,124,852,599
Deductions from Revenue	1,333,944,188	1,215,530,442	1,068,216,515	933,232,336	805,155,142
Net Patient Revenue	1,825,757,232	1,666,814,980	1,533,501,382	1,407,723,301	1,319,697,457
Other Operating Revenue	69,888,745	67,644,799	69,423,086	62,722,453	54,199,364
Other Nonoperating Revenue	54,093,518	43,783,036	40,895,332	9,609,816	11,449,900
Total Net Revenue	1,949,739,495	1,778,242,815	1,643,819,800	1,480,055,570	1,385,346,721
Total Expenses	1,800,736,855	1,648,588,537	1,528,310,065	1,440,703,717	1,328,470,349
HOSPITAL UNIT (Excludes Separate Nursing Home Units)					
Utilization - Inpatient					
Beds	2,484	2,421	2,453	2,414	2,281
Admissions	103,686	103,371	103,105	103,517	102,888
Inpatient Days	471,793	460,351	482,021	459,871	445,638
Average Length of Stay	4.6	4.5	4.7	4.4	4.3
Personnel					
Total Full Time	11,960	11,620	11,127	10,667	10,659
Total Part Time	6,352	6,403	5,771	5,838	5,944
Revenue and Expenses - Totals					
(Includes Inpatient and Outpatient)					
Total Net Revenue	$1,870,972,965	$1,700,302,201	$1,565,817,386	$1,401,772,970	$1,312,606,078
Total Expenses	1,727,928,485	1,578,014,372	1,458,411,635	1,364,748,522	1,254,156,946
COMMUNITY HEALTH INDICATORS PER 1000 POPULATION					
Total Population (in thousands)	945	935	926	917	910
Inpatient					
Beds	4.3	4.6	4.7	4.7	4.7
Admissions	113.1	113.9	115.1	116.7	117.3
Inpatient Days	1,032.6	1,094.7	1,125.4	1,144.4	1,177.4
Inpatient Surgeries	34.0	34.3	35.1	37.8	35.5
Births	11.3	11.2	11.2	11.2	10.9
Outpatient					
Emergency Outpatient Visits	353.1	332.9	317.8	329.0	304.1
Other Outpatient Visits	2,718.9	2,726.3	2,807.8	2,655.9	2,616.5
Total Outpatient Visits	3,072.0	3,059.1	3,125.5	2,984.9	2,920.5
Outpatient Surgeries	46.7	40.6	41.5	42.8	42.6
Expense per Capita (per person)	$1,906.3	$1,763.7	$1,649.8	$1,570.8	$1,459.3

States

TABLE 6

NEBRASKA

U.S. Registered Community Hospitals
(Nonfederal, short-term general and other special hospitals)

Overview 2002–2006

	2006	2005	2004	2003	2002
Total Community Hospitals in Nebraska.......	85	87	85	85	86
Bed Size Category					
6-24	19	22	22	22	19
25-49	24	23	22	22	30
50-99	23	22	20	19	16
100-199	8	8	10	11	9
200-299	6	7	6	6	6
300-399	3	3	3	2	2
400-499	1	1	1	1	0
500 + ...	1	1	1	2	4
Location					
Hospitals Urban..........................	16	17	13	13	14
Hospitals Rural	69	70	72	72	72
Control					
State and Local Government................	40	40	39	39	41
Not for Profit.............................	43	45	44	44	43
Investor owned	2	2	2	2	2
Physician Models					
Independent Practice Association	7	7	8	7	5
Group Practice without Walls................	3	3	3	1	2
Open Physician-Hospital Organization	13	13	11	12	14
Closed Physician-Hospital Organization	0	0	0	0	0
Management Service Organization	3	2	1	1	0
Integrated Salary Model....................	37	33	31	33	22
Equity Model.............................	0	0	0	0	0
Foundation...............................	0	2	1	2	1
Insurance Products					
Health Maintenance Organization	5	4	5	4	4
Preferred Provider Organization..............	20	19	19	16	17
Indemnity Fee for Service	3	3	3	2	2
Managed Care Contracts					
Health Maintenance Organization	23	23	21	25	21
Preferred Provider Organization..............	58	52	54	63	46
Affiliations					
Hospitals in a System*.....................	26	27	26	26	26
Hospitals in a Network.....................	44	42	43	45	33
Hospitals in a Group Purchasing Organization..	66	60	62	71	50

* Please note that system affiliate information for hospitals is derived from AHA membership. In years prior to 2003 the affiliation was derived from a question on the AHA Annual Survey of hospitals; therefore, non-responding hospitals were not included in the system affiliation counts. Years prior to 2003 have been updated to reflect this change, which now include affiliation for non-reporting hospitals.

States

TABLE 6

NEBRASKA

U.S. Registered Community Hospitals
(Nonfederal, short-term general and other special hospitals)

Utilization, Personnel, Revenue and Expenses, Community Health Indicators 2002–2006

	2006	2005	2004	2003	2002
TOTAL FACILITY (Includes Hospital and Nursing Home Units)					
Utilization - Inpatient					
Beds	7,375	7,566	7,336	7,467	8,106
Admissions	215,219	214,240	211,025	211,567	206,208
Inpatient Days	1,666,078	1,757,311	1,612,857	1,593,254	1,723,683
Average Length of Stay	7.7	8.2	7.6	7.5	8.4
Inpatient Surgeries	67,255	69,536	71,164	73,396	70,433
Births	26,226	25,725	25,986	25,796	24,030
Utilization - Outpatient					
Emergency Outpatient Visits	551,914	554,269	551,836	532,934	511,085
Other Outpatient Visits	3,497,191	3,336,135	3,397,641	3,143,164	2,955,952
Total Outpatient Visits	4,049,105	3,890,404	3,949,477	3,676,098	3,467,037
Outpatient Surgeries	131,698	133,477	125,001	131,898	132,704
Personnel					
Full Time RNs	6,799	6,249	5,851	5,592	5,548
Full Time LPNs	1,039	1,050	1,049	1,070	997
Part Time RNs	3,646	3,457	3,817	3,839	4,167
Part Time LPNs	590	624	657	689	678
Total Full Time	27,907	26,636	25,601	25,193	24,517
Total Part Time	13,082	12,871	14,200	13,994	14,665
Revenue - Inpatient					
Gross Inpatient Revenue	$5,152,084,912	$4,582,880,874	$4,120,664,079	$3,883,504,195	$3,420,226,799
Revenue - Outpatient					
Gross Outpatient Revenue	$3,474,072,754	$3,035,020,244	$2,616,253,431	$2,357,540,030	$2,180,716,982
Revenue and Expenses - Totals					
(Includes Inpatient and Outpatient)					
Total Gross Revenue	$8,626,157,666	$7,617,901,118	$6,736,917,510	$6,241,044,225	$5,600,943,781
Deductions from Revenue	4,630,561,170	3,976,606,980	3,385,802,954	3,091,883,586	2,630,090,894
Net Patient Revenue	3,995,596,496	3,641,294,138	3,351,114,556	3,149,160,639	2,970,852,887
Other Operating Revenue	192,326,079	184,632,186	157,573,205	160,550,119	146,854,319
Other Nonoperating Revenue	132,919,108	66,496,703	61,483,416	-19,986,175	23,940,303
Total Net Revenue	4,320,841,683	3,892,423,027	3,570,171,177	3,289,724,583	3,141,647,509
Total Expenses	3,862,460,549	3,568,319,403	3,254,039,649	3,072,367,016	2,892,566,453
HOSPITAL UNIT (Excludes Separate Nursing Home Units)					
Utilization - Inpatient					
Beds	5,734	6,043	5,795	5,647	6,414
Admissions	211,591	210,663	207,634	207,183	200,622
Inpatient Days	1,151,365	1,261,063	1,152,562	1,058,691	1,180,270
Average Length of Stay	5.4	6.0	5.6	5.1	5.9
Personnel					
Total Full Time	26,795	25,596	24,552	24,008	23,564
Total Part Time	12,430	12,086	13,421	13,080	13,873
Revenue and Expenses - Totals					
(Includes Inpatient and Outpatient)					
Total Net Revenue	$4,235,396,340	$3,814,957,460	$3,491,161,406	$3,205,088,933	$3,061,905,470
Total Expenses	3,778,967,078	3,489,172,670	3,172,415,483	2,987,801,196	2,805,501,875
COMMUNITY HEALTH INDICATORS PER 1000 POPULATION					
Total Population (in thousands)	1,768	1,758	1,747	1,737	1,727
Inpatient					
Beds	4.2	4.3	4.2	4.3	4.7
Admissions	121.7	121.9	120.8	121.8	119.4
Inpatient Days	942.2	999.5	923.2	917.2	998.1
Inpatient Surgeries	38.0	39.6	40.7	42.3	40.8
Births	14.8	14.6	14.9	14.9	13.9
Outpatient					
Emergency Outpatient Visits	312.1	315.3	315.9	306.8	295.9
Other Outpatient Visits	1,977.7	1,897.5	1,944.9	1,809.5	1,711.6
Total Outpatient Visits	2,289.8	2,212.8	2,260.7	2,116.3	2,007.5
Outpatient Surgeries	74.5	75.9	71.6	75.9	76.8
Expense per Capita (per person)	$2,184.2	$2,029.6	$1,862.7	$1,768.8	$1,674.9

States

TABLE 6

NEVADA

U.S. Registered Community Hospitals
(Nonfederal, short-term general and other special hospitals)

Overview 2002–2006

	2006	2005	2004	2003	2002
Total Community Hospitals in Nevada	33	32	30	25	26
Bed Size Category					
6-24	6	4	1	1	0
25-49	5	6	6	5	7
50-99	9	9	9	6	5
100-199	5	5	7	7	8
200-299	3	3	2	2	1
300-399	2	2	2	1	2
400-499	0	0	0	0	0
500 + ...	3	3	3	3	3
Location					
Hospitals Urban........................	22	22	21	16	17
Hospitals Rural	11	10	9	9	9
Control					
State and Local Government...............	7	6	6	7	6
Not for Profit...........................	11	11	10	9	9
Investor owned	15	15	14	9	11
Physician Models					
Independent Practice Association	4	3	2	3	5
Group Practice without Walls...............	0	0	1	1	0
Open Physician-Hospital Organization	3	3	2	2	1
Closed Physician-Hospital Organization	1	1	1	0	0
Management Service Organization	1	1	1	2	1
Integrated Salary Model...................	3	3	3	5	3
Equity Model	0	0	0	0	0
Foundation.............................	1	0	0	0	0
Insurance Products					
Health Maintenance Organization	3	4	4	4	3
Preferred Provider Organization..............	4	5	4	4	4
Indemnity Fee for Service	2	2	2	3	2
Managed Care Contracts					
Health Maintenance Organization	12	10	10	11	13
Preferred Provider Organization..............	16	10	13	13	14
Affiliations					
Hospitals in a System*	21	20	19	14	14
Hospitals in a Network	4	3	4	4	4
Hospitals in a Group Purchasing Organization..	17	14	11	15	14

* Please note that system affiliate information for hospitals is derived from AHA membership. In years prior to 2003 the affiliation was derived from a question on the AHA Annual Survey of hospitals; therefore, non-responding hospitals were not included in the system affiliation counts. Years prior to 2003 have been updated to reflect this change, which now include affiliation for non-reporting hospitals.

104 AHA Hospital Statistics © 2008 Health Forum LLC, an affiliate of the American Hospital Association

TABLE 6

NEVADA

U.S. Registered Community Hospitals
(Nonfederal, short-term general and other special hospitals)

Utilization, Personnel, Revenue and Expenses, Community Health Indicators 2002–2006

	2006	2005	2004	2003	2002
TOTAL FACILITY (Includes Hospital and Nursing Home Units)					
Utilization - Inpatient					
Beds	4,826	4,685	4,752	4,282	4,495
Admissions	245,649	240,596	232,603	212,821	211,657
Inpatient Days	1,307,303	1,268,272	1,246,727	1,111,624	1,110,583
Average Length of Stay	5.3	5.3	5.4	5.2	5.2
Inpatient Surgeries	71,718	71,701	71,927	66,661	75,406
Births	32,737	31,210	29,196	30,801	29,709
Utilization - Outpatient					
Emergency Outpatient Visits	697,906	712,484	606,094	626,686	626,330
Other Outpatient Visits	1,689,902	1,901,170	1,839,386	1,657,287	1,835,894
Total Outpatient Visits	2,387,808	2,613,654	2,445,480	2,283,973	2,462,224
Outpatient Surgeries	83,381	96,495	106,988	71,739	87,157
Personnel					
Full Time RNs	5,317	5,290	5,163	4,606	4,605
Full Time LPNs	452	504	540	460	422
Part Time RNs	1,633	1,390	1,429	1,552	1,398
Part Time LPNs	111	77	100	122	83
Total Full Time	17,567	18,716	17,751	16,859	16,340
Total Part Time	4,255	3,716	3,799	4,179	3,797
Revenue - Inpatient					
Gross Inpatient Revenue	$8,318,719,056	$7,471,884,853	$6,156,363,442	$5,787,996,156	$5,183,035,024
Revenue - Outpatient					
Gross Outpatient Revenue	$3,245,923,076	$2,899,874,111	$2,529,847,264	$2,115,614,370	$1,883,871,488
Revenue and Expenses - Totals					
(Includes Inpatient and Outpatient)					
Total Gross Revenue	$11,564,642,132	$10,371,758,964	$8,686,210,706	$7,903,610,526	$7,066,906,512
Deductions from Revenue	8,554,764,914	7,387,212,650	5,805,707,829	5,414,900,197	4,672,604,272
Net Patient Revenue	3,009,877,218	2,984,546,314	2,880,502,877	2,488,710,329	2,394,302,240
Other Operating Revenue	79,167,789	79,622,920	103,442,479	141,955,261	179,018,832
Other Nonoperating Revenue	31,991,694	12,140,050	17,918,332	15,230,192	16,877,884
Total Net Revenue	3,121,036,701	3,076,309,284	3,001,863,688	2,645,895,782	2,590,198,956
Total Expenses	2,930,773,692	3,105,816,107	2,787,592,070	2,583,114,447	2,257,000,776
HOSPITAL UNIT (Excludes Separate Nursing Home Units)					
Utilization - Inpatient					
Beds	4,670	4,655	4,673	4,141	4,416
Admissions	245,070	240,224	232,527	212,723	211,562
Inpatient Days	1,257,697	1,257,630	1,220,754	1,066,782	1,083,111
Average Length of Stay	5.1	5.2	5.2	5.0	5.1
Personnel					
Total Full Time	17,471	18,696	17,707	16,767	16,270
Total Part Time	4,236	3,712	3,788	4,159	3,779
Revenue and Expenses - Totals					
(Includes Inpatient and Outpatient)					
Total Net Revenue	$3,112,151,041	$3,073,496,634	$2,998,131,909	$2,640,298,685	$2,586,007,972
Total Expenses	2,922,980,821	3,104,642,195	2,786,047,490	2,578,395,080	2,254,904,246
COMMUNITY HEALTH INDICATORS PER 1000 POPULATION					
Total Population (in thousands)	2,496	2,412	2,332	2,241	2,169
Inpatient					
Beds	1.9	1.9	2.0	1.9	2.1
Admissions	98.4	99.7	99.7	95.0	97.6
Inpatient Days	523.9	525.8	534.5	496.0	512.0
Inpatient Surgeries	28.7	29.7	30.8	29.7	34.8
Births	13.1	12.9	12.5	13.7	13.7
Outpatient					
Emergency Outpatient Visits	279.7	295.4	259.8	279.6	288.7
Other Outpatient Visits	677.2	788.1	788.6	739.5	846.3
Total Outpatient Visits	956.8	1,083.5	1,048.4	1,019.1	1,135.1
Outpatient Surgeries	33.4	40.0	45.9	32.0	40.2
Expense per Capita (per person)	$1,174.4	$1,287.5	$1,195.1	$1,152.6	$1,040.5

States

TABLE 6

NEW HAMPSHIRE

U.S. Registered Community Hospitals
(Nonfederal, short-term general and other special hospitals)

Overview 2002–2006

	2006	2005	2004	2003	2002
Total Community Hospitals in New Hampshire	28	28	28	28	28
Bed Size Category					
6-24	1	1	1	1	1
25-49	8	8	7	7	6
50-99	9	9	10	10	11
100-199	6	6	6	7	6
200-299	3	3	3	2	3
300-399	1	1	1	1	1
400-499	0	0	0	0	0
500 +	0	0	0	0	0
Location					
Hospitals Urban	11	11	10	10	10
Hospitals Rural	17	17	18	18	18
Control					
State and Local Government	0	0	0	0	0
Not for Profit	24	24	24	24	24
Investor owned	4	4	4	4	4
Physician Models					
Independent Practice Association	3	4	4	3	2
Group Practice without Walls	0	0	0	1	2
Open Physician-Hospital Organization	10	10	10	10	10
Closed Physician-Hospital Organization	2	2	3	4	4
Management Service Organization	3	3	3	3	4
Integrated Salary Model	15	14	14	12	12
Equity Model	0	1	0	0	0
Foundation	1	2	1	1	1
Insurance Products					
Health Maintenance Organization	0	1	2	3	2
Preferred Provider Organization	0	1	1	1	1
Indemnity Fee for Service	0	1	1	1	1
Managed Care Contracts					
Health Maintenance Organization	24	23	24	25	26
Preferred Provider Organization	23	23	24	25	25
Affiliations					
Hospitals in a System*	6	7	7	5	5
Hospitals in a Network	12	11	11	9	8
Hospitals in a Group Purchasing Organization	26	25	26	26	25

* Please note that system affiliate information for hospitals is derived from AHA membership. In years prior to 2003 the affiliation was derived from a question on the AHA Annual Survey of hospitals; therefore, non-responding hospitals were not included in the system affiliation counts. Years prior to 2003 have been updated to reflect this change, which now include affiliation for non-reporting hospitals.

TABLE 6

NEW HAMPSHIRE

U.S. Registered Community Hospitals
(Nonfederal, short-term general and other special hospitals)

Utilization, Personnel, Revenue and Expenses, Community Health Indicators 2002–2006

	2006	2005	2004	2003	2002
TOTAL FACILITY (Includes Hospital and Nursing Home Units)					
Utilization - Inpatient					
Beds	2,825	2,843	2,807	2,796	2,879
Admissions	118,956	117,468	117,130	117,814	117,996
Inpatient Days	644,096	647,457	648,454	637,803	646,838
Average Length of Stay	5.4	5.5	5.5	5.4	5.5
Inpatient Surgeries	33,612	35,584	37,755	33,535	33,553
Births	13,615	13,696	14,043	13,634	13,748
Utilization - Outpatient					
Emergency Outpatient Visits	604,317	621,217	563,318	547,870	550,380
Other Outpatient Visits	3,266,700	3,160,825	2,403,954	2,523,260	2,472,527
Total Outpatient Visits	3,871,017	3,782,042	2,967,272	3,071,130	3,022,907
Outpatient Surgeries	86,761	90,385	94,192	87,795	85,056
Personnel					
Full Time RNs	3,852	3,775	3,423	3,248	3,053
Full Time LPNs	208	215	147	158	159
Part Time RNs	2,453	2,462	2,513	2,483	2,720
Part Time LPNs	123	136	135	139	135
Total Full Time	18,632	18,390	15,560	14,966	14,657
Total Part Time	8,674	8,459	8,314	7,981	8,522
Revenue - Inpatient					
Gross Inpatient Revenue	$2,702,075,606	$2,428,565,909	$2,020,888,964	$1,810,524,954	$1,631,730,543
Revenue - Outpatient					
Gross Outpatient Revenue	$3,488,005,564	$2,985,681,639	$2,373,162,075	$2,014,053,023	$1,730,622,946
Revenue and Expenses - Totals					
(Includes Inpatient and Outpatient)					
Total Gross Revenue	$6,190,081,170	$5,414,247,548	$4,394,051,039	$3,824,577,977	$3,362,353,489
Deductions from Revenue	3,195,298,030	2,798,961,017	2,142,869,543	1,779,776,571	1,525,457,983
Net Patient Revenue	2,994,783,140	2,615,286,531	2,251,181,496	2,044,801,406	1,836,895,506
Other Operating Revenue	79,223,066	80,767,166	63,792,812	70,604,056	58,980,628
Other Nonoperating Revenue	57,646,499	57,076,374	36,058,708	2,981,869	-13,731,846
Total Net Revenue	3,131,652,705	2,753,130,071	2,351,033,016	2,118,387,331	1,882,144,288
Total Expenses	2,848,299,424	2,548,210,216	2,188,643,072	1,994,793,981	1,830,377,475
HOSPITAL UNIT (Excludes Separate Nursing Home Units)					
Utilization - Inpatient					
Beds	2,645	2,655	2,627	2,616	2,691
Admissions	118,323	116,803	116,654	117,292	117,544
Inpatient Days	584,931	586,625	588,035	577,251	583,999
Average Length of Stay	4.9	5.0	5.0	4.9	5.0
Personnel					
Total Full Time	18,545	18,278	15,453	14,854	14,531
Total Part Time	8,594	8,372	8,246	7,905	8,468
Revenue and Expenses - Totals					
(Includes Inpatient and Outpatient)					
Total Net Revenue	$3,118,367,395	$2,741,511,410	$2,339,709,215	$2,107,902,639	$1,871,385,906
Total Expenses	2,837,832,481	2,537,711,796	2,178,924,493	1,985,755,739	1,823,178,785
COMMUNITY HEALTH INDICATORS PER 1000 POPULATION					
Total Population (in thousands)	1,315	1,307	1,298	1,286	1,274
Inpatient					
Beds	2.1	2.2	2.2	2.2	2.3
Admissions	90.5	89.9	90.2	91.6	92.6
Inpatient Days	489.8	495.4	499.6	496.0	507.7
Inpatient Surgeries	25.6	27.2	29.1	26.1	26.3
Births	10.4	10.5	10.8	10.6	10.8
Outpatient					
Emergency Outpatient Visits	459.6	475.4	434.0	426.1	432.0
Other Outpatient Visits	2,484.4	2,418.7	1,852.1	1,962.2	1,940.8
Total Outpatient Visits	2,944.0	2,894.1	2,286.1	2,388.3	2,372.8
Outpatient Surgeries	66.0	69.2	72.6	68.3	66.8
Expense per Capita (per person)	$2,166.2	$1,949.9	$1,686.2	$1,551.3	$1,436.8

States

TABLE 6

NEW JERSEY

U.S. Registered Community Hospitals
(Nonfederal, short-term general and other special hospitals)

Overview 2002–2006

	2006	2005	2004	2003	2002
Total Community Hospitals in New Jersey.....	79	80	80	78	81
Bed Size Category					
6-24	0	0	0	0	0
25-49	0	0	0	0	0
50-99	7	7	6	5	5
100-199	23	22	25	25	24
200-299	17	18	20	18	17
300-399	15	16	11	13	16
400-499	11	11	11	9	11
500 + ...	6	6	7	8	8
Location					
Hospitals Urban.............................	79	80	80	78	81
Hospitals Rural	0	0	0	0	0
Control					
State and Local Government.................	1	2	1	1	2
Not for Profit...............................	74	74	75	74	76
Investor owned	4	4	4	3	3
Physician Models					
Independent Practice Association	24	24	30	31	36
Group Practice without Walls................	2	2	3	3	3
Open Physician-Hospital Organization	5	9	10	13	14
Closed Physician-Hospital Organization	2	3	5	4	5
Management Service Organization	11	12	16	18	23
Integrated Salary Model.....................	17	15	15	11	15
Equity Model...............................	0	0	1	1	2
Foundation.................................	1	1	1	0	0
Insurance Products					
Health Maintenance Organization	10	7	8	9	10
Preferred Provider Organization..............	12	10	9	13	14
Indemnity Fee for Service	4	2	4	3	3
Managed Care Contracts					
Health Maintenance Organization	52	55	56	48	52
Preferred Provider Organization..............	49	55	53	47	50
Affiliations					
Hospitals in a System*.....................	45	44	46	44	42
Hospitals in a Network.....................	31	30	32	28	32
Hospitals in a Group Purchasing Organization..	52	55	53	55	61

* Please note that system affiliate information for hospitals is derived from AHA membership. In years prior to 2003 the affiliation was derived from a question on the AHA Annual Survey of hospitals; therefore, non-responding hospitals were not included in the system affiliation counts. Years prior to 2003 have been updated to reflect this change, which now include affiliation for non-reporting hospitals.

TABLE 6

NEW JERSEY

U.S. Registered Community Hospitals
(Nonfederal, short-term general and other special hospitals)

Utilization, Personnel, Revenue and Expenses, Community Health Indicators 2002–2006

	2006	2005	2004	2003	2002
TOTAL FACILITY (Includes Hospital and Nursing Home Units)					
Utilization - Inpatient					
Beds	22,094	22,090	21,952	22,807	24,094
Admissions	1,111,101	1,109,705	1,103,743	1,107,659	1,094,781
Inpatient Days	5,835,422	5,925,414	5,911,631	6,154,335	6,190,443
Average Length of Stay	5.3	5.3	5.4	5.6	5.7
Inpatient Surgeries	284,822	282,259	284,886	296,820	303,451
Births	108,995	109,227	108,029	113,420	112,900
Utilization - Outpatient					
Emergency Outpatient Visits	3,256,298	3,078,419	3,027,063	2,922,644	2,940,592
Other Outpatient Visits	13,734,887	13,748,497	14,695,340	11,763,785	12,957,409
Total Outpatient Visits	16,991,185	16,826,916	17,722,403	14,686,429	15,898,001
Outpatient Surgeries	407,085	417,084	423,269	419,982	416,709
Personnel					
Full Time RNs	26,071	25,241	23,858	22,984	21,384
Full Time LPNs	1,400	1,652	1,675	1,714	1,929
Part Time RNs	11,367	13,117	11,838	11,499	12,146
Part Time LPNs	478	624	577	662	770
Total Full Time	104,148	103,106	97,242	97,831	98,194
Total Part Time	37,053	39,603	37,057	36,109	38,591
Revenue - Inpatient					
Gross Inpatient Revenue	$45,310,317,960	$43,952,410,001	$40,437,203,818	$38,355,261,854	$29,788,891,087
Revenue - Outpatient					
Gross Outpatient Revenue	$17,267,735,947	$15,777,247,986	$14,458,714,520	$12,472,208,125	$10,149,816,977
Revenue and Expenses - Totals					
(Includes Inpatient and Outpatient)					
Total Gross Revenue	$62,578,053,907	$59,729,657,987	$54,895,918,338	$50,827,469,979	$39,938,708,064
Deductions from Revenue	47,643,352,686	45,310,599,793	41,382,302,648	37,708,618,723	27,488,534,367
Net Patient Revenue	14,934,701,221	14,419,058,194	13,513,615,690	13,118,851,256	12,450,173,697
Other Operating Revenue	1,010,071,748	922,878,762	738,399,866	645,599,155	667,392,368
Other Nonoperating Revenue	283,078,006	219,417,576	198,750,109	213,933,523	26,399,177
Total Net Revenue	16,227,850,975	15,561,354,532	14,450,765,665	13,978,383,934	13,143,965,242
Total Expenses	15,863,979,000	14,923,445,789	13,989,784,649	13,616,125,636	12,841,553,561
HOSPITAL UNIT (Excludes Separate Nursing Home Units)					
Utilization - Inpatient					
Beds	21,663	21,607	21,482	22,384	23,315
Admissions	1,107,354	1,104,354	1,099,223	1,104,636	1,091,471
Inpatient Days	5,706,480	5,766,665	5,755,885	6,013,949	5,921,584
Average Length of Stay	5.2	5.2	5.2	5.4	5.4
Personnel					
Total Full Time	103,669	102,583	96,664	97,114	97,573
Total Part Time	36,787	39,383	36,822	35,637	38,411
Revenue and Expenses - Totals					
(Includes Inpatient and Outpatient)					
Total Net Revenue	$16,177,529,982	$15,514,141,581	$14,399,602,815	$13,942,159,660	$13,070,208,862
Total Expenses	15,839,497,100	14,885,121,726	13,940,628,001	13,586,472,196	12,781,447,599
COMMUNITY HEALTH INDICATORS PER 1000 POPULATION					
Total Population (in thousands)	8,725	8,703	8,676	8,633	8,578
Inpatient					
Beds	2.5	2.5	2.5	2.6	2.8
Admissions	127.4	127.5	127.2	128.3	127.6
Inpatient Days	668.9	680.8	681.4	712.9	721.7
Inpatient Surgeries	32.6	32.4	32.8	34.4	35.4
Births	12.5	12.6	12.5	13.1	13.2
Outpatient					
Emergency Outpatient Visits	373.2	353.7	348.9	338.6	342.8
Other Outpatient Visits	1,574.3	1,579.7	1,693.8	1,362.7	1,510.6
Total Outpatient Visits	1,947.5	1,933.4	2,042.7	1,701.3	1,853.5
Outpatient Surgeries	46.7	47.9	48.8	48.7	48.6
Expense per Capita (per person)	$1,818.3	$1,714.7	$1,612.5	$1,577.3	$1,497.1

States

TABLE **6**

NEW MEXICO

U.S. Registered Community Hospitals
(Nonfederal, short-term general and other special hospitals)

Overview 2002–2006

	2006	2005	2004	2003	2002
Total Community Hospitals in New Mexico	36	37	37	37	36
Bed Size Category					
6-24	6	4	4	4	3
25-49	8	10	9	9	11
50-99	9	10	10	9	8
100-199	10	9	9	10	9
200-299	1	3	4	4	4
300-399	1	1	1	1	0
400-499	0	0	0	0	1
500 + ...	1	0	0	0	0
Location					
Hospitals Urban...........................	14	15	15	15	14
Hospitals Rural	22	22	22	22	22
Control					
State and Local Government...............	8	8	9	9	9
Not for Profit	15	15	18	19	19
Investor owned	13	14	10	9	8
Physician Models					
Independent Practice Association	8	6	8	7	6
Group Practice without Walls...............	0	0	0	0	0
Open Physician-Hospital Organization	4	6	6	7	5
Closed Physician-Hospital Organization	0	0	0	1	2
Management Service Organization	0	0	0	0	1
Integrated Salary Model....................	9	11	8	7	6
Equity Model	1	2	1	0	0
Foundation................................	2	2	1	0	2
Insurance Products					
Health Maintenance Organization	8	7	6	8	8
Preferred Provider Organization.............	6	6	5	6	7
Indemnity Fee for Service	4	4	2	3	5
Managed Care Contracts					
Health Maintenance Organization	21	22	18	17	22
Preferred Provider Organization.............	23	23	19	16	20
Affiliations					
Hospitals in a System*.....................	29	30	30	31	28
Hospitals in a Network.....................	6	6	5	4	4
Hospitals in a Group Purchasing Organization..	24	26	23	20	24

* Please note that system affiliate information for hospitals is derived from AHA membership. In years prior to 2003 the affiliation was derived from a question on the AHA Annual Survey of hospitals; therefore, non-responding hospitals were not included in the system affiliation counts. Years prior to 2003 have been updated to reflect this change, which now include affiliation for non-reporting hospitals.

TABLE 6

NEW MEXICO

U.S. Registered Community Hospitals
(Nonfederal, short-term general and other special hospitals)

Utilization, Personnel, Revenue and Expenses, Community Health Indicators 2002–2006

	2006	2005	2004	2003	2002
TOTAL FACILITY (Includes Hospital and Nursing Home Units)					
Utilization - Inpatient					
Beds	3,525	3,505	3,678	3,680	3,602
Admissions	160,792	171,547	163,416	165,709	180,041
Inpatient Days	762,267	807,324	781,150	780,895	849,396
Average Length of Stay	4.7	4.7	4.8	4.7	4.7
Inpatient Surgeries	57,642	52,087	48,648	50,772	59,388
Births	24,275	24,477	24,571	27,950	28,178
Utilization - Outpatient					
Emergency Outpatient Visits	777,671	742,439	725,603	675,058	705,643
Other Outpatient Visits	3,566,448	3,971,938	4,315,563	3,827,511	3,482,019
Total Outpatient Visits	4,344,119	4,714,377	5,041,166	4,502,569	4,187,662
Outpatient Surgeries	78,948	81,852	81,127	81,825	103,434
Personnel					
Full Time RNs	4,555	4,890	4,955	4,332	4,300
Full Time LPNs	484	545	588	681	626
Part Time RNs	2,726	2,415	2,183	2,731	2,365
Part Time LPNs	338	312	299	282	260
Total Full Time	18,746	20,955	20,275	23,248	20,133
Total Part Time	8,132	7,273	6,348	8,001	7,114
Revenue - Inpatient					
Gross Inpatient Revenue	$3,696,095,782	$3,740,792,937	$3,213,735,333	$2,694,623,925	$2,660,033,608
Revenue - Outpatient					
Gross Outpatient Revenue	$3,022,732,688	$2,754,519,275	$2,383,978,355	$1,853,344,484	$1,848,890,309
Revenue and Expenses - Totals					
(Includes Inpatient and Outpatient)					
Total Gross Revenue	$6,718,828,470	$6,495,312,212	$5,597,713,688	$4,547,968,409	$4,508,923,917
Deductions from Revenue	4,102,007,203	3,950,367,545	3,293,098,514	2,600,953,693	2,451,800,462
Net Patient Revenue	2,616,821,267	2,544,944,667	2,304,615,174	1,947,014,716	2,057,123,455
Other Operating Revenue	141,948,486	147,448,779	125,469,086	135,028,348	142,673,861
Other Nonoperating Revenue	29,409,340	21,735,358	34,435,552	32,695,504	30,460,788
Total Net Revenue	2,788,179,093	2,714,128,804	2,464,519,812	2,114,738,568	2,230,258,104
Total Expenses	2,532,320,664	2,634,907,395	2,303,636,339	2,175,580,509	2,129,702,267
HOSPITAL UNIT (Excludes Separate Nursing Home Units)					
Utilization - Inpatient					
Beds	3,478	3,470	3,631	3,680	3,592
Admissions	160,746	171,494	163,374	165,709	179,996
Inpatient Days	751,554	798,081	772,542	780,895	849,127
Average Length of Stay	4.7	4.7	4.7	4.7	4.7
Personnel					
Total Full Time	18,692	20,900	20,175	23,248	20,133
Total Part Time	8,122	7,260	6,348	8,001	7,114
Revenue and Expenses - Totals					
(Includes Inpatient and Outpatient)					
Total Net Revenue	$2,785,047,800	$2,711,389,967	$2,462,884,622	$2,114,738,568	$2,230,225,516
Total Expenses	2,530,199,604	2,632,999,432	2,301,783,109	2,175,580,509	2,129,675,083
COMMUNITY HEALTH INDICATORS PER 1000 POPULATION					
Total Population (in thousands)	1,955	1,926	1,901	1,878	1,855
Inpatient					
Beds	1.8	1.8	1.9	2.0	1.9
Admissions	82.3	89.1	86.0	88.3	97.0
Inpatient Days	390.0	419.2	411.0	415.9	457.8
Inpatient Surgeries	29.5	27.0	25.6	27.0	32.0
Births	12.4	12.7	12.9	14.9	15.2
Outpatient					
Emergency Outpatient Visits	397.9	385.5	381.8	359.5	380.3
Other Outpatient Visits	1,824.6	2,062.3	2,270.6	2,038.5	1,876.7
Total Outpatient Visits	2,222.5	2,447.8	2,652.4	2,398.0	2,257.1
Outpatient Surgeries	40.4	42.5	42.7	43.6	55.7
Expense per Capita (per person)	$1,295.6	$1,368.1	$1,212.0	$1,158.7	$1,147.9

States

Overview 2002–2006

	2006	2005	2004	2003	2002
Total Community Hospitals in New York	203	203	206	207	211
Bed Size Category					
6-24	5	5	5	5	4
25-49	8	7	7	7	8
50-99	23	24	23	21	23
100-199	50	51	49	51	53
200-299	42	40	45	47	46
300-399	28	29	25	24	25
400-499	9	14	18	18	18
500 + ...	38	33	34	34	34
Location					
Hospitals Urban	163	163	170	170	173
Hospitals Rural	40	40	36	37	38
Control					
State and Local Government	23	22	23	26	26
Not for Profit	177	179	180	178	181
Investor owned	3	2	3	3	4
Physician Models					
Independent Practice Association	31	33	33	42	45
Group Practice without Walls	5	4	5	5	8
Open Physician-Hospital Organization	20	15	16	16	22
Closed Physician-Hospital Organization	7	8	5	11	11
Management Service Organization	14	9	11	12	13
Integrated Salary Model	54	50	49	55	46
Equity Model	3	4	2	2	3
Foundation	2	2	0	4	4
Insurance Products					
Health Maintenance Organization	35	35	41	52	47
Preferred Provider Organization	19	23	33	29	26
Indemnity Fee for Service	10	12	17	12	6
Managed Care Contracts					
Health Maintenance Organization	113	107	108	129	116
Preferred Provider Organization	106	101	102	118	107
Affiliations					
Hospitals in a System*	79	74	72	72	74
Hospitals in a Network	68	65	66	74	67
Hospitals in a Group Purchasing Organization ..	130	124	118	140	128

* Please note that system affiliate information for hospitals is derived from AHA membership. In years prior to 2003 the affiliation was derived from a question on the AHA Annual Survey of hospitals; therefore, non-responding hospitals were not included in the system affiliation counts. Years prior to 2003 have been updated to reflect this change, which now include affiliation for non-reporting hospitals.

States

TABLE 6

NEW YORK

U.S. Registered Community Hospitals
(Nonfederal, short-term general and other special hospitals)

Utilization, Personnel, Revenue and Expenses, Community Health Indicators 2002–2006

	2006	2005	2004	2003	2002
TOTAL FACILITY (Includes Hospital and Nursing Home Units)					
Utilization - Inpatient					
Beds	63,591	63,068	64,205	64,705	65,570
Admissions	2,571,572	2,537,762	2,525,777	2,499,137	2,463,447
Inpatient Days	18,510,969	18,277,363	18,482,900	18,455,619	18,394,472
Average Length of Stay.	7.2	7.2	7.3	7.4	7.5
Inpatient Surgeries.	698,078	668,566	668,644	663,390	698,796
Births.	249,648	250,417	250,456	253,244	251,311
Utilization - Outpatient					
Emergency Outpatient Visits	7,924,843	7,639,381	7,612,589	7,483,787	7,474,440
Other Outpatient Visits.	46,104,567	43,898,912	42,117,477	40,752,129	39,286,094
Total Outpatient Visits	54,029,410	51,538,293	49,730,066	48,235,916	46,760,534
Outpatient Surgeries	1,354,724	1,259,196	1,288,074	1,331,027	1,379,645
Personnel					
Full Time RNs	72,165	67,837	67,182	63,439	62,771
Full Time LPNs	6,174	6,423	6,792	6,957	7,361
Part Time RNs.	22,604	23,521	23,412	22,574	21,022
Part Time LPNs	1,850	2,036	2,135	2,288	2,240
Total Full Time.	319,765	311,322	313,844	305,826	307,318
Total Part Time	74,473	74,617	75,365	76,403	69,818
Revenue - Inpatient					
Gross Inpatient Revenue.	$71,010,568,325	$66,080,727,158	$59,845,203,393	$55,082,083,246	$47,822,780,230
Revenue - Outpatient					
Gross Outpatient Revenue	$37,230,180,894	$33,027,420,524	$30,028,806,702	$25,788,229,994	$22,679,522,539
Revenue and Expenses - Totals					
(Includes Inpatient and Outpatient)					
Total Gross Revenue.	$108,240,749,219	$99,108,147,682	$89,874,010,095	$80,870,313,240	$70,502,302,769
Deductions from Revenue.	64,798,876,462	58,467,022,570	51,448,977,266	44,899,282,816	37,481,624,861
Net Patient Revenue	43,441,872,757	40,641,125,112	38,425,032,829	35,971,030,424	33,020,677,908
Other Operating Revenue	4,156,988,495	3,738,648,013	3,735,758,067	3,282,754,959	3,204,465,501
Other Nonoperating Revenue	959,995,822	636,663,624	736,713,307	812,355,098	338,322,872
Total Net Revenue.	48,558,857,074	45,016,436,749	42,897,504,203	40,066,140,481	36,563,466,281
Total Expenses.	47,808,815,271	44,701,048,591	42,332,666,603	39,939,711,060	36,549,754,047
HOSPITAL UNIT (Excludes Separate Nursing Home Units)					
Utilization - Inpatient					
Beds	58,005	58,596	58,524	57,780	57,534
Admissions	2,557,311	2,527,409	2,513,339	2,484,569	2,448,584
Inpatient Days	16,556,677	16,772,641	16,471,866	16,087,573	15,627,829
Average Length of Stay.	6.5	6.6	6.6	6.5	6.4
Personnel					
Total Full Time.	315,355	307,991	303,125	300,715	301,508
Total Part Time	72,457	71,379	72,486	74,293	67,801
Revenue and Expenses - Totals					
(Includes Inpatient and Outpatient)					
Total Net Revenue.	$48,111,502,694	$44,687,516,050	$42,533,180,009	$39,473,173,917	$35,990,827,886
Total Expenses.	47,414,611,530	44,410,483,707	42,017,458,035	39,358,980,608	35,915,200,955
COMMUNITY HEALTH INDICATORS PER 1000 POPULATION					
Total Population (in thousands)	19,306	19,316	19,292	19,238	19,168
Inpatient					
Beds	3.3	3.3	3.3	3.4	3.4
Admissions	133.2	131.4	130.9	129.9	128.5
Inpatient Days	958.8	946.2	958.1	959.3	959.7
Inpatient Surgeries.	36.2	34.6	34.7	34.5	36.5
Births.	12.9	13.0	13.0	13.2	13.1
Outpatient					
Emergency Outpatient Visits	410.5	395.5	394.6	389.0	390.0
Other Outpatient Visits.	2,388.1	2,272.7	2,183.2	2,118.3	2,049.6
Total Outpatient Visits	2,798.6	2,668.2	2,577.8	2,507.3	2,439.6
Outpatient Surgeries	70.2	65.2	66.8	69.2	72.0
Expense per Capita (per person). . . .	$2,476.3	$2,314.2	$2,194.4	$2,076.1	$1,906.9

TABLE 6

NORTH CAROLINA

U.S. Registered Community Hospitals
(Nonfederal, short-term general and other special hospitals)

Overview 2002–2006

	2006	2005	2004	2003	2002
Total Community Hospitals in North Carolina ..	114	115	115	113	113
Bed Size Category					
6-24	3	4	4	4	4
25-49	15	16	12	10	10
50-99	22	22	25	24	27
100-199	38	37	38	39	37
200-299	13	15	15	14	13
300-399	9	7	7	8	8
400-499	1	2	1	2	1
500 + ...	13	12	13	12	13
Location					
Hospitals Urban	56	56	53	51	51
Hospitals Rural	58	59	62	62	62
Control					
State and Local Government	32	32	32	29	30
Not for Profit	75	75	74	76	75
Investor owned	7	8	9	8	8
Physician Models					
Independent Practice Association	13	14	15	12	10
Group Practice without Walls	3	3	4	6	4
Open Physician-Hospital Organization	14	17	20	23	25
Closed Physician-Hospital Organization	8	8	6	7	4
Management Service Organization	14	10	11	15	16
Integrated Salary Model	45	38	37	38	35
Equity Model	3	2	2	2	1
Foundation	4	4	4	8	7
Insurance Products					
Health Maintenance Organization	12	9	11	11	10
Preferred Provider Organization	21	19	19	21	22
Indemnity Fee for Service	4	4	6	7	5
Managed Care Contracts					
Health Maintenance Organization	74	70	71	72	66
Preferred Provider Organization	86	80	85	84	81
Affiliations					
Hospitals in a System*	59	65	65	62	63
Hospitals in a Network	43	37	43	45	41
Hospitals in a Group Purchasing Organization ..	102	90	89	93	86

* Please note that system affiliate information for hospitals is derived from AHA membership. In years prior to 2003 the affiliation was derived from a question on the AHA Annual Survey of hospitals; therefore, non-responding hospitals were not included in the system affiliation counts. Years prior to 2003 have been updated to reflect this change, which now include affiliation for non-reporting hospitals.

TABLE 6

NORTH CAROLINA

U.S. Registered Community Hospitals
(Nonfederal, short-term general and other special hospitals)

Utilization, Personnel, Revenue and Expenses, Community Health Indicators 2002–2006

	2006	2005	2004	2003	2002
TOTAL FACILITY (Includes Hospital and Nursing Home Units)					
Utilization - Inpatient					
Beds	23,441	23,344	23,498	23,285	23,583
Admissions	1,015,594	1,013,094	1,005,965	987,209	966,722
Inpatient Days	6,131,924	6,089,400	6,115,774	6,053,100	5,929,916
Average Length of Stay	6.0	6.0	6.1	6.1	6.1
Inpatient Surgeries	294,298	301,188	304,921	295,672	291,914
Births	120,778	117,137	114,108	110,364	108,967
Utilization - Outpatient					
Emergency Outpatient Visits	3,849,736	3,784,070	3,483,332	3,433,432	3,322,226
Other Outpatient Visits	13,363,083	13,017,649	11,831,202	11,107,315	10,500,582
Total Outpatient Visits	17,212,819	16,801,719	15,314,534	14,540,747	13,822,808
Outpatient Surgeries	561,285	588,276	608,488	556,577	519,494
Personnel					
Full Time RNs	31,642	29,786	28,825	26,344	26,990
Full Time LPNs	2,000	2,215	2,157	2,114	2,221
Part Time RNs	13,498	13,730	12,470	12,378	11,510
Part Time LPNs	761	834	828	766	738
Total Full Time	121,023	118,275	116,111	107,326	107,239
Total Part Time	36,764	37,399	34,438	34,498	32,029
Revenue - Inpatient					
Gross Inpatient Revenue	$20,338,755,428	$18,580,679,238	$17,237,298,617	$15,414,708,940	$13,579,832,889
Revenue - Outpatient					
Gross Outpatient Revenue	$15,852,323,132	$13,815,373,836	$11,892,189,064	$9,605,613,777	$8,591,785,373
Revenue and Expenses - Totals (Includes Inpatient and Outpatient)					
Total Gross Revenue	$36,191,078,560	$32,396,053,074	$29,129,487,681	$25,020,322,717	$22,171,618,262
Deductions from Revenue	20,163,280,987	17,752,655,424	15,475,967,403	12,727,067,302	10,719,115,151
Net Patient Revenue	16,027,797,573	14,643,397,650	13,653,520,278	12,293,255,415	11,452,503,111
Other Operating Revenue	774,858,487	723,646,759	725,740,871	678,356,147	645,286,961
Other Nonoperating Revenue	556,662,511	340,797,263	357,649,552	385,414,921	81,728,986
Total Net Revenue	17,359,318,571	15,707,841,672	14,736,910,701	13,357,026,483	12,179,519,058
Total Expenses	15,721,863,715	14,661,849,081	13,310,632,196	12,369,931,674	11,563,648,159
HOSPITAL UNIT (Excludes Separate Nursing Home Units)					
Utilization - Inpatient					
Beds	20,428	20,767	20,739	20,759	20,627
Admissions	1,004,707	1,003,543	995,794	977,527	957,259
Inpatient Days	5,164,167	5,253,458	5,203,268	5,215,187	4,968,309
Average Length of Stay	5.1	5.2	5.2	5.3	5.2
Personnel					
Total Full Time	118,627	116,358	113,268	105,215	105,030
Total Part Time	35,802	36,432	33,255	33,515	31,000
Revenue and Expenses - Totals (Includes Inpatient and Outpatient)					
Total Net Revenue	$17,183,454,204	$15,559,562,668	$14,590,640,384	$13,232,487,962	$12,041,087,073
Total Expenses	15,526,247,079	14,505,827,063	13,163,805,794	12,242,509,865	11,418,905,299
COMMUNITY HEALTH INDICATORS PER 1000 POPULATION					
Total Population (in thousands)	8,857	8,672	8,531	8,416	8,313
Inpatient					
Beds	2.6	2.7	2.8	2.8	2.8
Admissions	114.7	116.8	117.9	117.3	116.3
Inpatient Days	692.4	702.2	716.9	719.3	713.3
Inpatient Surgeries	33.2	34.7	35.7	35.1	35.1
Births	13.6	13.5	13.4	13.1	13.1
Outpatient					
Emergency Outpatient Visits	434.7	436.3	408.3	408.0	399.6
Other Outpatient Visits	1,508.8	1,501.0	1,386.8	1,319.8	1,263.1
Total Outpatient Visits	1,943.5	1,937.4	1,795.2	1,727.8	1,662.7
Outpatient Surgeries	63.4	67.8	71.3	66.1	62.5
Expense per Capita (per person)	$1,775.2	$1,690.6	$1,560.3	$1,469.9	$1,390.9

States

TABLE 6

NORTH DAKOTA

U.S. Registered Community Hospitals
(Nonfederal, short-term general and other special hospitals)

Overview 2002–2006

	2006	2005	2004	2003	2002
Total Community Hospitals in North Dakota ...	41	40	40	40	42
Bed Size Category					
6-24	9	8	8	7	7
25-49	13	13	14	14	11
50-99	12	12	11	11	16
100-199	2	3	3	4	2
200-299	3	2	2	2	4
300-399	0	0	0	0	0
400-499	1	1	0	1	1
500 + ...	1	1	2	1	1
Location					
Hospitals Urban........................	6	6	6	6	7
Hospitals Rural	35	34	34	34	35
Control					
State and Local Government..............	0	0	0	0	0
Not for Profit...........................	41	40	40	40	41
Investor owned	0	0	0	0	1
Physician Models					
Independent Practice Association	4	4	4	4	4
Group Practice without Walls...............	1	3	2	1	1
Open Physician-Hospital Organization	2	1	1	1	2
Closed Physician-Hospital Organization	2	2	1	3	2
Management Service Organization	0	0	1	0	0
Integrated Salary Model...................	16	16	10	10	13
Equity Model............................	1	1	1	1	1
Foundation.............................	5	4	1	1	2
Insurance Products					
Health Maintenance Organization	1	0	0	0	0
Preferred Provider Organization.............	5	5	3	6	4
Indemnity Fee for Service	1	0	0	2	1
Managed Care Contracts					
Health Maintenance Organization	4	6	4	4	5
Preferred Provider Organization.............	19	19	18	16	19
Affiliations					
Hospitals in a System*....................	14	13	12	13	12
Hospitals in a Network....................	10	10	10	11	9
Hospitals in a Group Purchasing Organization..	32	28	24	25	27

* Please note that system affiliate information for hospitals is derived from AHA membership. In years prior to 2003 the affiliation was derived from a question on the AHA Annual Survey of hospitals; therefore, non-responding hospitals were not included in the system affiliation counts. Years prior to 2003 have been updated to reflect this change, which now include affiliation for non-reporting hospitals.

States

TABLE 6

NORTH DAKOTA

U.S. Registered Community Hospitals
(Nonfederal, short-term general and other special hospitals)

Utilization, Personnel, Revenue and Expenses, Community Health Indicators 2002–2006

	2006	2005	2004	2003	2002
TOTAL FACILITY (Includes Hospital and Nursing Home Units)					
Utilization - Inpatient					
Beds	3,550	3,494	3,567	3,595	3,880
Admissions	88,737	87,485	88,004	88,132	94,630
Inpatient Days	762,500	767,324	769,880	774,175	845,194
Average Length of Stay	8.6	8.8	8.7	8.8	8.9
Inpatient Surgeries	28,577	27,730	28,678	28,325	27,650
Births	9,587	9,281	9,238	9,143	9,337
Utilization - Outpatient					
Emergency Outpatient Visits	263,144	263,489	254,409	261,714	295,074
Other Outpatient Visits	1,446,140	1,599,948	1,594,764	1,551,282	1,621,700
Total Outpatient Visits	1,709,284	1,863,437	1,849,173	1,812,996	1,916,774
Outpatient Surgeries	44,257	42,892	47,079	47,969	48,213
Personnel					
Full Time RNs	2,110	2,089	2,296	1,836	1,884
Full Time LPNs	544	521	584	534	531
Part Time RNs	2,244	2,153	1,756	2,145	2,453
Part Time LPNs	602	571	424	538	583
Total Full Time	11,623	11,714	11,744	10,892	11,676
Total Part Time	8,050	7,866	6,776	8,236	9,379
Revenue - Inpatient					
Gross Inpatient Revenue	$1,334,432,797	$1,265,396,292	$1,188,078,532	$1,104,753,788	$1,302,289,738
Revenue - Outpatient					
Gross Outpatient Revenue	$1,527,971,411	$1,411,506,368	$1,261,112,345	$1,127,663,697	$1,134,691,244
Revenue and Expenses - Totals					
(Includes Inpatient and Outpatient)					
Total Gross Revenue	$2,862,404,208	$2,676,902,660	$2,449,190,877	$2,232,417,485	$2,436,980,982
Deductions from Revenue	1,303,212,416	1,204,587,282	1,070,387,845	941,238,095	1,094,215,330
Net Patient Revenue	1,559,191,792	1,472,315,378	1,378,803,032	1,291,179,390	1,342,765,652
Other Operating Revenue	78,157,365	79,881,629	70,301,224	64,972,544	63,807,911
Other Nonoperating Revenue	38,911,418	23,059,817	25,078,701	22,182,704	8,085,712
Total Net Revenue	1,676,260,575	1,575,256,824	1,474,182,957	1,378,334,638	1,414,659,275
Total Expenses	1,630,169,448	1,508,285,775	1,414,152,181	1,347,844,373	1,351,763,031
HOSPITAL UNIT (Excludes Separate Nursing Home Units)					
Utilization - Inpatient					
Beds	2,589	2,497	2,559	2,656	2,883
Admissions	85,589	84,778	85,546	85,822	92,446
Inpatient Days	446,177	446,887	439,666	466,368	515,332
Average Length of Stay	5.2	5.3	5.1	5.4	5.6
Personnel					
Total Full Time	10,927	11,072	10,773	10,281	11,066
Total Part Time	7,481	7,274	6,153	7,671	8,878
Revenue and Expenses - Totals					
(Includes Inpatient and Outpatient)					
Total Net Revenue	$1,621,940,757	$1,525,993,700	$1,423,651,440	$1,329,671,873	$1,365,837,644
Total Expenses	1,587,820,886	1,470,178,178	1,373,930,577	1,307,814,219	1,314,789,098
COMMUNITY HEALTH INDICATORS PER 1000 POPULATION					
Total Population (in thousands)	636	635	636	633	634
Inpatient					
Beds	5.6	5.5	5.6	5.7	6.1
Admissions	139.6	137.9	138.4	139.3	149.3
Inpatient Days	1,199.2	1,209.1	1,210.8	1,223.8	1,333.9
Inpatient Surgeries	44.9	43.7	45.1	44.8	43.6
Births	15.1	14.6	14.5	14.5	14.7
Outpatient					
Emergency Outpatient Visits	413.8	415.2	400.1	413.7	465.7
Other Outpatient Visits	2,274.3	2,521.2	2,508.1	2,452.2	2,559.3
Total Outpatient Visits	2,688.1	2,936.4	2,908.2	2,865.9	3,025.0
Outpatient Surgeries	69.6	67.6	74.0	75.8	76.1
Expense per Capita (per person)	$2,563.7	$2,376.7	$2,224.0	$2,130.6	$2,133.3

TABLE **6**

OHIO

U.S. Registered Community Hospitals
(Nonfederal, short-term general and other special hospitals)

Overview 2002–2006

	2006	2005	2004	2003	2002
Total Community Hospitals in Ohio...........	171	170	166	163	168
Bed Size Category					
6-24	4	5	3	0	2
25-49	36	32	31	29	27
50-99	26	27	23	26	27
100-199	45	43	47	49	50
200-299	26	25	24	24	27
300-399	14	19	17	16	16
400-499	8	8	10	9	9
500 + ...	12	11	11	10	10
Location					
Hospitals Urban.........................	117	116	117	113	116
Hospitals Rural	54	54	49	50	52
Control					
State and Local Government................	23	23	23	23	23
Not for Profit	136	137	138	136	141
Investor owned	12	10	5	4	4
Physician Models					
Independent Practice Association	26	19	20	20	17
Group Practice without Walls...............	11	11	7	9	11
Open Physician-Hospital Organization	45	47	45	43	47
Closed Physician-Hospital Organization	24	24	25	25	18
Management Service Organization	38	39	37	35	33
Integrated Salary Model	64	58	56	55	44
Equity Model	7	7	5	2	7
Foundation...............................	25	22	23	20	14
Insurance Products					
Health Maintenance Organization	35	23	27	28	27
Preferred Provider Organization..............	45	32	33	34	32
Indemnity Fee for Service	17	14	19	14	12
Managed Care Contracts					
Health Maintenance Organization	109	110	107	114	104
Preferred Provider Organization..............	122	127	117	123	112
Affiliations					
Hospitals in a System*.....................	93	92	88	83	84
Hospitals in a Network	74	66	67	67	60
Hospitals in a Group Purchasing Organization..	144	144	133	140	126

* Please note that system affiliate information for hospitals is derived from AHA membership. In years prior to 2003 the affiliation was derived from a question on the AHA Annual Survey of hospitals; therefore, non-responding hospitals were not included in the system affiliation counts. Years prior to 2003 have been updated to reflect this change, which now include affiliation for non-reporting hospitals.

TABLE 6

OHIO

U.S. Registered Community Hospitals
(Nonfederal, short-term general and other special hospitals)

Utilization, Personnel, Revenue and Expenses, Community Health Indicators 2002–2006

	2006	2005	2004	2003	2002
TOTAL FACILITY (Includes Hospital and Nursing Home Units)					
Utilization - Inpatient					
Beds	32,822	33,250	33,398	32,981	33,706
Admissions	1,542,333	1,511,171	1,474,876	1,457,933	1,475,630
Inpatient Days	7,742,312	7,801,663	7,718,229	7,501,323	7,657,394
Average Length of Stay...........	5.0	5.2	5.2	5.1	5.2
Inpatient Surgeries..............	414,838	414,613	415,641	416,945	431,329
Births.........................	147,992	146,625	147,087	147,253	150,298
Utilization - Outpatient					
Emergency Outpatient Visits	5,840,398	5,593,421	5,401,226	5,354,136	5,125,829
Other Outpatient Visits...........	26,846,119	25,756,970	25,145,977	24,668,217	23,229,558
Total Outpatient Visits	32,686,517	31,350,391	30,547,203	30,022,353	28,355,387
Outpatient Surgeries	782,568	806,211	791,207	798,612	810,253
Personnel					
Full Time RNs	43,114	42,180	39,184	38,391	35,036
Full Time LPNs	4,279	4,510	4,325	4,319	4,011
Part Time RNs..................	23,277	22,608	22,851	22,823	22,467
Part Time LPNs	2,122	2,278	2,311	2,227	2,211
Total Full Time.................	181,475	183,355	171,655	168,483	161,392
Total Part Time	70,557	67,961	67,388	69,146	66,399
Revenue - Inpatient					
Gross Inpatient Revenue..........	$35,776,947,886	$32,838,049,256	$29,068,190,645	$25,399,812,064	$23,112,708,865
Revenue - Outpatient					
Gross Outpatient Revenue	$28,562,090,312	$25,659,811,203	$22,371,774,845	$19,459,508,400	$16,391,385,950
Revenue and Expenses - Totals					
(Includes Inpatient and Outpatient)					
Total Gross Revenue..............	$64,339,038,198	$58,497,860,459	$51,439,965,490	$44,859,320,464	$39,504,094,815
Deductions from Revenue.........	39,005,578,638	34,669,271,066	29,452,662,017	24,821,741,430	20,841,549,318
Net Patient Revenue	25,333,459,560	23,828,589,393	21,987,303,473	20,037,579,034	18,662,545,497
Other Operating Revenue	1,572,944,936	1,418,198,645	1,271,069,402	1,114,390,509	1,069,165,656
Other Nonoperating Revenue	665,928,838	405,904,678	360,710,829	252,611,257	60,979,408
Total Net Revenue...............	27,572,333,334	25,652,692,716	23,619,083,704	21,404,580,800	19,792,690,561
Total Expenses..................	25,712,641,988	24,084,934,719	22,138,349,794	20,465,149,310	19,132,292,794
HOSPITAL UNIT (Excludes Separate Nursing Home Units)					
Utilization - Inpatient					
Beds	30,827	31,422	31,516	31,260	31,729
Admissions	1,521,553	1,493,794	1,459,452	1,440,323	1,458,479
Inpatient Days	7,158,331	7,246,049	7,127,973	6,977,632	7,051,923
Average Length of Stay...........	4.7	4.9	4.9	4.8	4.8
Personnel					
Total Full Time.................	179,982	182,022	162,601	167,029	159,965
Total Part Time	69,778	67,196	62,931	68,267	65,646
Revenue and Expenses - Totals					
(Includes Inpatient and Outpatient)					
Total Net Revenue...............	$27,333,636,562	$25,417,810,898	$23,467,323,085	$21,161,469,394	$19,619,443,053
Total Expenses..................	25,525,939,444	23,846,822,087	22,008,158,681	20,242,498,362	18,970,939,986
COMMUNITY HEALTH INDICATORS PER 1000 POPULATION					
Total Population (in thousands)	11,478	11,471	11,461	11,438	11,415
Inpatient					
Beds	2.9	2.9	2.9	2.9	3.0
Admissions	134.4	131.7	128.7	127.5	129.3
Inpatient Days	674.5	680.1	673.4	655.8	670.8
Inpatient Surgeries..............	36.1	36.1	36.3	36.5	37.8
Births.........................	12.9	12.8	12.8	12.9	13.2
Outpatient					
Emergency Outpatient Visits	508.8	487.6	471.3	468.1	449.1
Other Outpatient Visits...........	2,338.9	2,245.5	2,194.0	2,156.7	2,035.1
Total Outpatient Visits	2,847.8	2,733.1	2,665.2	2,624.8	2,484.1
Outpatient Surgeries	68.2	70.3	69.0	69.8	71.0
Expense per Capita (per person)....	$2,240.2	$2,099.7	$1,931.6	$1,789.2	$1,676.1

States

TABLE 6

OKLAHOMA

U.S. Registered Community Hospitals
(Nonfederal, short-term general and other special hospitals)

Overview 2002–2006

	2006	2005	2004	2003	2002
Total Community Hospitals in Oklahoma	112	110	109	108	105
Bed Size Category					
6-24	23	18	18	17	15
25-49	37	38	40	40	36
50-99	25	25	21	21	24
100-199	13	15	16	16	15
200-299	3	5	5	6	6
300-399	5	3	3	2	3
400-499	2	1	2	1	2
500 + ...	4	5	4	5	4
Location					
Hospitals Urban	46	45	41	41	38
Hospitals Rural	66	65	68	67	67
Control					
State and Local Government	44	41	45	47	44
Not for Profit	35	39	42	46	46
Investor owned	33	30	22	15	15
Physician Models					
Independent Practice Association	15	17	11	16	14
Group Practice without Walls	3	4	3	3	3
Open Physician-Hospital Organization	17	14	14	16	15
Closed Physician-Hospital Organization	5	9	7	8	8
Management Service Organization	10	13	15	14	11
Integrated Salary Model	25	22	26	34	22
Equity Model	1	4	1	1	0
Foundation	1	4	2	4	0
Insurance Products					
Health Maintenance Organization	7	8	10	11	11
Preferred Provider Organization	13	11	14	24	17
Indemnity Fee for Service	3	3	4	10	6
Managed Care Contracts					
Health Maintenance Organization	35	32	28	39	37
Preferred Provider Organization	60	63	50	65	54
Affiliations					
Hospitals in a System*	56	58	53	56	55
Hospitals in a Network	24	22	22	22	17
Hospitals in a Group Purchasing Organization . .	85	81	76	80	66

* Please note that system affiliate information for hospitals is derived from AHA membership. In years prior to 2003 the affiliation was derived from a question on the AHA Annual Survey of hospitals; therefore, non-responding hospitals were not included in the system affiliation counts. Years prior to 2003 have been updated to reflect this change, which now include affiliation for non-reporting hospitals.

TABLE 6

OKLAHOMA

U.S. Registered Community Hospitals
(Nonfederal, short-term general and other special hospitals)

Utilization, Personnel, Revenue and Expenses, Community Health Indicators 2002–2006

	2006	2005	2004	2003	2002
TOTAL FACILITY (Includes Hospital and Nursing Home Units)					
Utilization - Inpatient					
Beds	10,773	10,814	10,804	11,018	11,122
Admissions	454,085	456,759	454,875	449,936	445,952
Inpatient Days	2,307,539	2,341,597	2,370,273	2,380,232	2,371,009
Average Length of Stay	5.1	5.1	5.2	5.3	5.3
Inpatient Surgeries	112,716	114,376	127,837	116,951	109,770
Births	47,489	45,225	43,167	44,736	43,564
Utilization - Outpatient					
Emergency Outpatient Visits	1,554,914	1,428,028	1,358,288	1,386,848	1,292,652
Other Outpatient Visits	3,779,892	3,983,463	3,972,073	4,102,880	3,510,111
Total Outpatient Visits	5,334,806	5,411,491	5,330,361	5,489,728	4,802,763
Outpatient Surgeries	188,902	189,427	189,338	180,442	173,030
Personnel					
Full Time RNs	9,638	9,382	8,571	8,867	8,738
Full Time LPNs	2,209	2,246	2,553	2,393	2,302
Part Time RNs	3,508	2,746	3,223	3,110	3,469
Part Time LPNs	690	642	678	769	698
Total Full Time	42,811	42,957	39,573	42,527	41,470
Total Part Time	12,270	9,893	12,209	12,063	13,105
Revenue - Inpatient					
Gross Inpatient Revenue	$9,412,503,176	$8,557,722,404	$7,876,618,375	$7,071,793,695	$6,358,250,635
Revenue - Outpatient					
Gross Outpatient Revenue	$5,508,080,380	$4,920,113,693	$4,120,562,889	$3,555,834,680	$3,123,729,308
Revenue and Expenses - Totals					
(Includes Inpatient and Outpatient)					
Total Gross Revenue	$14,920,583,556	$13,477,836,097	$11,997,181,264	$10,627,628,375	$9,481,979,943
Deductions from Revenue	9,331,819,127	8,181,135,336	7,260,891,202	6,294,574,391	5,455,901,182
Net Patient Revenue	5,588,764,429	5,296,700,761	4,736,290,062	4,333,053,984	4,026,078,761
Other Operating Revenue	247,484,700	246,057,846	286,260,545	336,044,566	253,147,564
Other Nonoperating Revenue	86,916,871	60,680,859	51,828,639	55,328,125	26,110,536
Total Net Revenue	5,923,166,000	5,603,439,466	5,074,379,246	4,724,426,675	4,305,336,861
Total Expenses	5,384,898,786	5,189,657,883	4,731,185,235	4,427,836,412	3,986,180,785
HOSPITAL UNIT (Excludes Separate Nursing Home Units)					
Utilization - Inpatient					
Beds	10,392	10,533	10,465	10,669	10,877
Admissions	451,626	453,877	451,720	445,825	443,327
Inpatient Days	2,204,009	2,260,754	2,268,446	2,274,063	2,295,445
Average Length of Stay	4.9	5.0	5.0	5.1	5.2
Personnel					
Total Full Time	42,351	42,764	39,420	42,093	41,248
Total Part Time	12,075	9,815	12,159	11,939	13,022
Revenue and Expenses - Totals					
(Includes Inpatient and Outpatient)					
Total Net Revenue	$5,904,273,214	$5,578,528,213	$5,045,401,661	$4,704,868,435	$4,290,663,306
Total Expenses	5,367,863,128	5,158,908,800	4,712,397,152	4,411,790,782	3,977,214,712
COMMUNITY HEALTH INDICATORS PER 1000 POPULATION					
Total Population (in thousands)	3,579	3,543	3,523	3,504	3,488
Inpatient					
Beds	3.0	3.1	3.1	3.1	3.2
Admissions	126.9	128.9	129.1	128.4	127.8
Inpatient Days	644.7	660.8	672.8	679.2	679.7
Inpatient Surgeries	31.5	32.3	36.3	33.4	31.5
Births	13.3	12.8	12.3	12.8	12.5
Outpatient					
Emergency Outpatient Visits	434.4	403.0	385.6	395.8	370.6
Other Outpatient Visits	1,056.1	1,124.2	1,127.5	1,170.8	1,006.2
Total Outpatient Visits	1,490.5	1,527.2	1,513.1	1,566.5	1,376.8
Outpatient Surgeries	52.8	53.5	53.7	51.5	49.6
Expense per Capita (per person)	$1,504.5	$1,464.6	$1,343.0	$1,263.5	$1,142.7

States

TABLE 6

OREGON

U.S. Registered Community Hospitals
(Nonfederal, short-term general and other special hospitals)

Overview 2002–2006

	2006	2005	2004	2003	2002
Total Community Hospitals in Oregon	58	58	58	58	60
Bed Size Category					
6-24	8	8	8	6	5
25-49	19	19	19	20	18
50-99	12	12	12	12	17
100-199	9	9	10	10	11
200-299	4	4	3	4	3
300-399	0	0	0	1	3
400-499	5	6	6	5	3
500 + ...	1	0	0	0	0
Location					
Hospitals Urban	29	29	26	27	29
Hospitals Rural	29	29	32	31	31
Control					
State and Local Government	13	12	12	12	12
Not for Profit	42	43	43	43	44
Investor owned	3	3	3	3	4
Physician Models					
Independent Practice Association	14	17	13	14	26
Group Practice without Walls	6	6	4	4	3
Open Physician-Hospital Organization	10	10	4	6	4
Closed Physician-Hospital Organization	3	3	3	4	4
Management Service Organization	9	9	7	5	7
Integrated Salary Model	31	29	21	17	21
Equity Model	1	1	0	0	0
Foundation	4	3	1	1	2
Insurance Products					
Health Maintenance Organization	13	14	10	12	14
Preferred Provider Organization	19	20	15	15	15
Indemnity Fee for Service	6	6	3	6	2
Managed Care Contracts					
Health Maintenance Organization	34	36	31	30	41
Preferred Provider Organization	46	45	35	35	47
Affiliations					
Hospitals in a System*	34	34	34	34	35
Hospitals in a Network	22	22	19	12	19
Hospitals in a Group Purchasing Organization . .	57	57	45	39	53

* Please note that system affiliate information for hospitals is derived from AHA membership. In years prior to 2003 the affiliation was derived from a question on the AHA Annual Survey of hospitals; therefore, non-responding hospitals were not included in the system affiliation counts. Years prior to 2003 have been updated to reflect this change, which now include affiliation for non-reporting hospitals.

TABLE 6

OREGON

U.S. Registered Community Hospitals
(Nonfederal, short-term general and other special hospitals)

Utilization, Personnel, Revenue and Expenses, Community Health Indicators 2002–2006

	2006	2005	2004	2003	2002
TOTAL FACILITY (Includes Hospital and Nursing Home Units)					
Utilization - Inpatient					
Beds	6,609	6,515	6,505	6,757	6,798
Admissions	341,540	336,173	341,307	342,282	345,193
Inpatient Days	1,508,314	1,490,898	1,461,923	1,455,069	1,511,420
Average Length of Stay	4.4	4.4	4.3	4.3	4.4
Inpatient Surgeries	117,402	114,513	114,611	114,111	113,669
Births	47,369	45,475	45,957	45,704	45,409
Utilization - Outpatient					
Emergency Outpatient Visits	1,250,008	1,216,163	1,147,196	1,113,166	1,117,313
Other Outpatient Visits	7,007,868	6,757,046	6,712,041	7,073,918	7,058,865
Total Outpatient Visits	8,257,876	7,973,209	7,859,237	8,187,084	8,176,178
Outpatient Surgeries	206,125	197,263	188,638	196,364	191,717
Personnel					
Full Time RNs	8,633	8,404	8,144	8,074	7,114
Full Time LPNs	219	251	431	532	547
Part Time RNs	7,901	7,976	7,510	6,582	7,454
Part Time LPNs	240	259	260	287	568
Total Full Time	35,767	34,474	33,571	33,648	32,765
Total Part Time	20,862	21,368	20,868	18,250	22,952
Revenue - Inpatient					
Gross Inpatient Revenue	$6,636,156,491	$6,178,760,391	$5,702,413,613	$5,042,552,776	$4,563,875,879
Revenue - Outpatient					
Gross Outpatient Revenue	$5,193,062,718	$4,697,819,458	$4,128,678,383	$3,652,443,825	$3,183,571,829
Revenue and Expenses - Totals					
(Includes Inpatient and Outpatient)					
Total Gross Revenue	$11,829,219,209	$10,876,579,849	$9,831,091,996	$8,694,996,601	$7,747,447,708
Deductions from Revenue	5,737,941,726	5,249,271,986	4,651,055,624	3,877,092,481	3,206,030,580
Net Patient Revenue	6,091,277,483	5,627,307,863	5,180,036,372	4,817,904,120	4,541,417,128
Other Operating Revenue	299,687,588	255,942,976	260,818,230	245,884,763	220,287,872
Other Nonoperating Revenue	138,893,278	92,691,720	67,106,324	21,294,360	6,824,416
Total Net Revenue	6,529,858,349	5,975,942,559	5,507,960,926	5,085,083,243	4,768,529,416
Total Expenses	6,192,331,481	5,665,479,466	5,206,775,669	4,806,543,508	4,468,834,030
HOSPITAL UNIT (Excludes Separate Nursing Home Units)					
Utilization - Inpatient					
Beds	6,345	6,251	6,265	6,460	6,452
Admissions	341,242	335,831	340,958	341,317	344,564
Inpatient Days	1,437,308	1,418,888	1,398,492	1,380,053	1,406,690
Average Length of Stay	4.2	4.2	4.1	4.0	4.1
Personnel					
Total Full Time	35,615	34,331	33,429	33,506	32,601
Total Part Time	20,784	21,280	20,784	18,131	22,777
Revenue and Expenses - Totals					
(Includes Inpatient and Outpatient)					
Total Net Revenue	$6,520,330,928	$5,964,862,021	$5,498,352,090	$5,075,462,319	$4,756,252,635
Total Expenses	6,183,003,680	5,653,222,094	5,196,487,284	4,796,593,445	4,455,142,703
COMMUNITY HEALTH INDICATORS PER 1000 POPULATION					
Total Population (in thousands)	3,701	3,639	3,589	3,561	3,524
Inpatient					
Beds	1.8	1.8	1.8	1.9	1.9
Admissions	92.3	92.4	95.1	96.1	98.0
Inpatient Days	407.6	409.7	407.3	408.6	429.0
Inpatient Surgeries	31.7	31.5	31.9	32.0	32.3
Births	12.8	12.5	12.8	12.8	12.9
Outpatient					
Emergency Outpatient Visits	337.8	334.2	319.6	312.6	317.1
Other Outpatient Visits	1,893.6	1,856.9	1,870.1	1,986.4	2,003.4
Total Outpatient Visits	2,231.4	2,191.1	2,189.7	2,299.0	2,320.5
Outpatient Surgeries	55.7	54.2	52.6	55.1	54.4
Expense per Capita (per person)	$1,673.3	$1,556.9	$1,450.7	$1,349.7	$1,268.3

TABLE 6

PENNSYLVANIA

U.S. Registered Community Hospitals
(Nonfederal, short-term general and other special hospitals)

Overview 2002–2006

	2006	2005	2004	2003	2002
Total Community Hospitals in Pennsylvania ...	188	191	197	201	201
Bed Size Category					
6-24	3	3	4	4	4
25-49	22	19	16	15	13
50-99	29	33	36	35	36
100-199	57	58	63	68	71
200-299	37	40	42	42	40
300-399	15	16	13	14	14
400-499	12	10	12	12	11
500 + ...	13	12	11	11	12
Location					
Hospitals Urban.............................	140	143	153	158	158
Hospitals Rural	48	48	44	43	43
Control					
State and Local Government.................	2	2	1	2	2
Not for Profit	161	165	172	177	184
Investor owned	25	24	24	22	15
Physician Models					
Independent Practice Association	9	9	12	19	18
Group Practice without Walls................	12	13	15	14	10
Open Physician-Hospital Organization	30	31	37	41	40
Closed Physician-Hospital Organization	6	7	5	4	10
Management Service Organization	30	26	27	26	28
Integrated Salary Model.....................	72	69	66	66	57
Equity Model	4	4	5	6	4
Foundation.................................	5	6	9	8	7
Insurance Products					
Health Maintenance Organization	29	28	30	26	25
Preferred Provider Organization..............	39	41	42	43	39
Indemnity Fee for Service	13	11	11	9	8
Managed Care Contracts					
Health Maintenance Organization	125	115	138	142	149
Preferred Provider Organization..............	121	109	131	139	143
Affiliations					
Hospitals in a System*......................	107	106	104	104	99
Hospitals in a Network......................	52	39	48	45	53
Hospitals in a Group Purchasing Organization..	142	124	143	156	161

* Please note that system affiliate information for hospitals is derived from AHA membership. In years prior to 2003 the affiliation was derived from a question on the AHA Annual Survey of hospitals; therefore, non-responding hospitals were not included in the system affiliation counts. Years prior to 2003 have been updated to reflect this change, which now include affiliation for non-reporting hospitals.

TABLE 6

PENNSYLVANIA

U.S. Registered Community Hospitals
(Nonfederal, short-term general and other special hospitals)

Utilization, Personnel, Revenue and Expenses, Community Health Indicators 2002–2006

	2006	2005	2004	2003	2002
TOTAL FACILITY (Includes Hospital and Nursing Home Units)					
Utilization - Inpatient					
Beds	39,567	39,602	40,079	40,908	40,534
Admissions	1,866,261	1,863,299	1,846,702	1,824,132	1,798,243
Inpatient Days	10,110,336	10,170,812	10,259,088	10,300,758	10,340,276
Average Length of Stay.	5.4	5.5	5.6	5.6	5.8
Inpatient Surgeries.	553,061	550,986	546,837	531,212	537,857
Births.	141,971	140,089	134,864	137,718	139,489
Utilization - Outpatient					
Emergency Outpatient Visits	5,583,228	5,379,119	5,277,055	5,160,713	5,059,150
Other Outpatient Visits.	30,127,411	29,531,995	28,135,789	28,124,567	27,349,887
Total Outpatient Visits	35,710,639	34,911,114	33,412,844	33,285,280	32,409,037
Outpatient Surgeries	998,156	1,000,746	993,636	966,727	983,477
Personnel					
Full Time RNs	47,217	46,105	43,382	41,791	40,679
Full Time LPNs	4,342	4,703	4,727	4,803	4,910
Part Time RNs	25,541	24,832	25,620	25,123	24,880
Part Time LPNs	2,105	2,256	2,431	2,494	2,557
Total Full Time	200,061	196,471	190,861	186,132	185,944
Total Part Time	75,335	73,870	74,959	73,239	74,311
Revenue - Inpatient					
Gross Inpatient Revenue.	$61,367,161,956	$57,094,838,770	$50,833,106,752	$46,206,502,599	$36,887,336,442
Revenue - Outpatient					
Gross Outpatient Revenue	$35,511,165,044	$31,755,327,351	$27,569,043,380	$24,363,370,431	$20,349,623,193
Revenue and Expenses - Totals					
(Includes Inpatient and Outpatient)					
Total Gross Revenue.	$96,878,327,000	$88,850,166,121	$78,402,150,132	$70,569,873,030	$57,236,959,635
Deductions from Revenue	69,114,526,615	63,021,240,504	54,797,070,047	48,563,663,012	36,862,617,072
Net Patient Revenue	27,763,800,385	25,828,925,617	23,605,080,085	22,006,210,018	20,374,342,563
Other Operating Revenue	1,410,478,499	1,277,949,356	1,141,606,635	1,114,923,665	1,073,805,639
Other Nonoperating Revenue	521,348,733	349,212,193	345,413,069	154,346,224	109,263,545
Total Net Revenue.	29,695,627,707	27,456,087,166	25,092,099,789	23,275,479,907	21,557,411,747
Total Expenses.	27,714,356,897	25,733,953,779	23,881,154,851	22,496,486,008	20,669,545,292
HOSPITAL UNIT (Excludes Separate Nursing Home Units)					
Utilization - Inpatient					
Beds	37,449	37,640	37,931	38,155	37,613
Admissions	1,843,785	1,840,409	1,820,785	1,793,209	1,765,118
Inpatient Days	9,458,378	9,565,533	9,585,201	9,470,572	9,427,742
Average Length of Stay.	5.1	5.2	5.3	5.3	5.3
Personnel					
Total Full Time	198,398	195,064	174,983	183,977	183,198
Total Part Time	74,360	72,851	72,378	71,902	72,709
Revenue and Expenses - Totals					
(Includes Inpatient and Outpatient)					
Total Net Revenue.	$29,511,480,040	$27,289,851,511	$24,903,242,365	$23,039,479,349	$21,296,239,697
Total Expenses.	27,484,488,144	25,604,477,946	23,719,764,958	22,296,561,994	20,474,291,752
COMMUNITY HEALTH INDICATORS PER 1000 POPULATION					
Total Population (in thousands)	12,441	12,405	12,377	12,351	12,322
Inpatient					
Beds	3.2	3.2	3.2	3.3	3.3
Admissions	150.0	150.2	149.2	147.7	145.9
Inpatient Days	812.7	819.9	828.9	834.0	839.2
Inpatient Surgeries.	44.5	44.4	44.2	43.0	43.7
Births.	11.4	11.3	10.9	11.2	11.3
Outpatient					
Emergency Outpatient Visits	448.8	433.6	426.3	417.8	410.6
Other Outpatient Visits.	2,421.7	2,380.6	2,273.2	2,277.0	2,219.7
Total Outpatient Visits	2,870.5	2,814.2	2,699.5	2,694.9	2,630.3
Outpatient Surgeries	80.2	80.7	80.3	78.3	79.8
Expense per Capita (per person). . . .	$2,227.7	$2,074.4	$1,929.4	$1,821.4	$1,677.5

TABLE 6

RHODE ISLAND

U.S. Registered Community Hospitals
(Nonfederal, short-term general and other special hospitals)

Overview 2002–2006

	2006	2005	2004	2003	2002
Total Community Hospitals in Rhode Island . . .	11	11	11	11	11
Bed Size Category					
6-24	0	0	0	0	0
25-49	0	0	0	0	0
50-99	1	1	1	1	1
100-199	6	6	6	6	5
200-299	2	2	2	2	3
300-399	1	1	1	1	1
400-499	0	0	0	0	0
500 + ...	1	1	1	1	1
Location					
Hospitals Urban	11	11	10	10	10
Hospitals Rural	0	0	1	1	1
Control					
State and Local Government	0	0	0	0	0
Not for Profit	11	11	11	11	11
Investor owned	0	0	0	0	0
Physician Models					
Independent Practice Association	6	6	6	7	7
Group Practice without Walls	0	0	0	1	1
Open Physician-Hospital Organization	7	7	6	6	6
Closed Physician-Hospital Organization	1	1	1	1	2
Management Service Organization	2	1	2	1	2
Integrated Salary Model	5	5	5	5	4
Equity Model	0	0	0	1	1
Foundation	3	3	3	3	3
Insurance Products					
Health Maintenance Organization	2	2	3	2	2
Preferred Provider Organization	2	2	3	2	2
Indemnity Fee for Service	1	1	2	1	1
Managed Care Contracts					
Health Maintenance Organization	10	10	9	9	10
Preferred Provider Organization	10	10	9	8	8
Affiliations					
Hospitals in a System*	5	5	5	5	5
Hospitals in a Network	3	3	1	1	1
Hospitals in a Group Purchasing Organization . .	10	10	9	9	10

* Please note that system affiliate information for hospitals is derived from AHA membership. In years prior to 2003 the affiliation was derived from a question on the AHA Annual Survey of hospitals; therefore, non-responding hospitals were not included in the system affiliation counts. Years prior to 2003 have been updated to reflect this change, which now include affiliation for non-reporting hospitals.

TABLE 6

RHODE ISLAND

U.S. Registered Community Hospitals
(Nonfederal, short-term general and other special hospitals)

Utilization, Personnel, Revenue and Expenses, Community Health Indicators 2002–2006

	2006	2005	2004	2003	2002
TOTAL FACILITY (Includes Hospital and Nursing Home Units)					
Utilization - Inpatient					
Beds	2,394	2,405	2,397	2,410	2,428
Admissions	127,179	126,619	125,308	122,692	122,741
Inpatient Days	680,881	684,067	663,734	657,057	649,451
Average Length of Stay	5.4	5.4	5.3	5.4	5.3
Inpatient Surgeries	36,517	36,321	38,190	38,196	36,943
Births	13,171	13,408	13,662	13,681	13,328
Utilization - Outpatient					
Emergency Outpatient Visits	466,720	454,840	431,433	463,961	468,530
Other Outpatient Visits	1,973,903	2,027,908	1,712,231	1,647,644	1,743,459
Total Outpatient Visits	2,440,623	2,482,748	2,143,664	2,111,605	2,211,989
Outpatient Surgeries	92,416	93,706	89,784	99,075	105,833
Personnel					
Full Time RNs	2,074	1,849	1,804	1,799	1,583
Full Time LPNs	128	143	146	180	183
Part Time RNs	2,862	2,823	2,757	2,703	2,720
Part Time LPNs	148	173	195	191	200
Total Full Time	12,612	13,006	12,218	11,265	11,440
Total Part Time	8,239	7,966	8,180	8,036	8,071
Revenue - Inpatient					
Gross Inpatient Revenue	$2,969,325,063	$2,782,209,685	$2,503,098,985	$2,217,386,561	$1,954,502,575
Revenue - Outpatient					
Gross Outpatient Revenue	$2,667,727,132	$2,431,758,707	$2,159,431,575	$1,867,182,587	$1,625,894,089
Revenue and Expenses - Totals					
(Includes Inpatient and Outpatient)					
Total Gross Revenue	$5,637,052,195	$5,213,968,392	$4,662,530,560	$4,084,569,148	$3,580,396,664
Deductions from Revenue	3,451,826,897	3,165,053,391	2,761,763,453	2,318,336,255	1,965,189,964
Net Patient Revenue	2,185,225,298	2,048,915,001	1,900,767,107	1,766,232,893	1,615,206,700
Other Operating Revenue	233,392,317	217,801,657	194,307,111	177,983,705	113,085,707
Other Nonoperating Revenue	15,205,663	14,066,548	13,381,409	7,490,446	45,373,163
Total Net Revenue	2,433,823,278	2,280,783,206	2,108,455,627	1,951,707,044	1,773,665,570
Total Expenses	2,395,122,194	2,242,386,790	2,084,652,695	1,941,065,141	1,791,383,545
HOSPITAL UNIT (Excludes Separate Nursing Home Units)					
Utilization - Inpatient					
Beds	2,370	2,346	2,354	2,348	2,373
Admissions	126,326	125,280	124,322	121,235	121,485
Inpatient Days	669,632	667,664	651,049	639,795	633,715
Average Length of Stay	5.3	5.3	5.2	5.3	5.2
Personnel					
Total Full Time	12,601	12,967	10,959	11,240	11,421
Total Part Time	8,231	7,931	8,001	7,996	8,010
Revenue and Expenses - Totals					
(Includes Inpatient and Outpatient)					
Total Net Revenue	$2,429,083,387	$2,265,259,405	$2,100,669,005	$1,936,762,614	$1,761,520,237
Total Expenses	2,391,044,858	2,231,955,395	2,081,390,651	1,925,735,374	1,780,279,260
COMMUNITY HEALTH INDICATORS PER 1000 POPULATION					
Total Population (in thousands)	1,068	1,074	1,079	1,075	1,069
Inpatient					
Beds	2.2	2.2	2.2	2.2	2.3
Admissions	119.1	117.9	116.1	114.2	114.9
Inpatient Days	637.8	637.2	615.2	611.3	607.8
Inpatient Surgeries	34.2	33.8	35.4	35.5	34.6
Births	12.3	12.5	12.7	12.7	12.5
Outpatient					
Emergency Outpatient Visits	437.2	423.7	399.9	431.7	438.5
Other Outpatient Visits	1,848.9	1,888.9	1,587.0	1,533.0	1,631.6
Total Outpatient Visits	2,286.1	2,312.6	1,986.8	1,964.7	2,070.0
Outpatient Surgeries	86.6	87.3	83.2	92.2	99.0
Expense per Capita (per person)	$2,243.4	$2,088.7	$1,932.1	$1,806.0	$1,676.4

States

TABLE 6

SOUTH CAROLINA

U.S. Registered Community Hospitals
(Nonfederal, short-term general and other special hospitals)

Overview 2002–2006

	2006	2005	2004	2003	2002
Total Community Hospitals in South Carolina..	66	63	62	61	62
Bed Size Category					
6-24	0	0	1	2	2
25-49	16	13	10	9	10
50-99	11	12	16	14	14
100-199	15	14	14	15	14
200-299	12	14	11	11	13
300-399	7	5	3	4	4
400-499	1	2	4	3	2
500 + ...	4	3	3	3	3
Location					
Hospitals Urban	41	39	35	35	35
Hospitals Rural	25	24	27	26	27
Control					
State and Local Government	19	19	19	20	21
Not for Profit	22	23	24	23	23
Investor owned	25	21	19	18	18
Physician Models					
Independent Practice Association	2	2	4	1	3
Group Practice without Walls	2	4	0	0	0
Open Physician-Hospital Organization	9	9	12	11	11
Closed Physician-Hospital Organization	1	6	1	1	1
Management Service Organization	4	4	6	6	8
Integrated Salary Model	12	10	7	10	8
Equity Model	0	0	0	1	5
Foundation	0	0	0	0	0
Insurance Products					
Health Maintenance Organization	4	2	2	0	4
Preferred Provider Organization	9	6	7	1	10
Indemnity Fee for Service	2	1	0	0	1
Managed Care Contracts					
Health Maintenance Organization	40	40	40	2	37
Preferred Provider Organization	46	46	44	2	42
Affiliations					
Hospitals in a System*	42	40	40	39	41
Hospitals in a Network	14	13	18	21	22
Hospitals in a Group Purchasing Organization . .	0	0	0	1	0

States

* Please note that system affiliate information for hospitals is derived from AHA membership. In years prior to 2003 the affiliation was derived from a question on the AHA Annual Survey of hospitals; therefore, non-responding hospitals were not included in the system affiliation counts. Years prior to 2003 have been updated to reflect this change, which now include affiliation for non-reporting hospitals.

TABLE 6

SOUTH CAROLINA

U.S. Registered Community Hospitals
(Nonfederal, short-term general and other special hospitals)

Utilization, Personnel, Revenue and Expenses, Community Health Indicators 2002–2006

	2006	2005	2004	2003	2002
TOTAL FACILITY (Includes Hospital and Nursing Home Units)					
Utilization - Inpatient					
Beds.........................	11,790	11,458	11,222	11,115	11,107
Admissions....................	521,773	528,122	512,908	506,488	513,136
Inpatient Days................	3,083,647	3,079,884	2,921,052	2,949,736	2,914,964
Average Length of Stay...........	5.9	5.8	5.7	5.8	5.7
Inpatient Surgeries...............	189,509	193,467	178,005	180,301	179,098
Births........................	52,676	51,142	50,634	48,497	48,864
Utilization - Outpatient					
Emergency Outpatient Visits.......	1,893,605	1,739,487	1,694,314	1,807,580	1,799,127
Other Outpatient Visits............	4,200,091	4,086,965	5,350,857	5,593,826	5,467,718
Total Outpatient Visits	6,093,696	5,826,452	7,045,171	7,401,406	7,266,845
Outpatient Surgeries	288,804	291,119	273,128	288,576	278,897
Personnel					
Full Time RNs	14,900	14,139	13,281	13,113	12,161
Full Time LPNs	1,462	1,417	1,420	1,603	1,545
Part Time RNs.................	5,429	5,406	5,474	5,570	5,116
Part Time LPNs................	491	449	507	1,593	648
Total Full Time.................	53,886	51,545	49,087	50,477	48,661
Total Part Time	15,478	15,267	15,768	17,938	15,356
Revenue - Inpatient					
Gross Inpatient Revenue..........	$13,760,712,078	$12,608,535,831	$11,113,931,424	$10,349,908,301	$9,137,079,254
Revenue - Outpatient					
Gross Outpatient Revenue	$7,918,853,975	$7,126,463,984	$6,244,132,865	$5,396,627,841	$4,772,097,600
Revenue and Expenses - Totals					
(Includes Inpatient and Outpatient)					
Total Gross Revenue.............	$21,679,566,053	$19,734,999,815	$17,358,064,289	$15,746,536,142	$13,909,176,854
Deductions from Revenue.........	13,957,650,045	12,554,885,094	10,562,293,848	9,466,073,391	7,966,264,098
Net Patient Revenue.............	7,721,916,008	7,180,114,721	6,795,770,441	6,280,462,751	5,942,912,756
Other Operating Revenue	222,065,204	230,677,665	215,550,499	331,921,316	221,416,734
Other Nonoperating Revenue	12,894,836	89,246,136	76,686,995	137,051,311	48,721,284
Total Net Revenue..............	7,956,876,048	7,500,038,522	7,088,007,935	6,749,435,378	6,213,050,774
Total Expenses.................	7,522,995,957	7,322,103,356	6,779,371,913	6,271,306,129	5,829,536,908
HOSPITAL UNIT (Excludes Separate Nursing Home Units)					
Utilization - Inpatient					
Beds.........................	10,695	11,089	10,594	10,190	10,182
Admissions....................	516,307	526,296	508,769	500,406	506,957
Inpatient Days	2,717,463	2,983,107	2,704,771	2,636,965	2,603,383
Average Length of Stay...........	5.3	5.7	5.3	5.3	5.1
Personnel					
Total Full Time.................	52,914	51,010	47,198	49,634	47,852
Total Part Time	15,161	15,177	15,470	17,694	15,120
Revenue and Expenses - Totals					
(Includes Inpatient and Outpatient)					
Total Net Revenue..............	$5,684,998,987	$7,466,733,849	$6,977,895,609	$6,614,628,560	$6,100,277,342
Total Expenses.................	7,443,633,754	7,304,244,135	6,701,411,300	6,191,999,092	5,764,072,107
COMMUNITY HEALTH INDICATORS PER 1000 POPULATION					
Total Population (in thousands)	4,321	4,247	4,195	4,142	4,101
Inpatient					
Beds.........................	2.7	2.7	2.7	2.7	2.7
Admissions....................	120.7	124.4	122.3	122.3	125.1
Inpatient Days	713.6	725.2	696.4	712.1	710.8
Inpatient Surgeries...............	43.9	45.6	42.4	43.5	43.7
Births........................	12.2	12.0	12.1	11.7	11.9
Outpatient					
Emergency Outpatient Visits.......	438.2	409.6	403.9	436.4	438.7
Other Outpatient Visits............	972.0	962.3	1,275.6	1,350.4	1,333.2
Total Outpatient Visits	1,410.2	1,371.9	1,679.5	1,786.8	1,771.9
Outpatient Surgeries	66.8	68.5	65.1	69.7	68.0
Expense per Capita (per person)....	$1,740.9	$1,724.1	$1,616.2	$1,513.9	$1,421.4

States

TABLE 6

SOUTH DAKOTA

U.S. Registered Community Hospitals
(Nonfederal, short-term general and other special hospitals)

Overview 2002–2006

	2006	2005	2004	2003	2002
Total Community Hospitals in South Dakota...	52	52	51	50	51
Bed Size Category					
6-24	15	13	13	13	12
25-49	14	15	13	12	13
50-99	10	12	12	12	12
100-199	8	7	7	7	9
200-299	2	2	3	3	2
300-399	1	1	1	1	1
400-499	1	1	1	1	1
500 + ...	1	1	1	1	1
Location					
Hospitals Urban.........................	10	10	6	6	6
Hospitals Rural	42	42	45	44	45
Control					
State and Local Government................	5	5	6	6	6
Not for Profit..........................	44	44	44	43	44
Investor owned	3	3	1	1	1
Physician Models					
Independent Practice Association	11	11	8	9	9
Group Practice without Walls................	3	4	2	3	3
Open Physician-Hospital Organization	6	6	5	4	5
Closed Physician-Hospital Organization	3	4	2	2	2
Management Service Organization	2	3	3	2	3
Integrated Salary Model....................	24	21	23	18	17
Equity Model...........................	2	2	1	0	1
Foundation.............................	1	1	1	0	1
Insurance Products					
Health Maintenance Organization	15	17	17	15	14
Preferred Provider Organization..............	18	20	19	20	21
Indemnity Fee for Service	6	7	5	5	6
Managed Care Contracts					
Health Maintenance Organization	23	22	21	23	24
Preferred Provider Organization..............	33	36	36	36	39
Affiliations					
Hospitals in a System*.....................	36	36	38	38	38
Hospitals in a Network	20	21	20	16	22
Hospitals in a Group Purchasing Organization..	46	48	47	46	46

* Please note that system affiliate information for hospitals is derived from AHA membership. In years prior to 2003 the affiliation was derived from a question on the AHA Annual Survey of hospitals; therefore, non-responding hospitals were not included in the system affiliation counts. Years prior to 2003 have been updated to reflect this change, which now include affiliation for non-reporting hospitals.

130 AHA Hospital Statistics © 2008 Health Forum LLC, an affiliate of the American Hospital Association

States

TABLE 6

SOUTH DAKOTA

U.S. Registered Community Hospitals
(Nonfederal, short-term general and other special hospitals)

Utilization, Personnel, Revenue and Expenses, Community Health Indicators 2002–2006

	2006	2005	2004	2003	2002
TOTAL FACILITY (Includes Hospital and Nursing Home Units)					
Utilization - Inpatient					
Beds	4,326	4,325	4,611	4,418	4,624
Admissions	96,964	102,127	103,495	102,984	100,141
Inpatient Days	1,022,716	1,027,776	1,039,983	994,529	1,001,800
Average Length of Stay.	10.5	10.1	10.0	9.7	10.0
Inpatient Surgeries.	35,010	34,546	33,384	35,226	38,478
Births.	11,380	11,357	11,235	10,588	9,537
Utilization - Outpatient					
Emergency Outpatient Visits	222,244	222,415	215,168	214,831	208,068
Other Outpatient Visits.	1,550,535	1,420,559	1,355,822	1,321,893	1,296,030
Total Outpatient Visits	1,772,779	1,642,974	1,570,990	1,536,724	1,504,098
Outpatient Surgeries	63,815	52,647	48,917	49,522	46,159
Personnel					
Full Time RNs	2,912	2,955	2,720	2,610	3,070
Full Time LPNs	203	212	229	234	307
Part Time RNs	1,987	1,907	1,913	1,851	1,390
Part Time LPNs	144	157	152	164	122
Total Full Time.	12,819	12,823	12,307	11,432	12,760
Total Part Time	7,449	7,186	7,321	7,286	6,209
Revenue - Inpatient					
Gross Inpatient Revenue.	$1,806,073,890	$1,742,221,313	$1,616,717,388	$1,452,307,627	$1,261,059,667
Revenue - Outpatient					
Gross Outpatient Revenue	$1,425,424,763	$1,183,690,864	$998,770,947	$863,523,142	$695,088,937
Revenue and Expenses - Totals					
(Includes Inpatient and Outpatient)					
Total Gross Revenue.	$3,231,498,653	$2,925,912,177	$2,615,488,335	$2,315,830,769	$1,956,148,604
Deductions from Revenue	1,533,819,613	1,368,023,876	1,189,382,034	980,153,650	772,856,470
Net Patient Revenue	1,697,679,040	1,557,888,301	1,426,106,301	1,335,677,119	1,183,292,134
Other Operating Revenue	140,692,507	99,897,462	103,911,665	92,587,786	86,084,094
Other Nonoperating Revenue	47,085,508	41,295,206	39,077,045	28,979,794	4,988,767
Total Net Revenue.	1,885,457,055	1,699,080,969	1,569,095,011	1,457,244,699	1,274,364,995
Total Expenses.	1,646,922,945	1,537,687,771	1,439,580,152	1,340,422,400	1,195,193,697
HOSPITAL UNIT (Excludes Separate Nursing Home Units)					
Utilization - Inpatient					
Beds	2,636	2,664	2,885	2,679	2,937
Admissions	95,183	100,240	101,758	101,431	98,694
Inpatient Days	442,682	457,739	492,821	446,442	519,705
Average Length of Stay.	4.7	4.6	4.8	4.4	5.3
Personnel					
Total Full Time.	11,863	11,843	11,315	10,472	11,801
Total Part Time	6,557	6,206	6,344	6,345	5,369
Revenue and Expenses - Totals					
(Includes Inpatient and Outpatient)					
Total Net Revenue.	$1,802,353,636	$1,621,139,772	$1,497,133,151	$1,390,873,445	$1,210,167,076
Total Expenses.	1,574,797,817	1,466,915,613	1,377,607,569	1,279,520,564	1,142,543,091
COMMUNITY HEALTH INDICATORS PER 1000 POPULATION					
Total Population (in thousands)	782	775	770	764	760
Inpatient					
Beds	5.5	5.6	6.0	5.8	6.1
Admissions	124.0	131.8	134.4	134.8	131.7
Inpatient Days	1,308.0	1,326.4	1,350.3	1,301.9	1,317.7
Inpatient Surgeries.	44.8	44.6	43.3	46.1	50.6
Births.	14.6	14.7	14.6	13.9	12.5
Outpatient					
Emergency Outpatient Visits	284.2	287.0	279.4	281.2	273.7
Other Outpatient Visits.	1,983.0	1,833.3	1,760.4	1,730.4	1,704.6
Total Outpatient Visits	2,267.2	2,120.3	2,039.7	2,011.6	1,978.3
Outpatient Surgeries	81.6	67.9	63.5	64.8	60.7
Expense per Capita (per person). . . .	$2,106.3	$1,984.4	$1,869.1	$1,754.7	$1,572.0

TABLE 6

TENNESSEE

U.S. Registered Community Hospitals
(Nonfederal, short-term general and other special hospitals)

Overview 2002–2006

	2006	2005	2004	2003	2002
Total Community Hospitals in Tennessee	130	130	127	125	125
Bed Size Category					
6-24	6	4	4	4	5
25-49	28	30	28	28	28
50-99	33	35	36	33	29
100-199	35	31	28	29	33
200-299	8	11	12	13	11
300-399	8	6	6	5	6
400-499	5	5	5	3	4
500 + ...	7	8	8	10	9
Location					
Hospitals Urban...........................	74	74	62	61	61
Hospitals Rural	56	56	65	64	64
Control					
State and Local Government................	24	24	24	25	26
Not for Profit	60	62	64	63	64
Investor owned	46	44	39	37	35
Physician Models					
Independent Practice Association	13	14	19	16	27
Group Practice without Walls...............	2	2	3	2	2
Open Physician-Hospital Organization	19	22	22	17	24
Closed Physician-Hospital Organization	3	2	2	9	9
Management Service Organization	18	17	22	26	32
Integrated Salary Model....................	11	14	13	19	22
Equity Model	0	0	0	0	2
Foundation...............................	4	7	4	5	2
Insurance Products					
Health Maintenance Organization	17	19	12	14	19
Preferred Provider Organization.............	26	31	24	35	44
Indemnity Fee for Service	15	14	9	10	13
Managed Care Contracts					
Health Maintenance Organization	75	77	70	74	82
Preferred Provider Organization.............	78	81	77	81	93
Affiliations					
Hospitals in a System*....................	98	98	94	93	89
Hospitals in a Network	41	40	40	39	41
Hospitals in a Group Purchasing Organization..	82	83	81	88	83

---

* Please note that system affiliate information for hospitals is derived from AHA membership. In years prior to 2003 the affiliation was derived from a question on the AHA Annual Survey of hospitals; therefore, non-responding hospitals were not included in the system affiliation counts. Years prior to 2003 have been updated to reflect this change, which now include affiliation for non-reporting hospitals.

TABLE 6

TENNESSEE

U.S. Registered Community Hospitals
(Nonfederal, short-term general and other special hospitals)

Utilization, Personnel, Revenue and Expenses, Community Health Indicators 2002–2006

	2006	2005	2004	2003	2002
TOTAL FACILITY (Includes Hospital and Nursing Home Units)					
Utilization - Inpatient					
Beds	20,328	20,578	20,363	20,313	20,446
Admissions	853,304	829,247	825,269	812,915	797,318
Inpatient Days	4,806,765	4,767,818	4,673,861	4,533,373	4,473,786
Average Length of Stay............	5.6	5.7	5.7	5.6	5.6
Inpatient Surgeries..............	231,102	253,509	235,406	233,939	227,882
Births.........................	81,067	81,454	81,088	79,022	77,090
Utilization - Outpatient					
Emergency Outpatient Visits.......	2,806,111	3,062,336	2,957,496	2,947,003	2,815,655
Other Outpatient Visits...........	8,055,773	8,603,983	7,304,854	7,209,449	7,136,086
Total Outpatient Visits	10,861,884	11,666,319	10,262,350	10,156,452	9,951,741
Outpatient Surgeries	380,827	386,061	376,841	393,996	391,725
Personnel					
Full Time RNs	23,420	21,295	20,374	19,389	18,073
Full Time LPNs	3,644	3,872	3,904	3,880	3,895
Part Time RNs..................	7,658	7,504	7,048	7,451	7,661
Part Time LPNs	989	996	1,033	1,051	1,154
Total Full Time.................	92,365	83,981	83,319	80,655	78,261
Total Part Time	23,142	21,350	20,385	20,875	23,695
Revenue - Inpatient					
Gross Inpatient Revenue..........	$19,934,787,410	$17,803,281,276	$16,239,786,328	$13,868,325,538	$11,947,904,647
Revenue - Outpatient					
Gross Outpatient Revenue	$13,015,442,619	$11,366,280,361	$10,132,787,849	$8,306,909,117	$7,268,386,224
Revenue and Expenses - Totals					
(Includes Inpatient and Outpatient)					
Total Gross Revenue.............	$32,950,230,029	$29,169,561,637	$26,372,574,177	$22,175,234,655	$19,216,290,871
Deductions from Revenue.........	21,525,822,289	18,614,613,384	16,471,811,012	13,155,043,109	10,705,040,668
Net Patient Revenue	11,424,407,740	10,554,948,253	9,900,763,165	9,020,191,546	8,511,250,203
Other Operating Revenue	415,142,709	360,314,741	392,768,909	606,002,225	340,382,627
Other Nonoperating Revenue	201,731,194	215,626,677	196,711,112	122,126,401	63,525,859
Total Net Revenue..............	12,041,281,643	11,130,889,671	10,490,243,186	9,748,320,172	8,915,158,689
Total Expenses.................	11,497,417,852	10,630,276,472	9,902,904,362	9,206,522,220	8,386,650,030
HOSPITAL UNIT (Excludes Separate Nursing Home Units)					
Utilization - Inpatient					
Beds	18,755	18,815	18,698	18,695	18,928
Admissions	841,956	815,516	811,465	798,996	784,003
Inpatient Days	4,300,755	4,191,641	4,123,042	4,022,663	3,902,204
Average Length of Stay...........	5.1	5.1	5.1	5.0	5.0
Personnel					
Total Full Time..................	91,079	82,566	81,915	79,171	76,883
Total Part Time	22,826	20,868	19,962	20,510	23,351
Revenue and Expenses - Totals					
(Includes Inpatient and Outpatient)					
Total Net Revenue..............	$11,933,067,685	$11,007,090,456	$10,363,793,823	$9,652,030,897	$8,781,164,810
Total Expenses.................	11,399,991,123	10,517,355,585	9,798,724,693	9,116,779,809	8,276,736,830
COMMUNITY HEALTH INDICATORS PER 1000 POPULATION					
Total Population (in thousands)	6,039	5,956	5,886	5,834	5,788
Inpatient					
Beds	3.4	3.5	3.5	3.5	3.5
Admissions	141.3	139.2	140.2	139.3	137.7
Inpatient Days	796.0	800.5	794.1	777.0	772.9
Inpatient Surgeries..............	38.3	42.6	40.0	40.1	39.4
Births.........................	13.4	13.7	13.8	13.5	13.3
Outpatient					
Emergency Outpatient Visits.......	464.7	514.2	502.5	505.1	486.4
Other Outpatient Visits...........	1,334.0	1,444.7	1,241.1	1,235.7	1,232.8
Total Outpatient Visits	1,798.7	1,958.8	1,743.6	1,740.8	1,719.3
Outpatient Surgeries	63.1	64.8	64.0	67.5	67.7
Expense per Capita (per person)....	$1,903.9	$1,784.9	$1,682.6	$1,578.0	$1,448.9

States

TABLE 6

TEXAS

U.S. Registered Community Hospitals
(Nonfederal, short-term general and other special hospitals)

Overview 2002–2006

	2006	2005	2004	2003	2002
Total Community Hospitals in Texas..........	**417**	**415**	**418**	**414**	**416**
Bed Size Category					
6-24	61	56	57	51	51
25-49	111	112	111	114	110
50-99	77	76	77	74	78
100-199	66	75	77	83	87
200-299	44	41	40	41	39
300-399	25	25	29	27	27
400-499	15	14	10	8	9
500 + ...	18	16	17	16	15
Location					
Hospitals Urban.........................	268	266	258	253	255
Hospitals Rural	149	149	160	161	161
Control					
State and Local Government................	120	124	126	129	129
Not for Profit	148	152	153	152	155
Investor owned	149	139	139	133	132
Physician Models					
Independent Practice Association	80	83	86	84	79
Group Practice without Walls...............	15	18	19	15	14
Open Physician-Hospital Organization	87	82	84	90	91
Closed Physician-Hospital Organization	15	16	13	17	20
Management Service Organization	55	49	45	50	53
Integrated Salary Model	89	79	74	69	62
Equity Model	7	8	6	7	7
Foundation...............................	34	38	29	29	30
Insurance Products					
Health Maintenance Organization	55	69	60	52	59
Preferred Provider Organization.............	88	103	89	87	85
Indemnity Fee for Service	22	31	22	16	23
Managed Care Contracts					
Health Maintenance Organization	308	310	308	304	311
Preferred Provider Organization.............	360	358	352	353	352
Affiliations					
Hospitals in a System*....................	257	248	253	245	242
Hospitals in a Network	111	108	106	94	94
Hospitals in a Group Purchasing Organization..	375	367	361	348	344

* Please note that system affiliate information for hospitals is derived from AHA membership. In years prior to 2003 the affiliation was derived from a question on the AHA Annual Survey of hospitals; therefore, non-responding hospitals were not included in the system affiliation counts. Years prior to 2003 have been updated to reflect this change, which now include affiliation for non-reporting hospitals.

TABLE 6

TEXAS

U.S. Registered Community Hospitals
(Nonfederal, short-term general and other special hospitals)

Utilization, Personnel, Revenue and Expenses, Community Health Indicators 2002–2006

	2006	2005	2004	2003	2002
TOTAL FACILITY (Includes Hospital and Nursing Home Units)					
Utilization - Inpatient					
Beds	58,964	58,153	58,116	57,374	56,833
Admissions	2,528,943	2,509,178	2,516,718	2,550,314	2,533,821
Inpatient Days	13,045,054	13,101,744	13,200,657	13,296,596	13,187,000
Average Length of Stay	5.2	5.2	5.2	5.2	5.2
Inpatient Surgeries	775,501	762,305	758,899	770,184	752,465
Births	384,775	374,254	370,341	370,572	371,677
Utilization - Outpatient					
Emergency Outpatient Visits	8,291,213	8,206,013	7,966,137	8,315,483	8,243,642
Other Outpatient Visits	23,647,835	24,123,153	24,475,723	24,379,552	25,258,993
Total Outpatient Visits	31,939,048	32,329,166	32,441,860	32,695,035	33,502,635
Outpatient Surgeries	1,009,948	1,031,651	1,048,977	1,094,832	1,093,705
Personnel					
Full Time RNs	67,758	66,243	63,316	60,518	58,370
Full Time LPNs	10,746	11,602	12,209	12,546	12,137
Part Time RNs	19,109	18,380	18,031	18,134	18,458
Part Time LPNs	2,827	3,066	3,047	3,396	3,396
Total Full Time	257,216	258,639	256,397	252,229	243,520
Total Part Time	58,940	58,600	56,596	57,159	58,389
Revenue - Inpatient					
Gross Inpatient Revenue	$72,387,591,622	$65,594,501,737	$60,347,518,071	$55,923,623,627	$48,954,346,337
Revenue - Outpatient					
Gross Outpatient Revenue	$39,341,027,194	$35,837,256,064	$31,294,217,216	$28,032,723,560	$24,518,438,912
Revenue and Expenses - Totals					
(Includes Inpatient and Outpatient)					
Total Gross Revenue	$111,728,618,816	$101,431,757,801	$91,641,735,287	$83,956,347,187	$73,472,785,249
Deductions from Revenue	76,907,991,231	68,258,928,090	60,659,781,049	54,205,639,586	45,004,634,205
Net Patient Revenue	34,820,627,585	33,172,829,711	30,981,954,238	29,750,707,601	28,468,151,044
Other Operating Revenue	3,850,147,633	3,246,953,907	3,177,637,345	2,888,147,540	2,760,139,848
Other Nonoperating Revenue	565,608,947	421,812,411	405,430,634	561,783,689	162,526,064
Total Net Revenue	39,236,384,165	36,841,596,029	34,565,022,217	33,200,638,830	31,390,816,956
Total Expenses	36,431,139,219	34,220,085,472	32,312,038,316	30,644,006,743	28,457,791,824
HOSPITAL UNIT (Excludes Separate Nursing Home Units)					
Utilization - Inpatient					
Beds	57,569	56,572	56,469	55,387	55,040
Admissions	2,513,704	2,491,171	2,499,152	2,527,209	2,508,127
Inpatient Days	12,657,778	12,630,818	12,710,867	12,803,387	12,719,345
Average Length of Stay	5.0	5.1	5.1	5.1	5.1
Personnel					
Total Full Time	256,004	257,474	245,760	250,202	241,964
Total Part Time	58,651	58,318	54,323	56,556	57,963
Revenue and Expenses - Totals					
(Includes Inpatient and Outpatient)					
Total Net Revenue	$39,069,726,193	$36,668,512,831	$34,450,802,001	$32,978,132,120	$31,211,712,467
Total Expenses	36,239,634,905	34,038,018,797	32,217,547,133	30,437,055,194	28,313,376,914
COMMUNITY HEALTH INDICATORS PER 1000 POPULATION					
Total Population (in thousands)	23,508	22,929	22,518	22,134	21,762
Inpatient					
Beds	2.5	2.5	2.6	2.6	2.6
Admissions	107.6	109.4	111.8	115.2	116.4
Inpatient Days	554.9	571.4	586.2	600.7	606.0
Inpatient Surgeries	33.0	33.2	33.7	34.8	34.6
Births	16.4	16.3	16.4	16.7	17.1
Outpatient					
Emergency Outpatient Visits	352.7	357.9	353.8	375.7	378.8
Other Outpatient Visits	1,006.0	1,052.1	1,086.9	1,101.5	1,160.7
Total Outpatient Visits	1,358.7	1,410.0	1,440.7	1,477.1	1,539.5
Outpatient Surgeries	43.0	45.0	46.6	49.5	50.3
Expense per Capita (per person)	$1,549.7	$1,492.5	$1,434.9	$1,384.5	$1,307.7

States

TABLE 6

UTAH

U.S. Registered Community Hospitals
(Nonfederal, short-term general and other special hospitals)

Overview 2002–2006

	2006	2005	2004	2003	2002
Total Community Hospitals in Utah...........	43	43	43	42	42
Bed Size Category					
6-24	6	6	8	7	6
25-49	14	13	10	12	13
50-99	8	9	10	8	8
100-199	8	8	8	9	9
200-299	4	4	4	3	3
300-399	1	1	2	2	2
400-499	2	2	1	1	1
500 + ...	0	0	0	0	0
Location					
Hospitals Urban.............................	25	25	20	21	21
Hospitals Rural	18	18	23	21	21
Control					
State and Local Government	6	6	6	6	6
Not for Profit	22	22	22	22	22
Investor owned	15	15	15	14	14
Physician Models					
Independent Practice Association	2	3	4	5	8
Group Practice without Walls................	1	0	0	0	2
Open Physician-Hospital Organization	3	3	3	3	4
Closed Physician-Hospital Organization	1	1	1	1	0
Management Service Organization	1	1	2	2	2
Integrated Salary Model	17	17	12	19	13
Equity Model	0	1	0	1	0
Foundation.................................	0	0	0	0	0
Insurance Products					
Health Maintenance Organization	20	18	16	19	15
Preferred Provider Organization.............	19	17	14	18	15
Indemnity Fee for Service	9	7	7	8	8
Managed Care Contracts					
Health Maintenance Organization	21	21	20	25	17
Preferred Provider Organization.............	21	20	19	25	20
Affiliations					
Hospitals in a System*	36	36	36	35	35
Hospitals in a Network	13	13	13	18	10
Hospitals in a Group Purchasing Organization..	27	25	25	31	26

States

* Please note that system affiliate information for hospitals is derived from AHA membership. In years prior to 2003 the affiliation was derived from a question on the AHA Annual Survey of hospitals; therefore, non-responding hospitals were not included in the system affiliation counts. Years prior to 2003 have been updated to reflect this change, which now include affiliation for non-reporting hospitals.

TABLE 6

UTAH

U.S. Registered Community Hospitals
(Nonfederal, short-term general and other special hospitals)

Utilization, Personnel, Revenue and Expenses, Community Health Indicators 2002–2006

	2006	2005	2004	2003	2002
TOTAL FACILITY (Includes Hospital and Nursing Home Units)					
Utilization - Inpatient					
Beds	4,528	4,555	4,517	4,406	4,403
Admissions	220,750	222,985	219,021	215,158	206,344
Inpatient Days	968,656	959,235	953,754	921,001	876,524
Average Length of Stay	4.4	4.3	4.4	4.3	4.2
Inpatient Surgeries	68,590	74,224	65,013	59,864	72,489
Births	53,194	51,094	50,626	49,824	48,792
Utilization - Outpatient					
Emergency Outpatient Visits	789,653	803,394	829,030	740,160	797,951
Other Outpatient Visits	4,192,042	3,995,682	3,890,088	3,805,509	4,016,360
Total Outpatient Visits	4,981,695	4,799,076	4,719,118	4,545,669	4,814,311
Outpatient Surgeries	149,004	170,810	156,181	155,803	156,769
Personnel					
Full Time RNs	6,125	6,227	6,106	5,506	4,939
Full Time LPNs	413	520	586	520	627
Part Time RNs	4,311	3,739	3,221	3,164	3,145
Part Time LPNs	359	341	368	381	405
Total Full Time	24,814	24,107	22,719	21,693	21,063
Total Part Time	13,536	12,056	10,887	11,760	10,564
Revenue - Inpatient					
Gross Inpatient Revenue	$4,396,532,960	$4,017,366,853	$3,952,050,264	$3,082,671,800	$3,062,158,326
Revenue - Outpatient					
Gross Outpatient Revenue	$3,068,647,875	$2,728,130,477	$2,511,704,075	$2,102,021,110	$1,897,673,822
Revenue and Expenses - Totals					
(Includes Inpatient and Outpatient)					
Total Gross Revenue	$7,465,180,835	$6,745,497,330	$6,463,754,339	$5,184,692,910	$4,959,832,148
Deductions from Revenue	3,754,113,535	3,286,143,364	3,247,500,404	2,355,358,986	2,384,893,655
Net Patient Revenue	3,711,067,300	3,459,353,966	3,216,253,935	2,829,333,924	2,574,938,493
Other Operating Revenue	175,237,458	173,824,984	145,434,265	123,232,186	139,121,419
Other Nonoperating Revenue	16,047,892	20,303,182	33,354,146	25,696,305	23,585,217
Total Net Revenue	3,902,352,650	3,653,482,132	3,395,042,346	2,978,262,415	2,737,645,129
Total Expenses	3,437,079,268	3,214,131,545	3,059,828,012	2,682,023,991	2,505,242,473
HOSPITAL UNIT (Excludes Separate Nursing Home Units)					
Utilization - Inpatient					
Beds	4,383	4,388	4,416	4,326	4,257
Admissions	218,711	221,525	217,621	213,834	204,612
Inpatient Days	929,668	911,303	928,859	898,863	831,512
Average Length of Stay	4.3	4.1	4.3	4.2	4.1
Personnel					
Total Full Time	24,704	23,933	22,612	21,616	21,007
Total Part Time	13,437	11,922	10,799	11,658	10,462
Revenue and Expenses - Totals					
(Includes Inpatient and Outpatient)					
Total Net Revenue	$3,892,595,169	$3,644,185,837	$3,388,971,273	$2,972,748,366	$2,728,571,258
Total Expenses	3,430,215,718	3,207,843,710	3,055,918,500	2,678,937,711	2,500,424,658
COMMUNITY HEALTH INDICATORS PER 1000 POPULATION					
Total Population (in thousands)	2,550	2,490	2,422	2,356	2,326
Inpatient					
Beds	1.8	1.8	1.9	1.9	1.9
Admissions	86.6	89.5	90.4	91.3	88.7
Inpatient Days	379.9	385.2	393.9	391.0	376.9
Inpatient Surgeries	26.9	29.8	26.8	25.4	31.2
Births	20.9	20.5	20.9	21.1	21.0
Outpatient					
Emergency Outpatient Visits	309.7	322.6	342.4	314.2	343.1
Other Outpatient Visits	1,643.9	1,604.5	1,606.5	1,615.4	1,726.8
Total Outpatient Visits	1,953.6	1,927.1	1,948.8	1,929.6	2,069.9
Outpatient Surgeries	58.4	68.6	64.5	66.1	67.4
Expense per Capita (per person)	$1,347.8	$1,290.6	$1,263.6	$1,138.5	$1,077.1

States

TABLE **6**

VERMONT

U.S. Registered Community Hospitals
(Nonfederal, short-term general and other special hospitals)

Overview 2002–2006

	2006	2005	2004	2003	2002
Total Community Hospitals in Vermont	14	14	14	14	14
Bed Size Category					
6-24	0	0	0	0	0
25-49	7	7	7	7	6
50-99	4	4	4	4	5
100-199	1	1	1	1	1
200-299	1	1	1	1	1
300-399	0	0	0	0	0
400-499	1	1	0	0	0
500 + ...	0	0	1	1	1
Location					
Hospitals Urban	2	2	2	2	2
Hospitals Rural	12	12	12	12	12
Control					
State and Local Government	0	0	0	0	0
Not for Profit	14	14	14	14	14
Investor owned	0	0	0	0	0
Physician Models					
Independent Practice Association	1	0	1	0	1
Group Practice without Walls	0	1	1	1	2
Open Physician-Hospital Organization	3	4	4	6	5
Closed Physician-Hospital Organization	1	1	1	0	1
Management Service Organization	1	1	1	2	3
Integrated Salary Model	9	9	9	8	7
Equity Model	0	0	0	0	0
Foundation	0	0	0	0	1
Insurance Products					
Health Maintenance Organization	3	3	5	5	5
Preferred Provider Organization	2	2	4	6	4
Indemnity Fee for Service	1	1	1	2	0
Managed Care Contracts					
Health Maintenance Organization	8	9	9	9	9
Preferred Provider Organization	8	9	10	11	7
Affiliations					
Hospitals in a System*	1	1	1	1	1
Hospitals in a Network	5	5	5	5	2
Hospitals in a Group Purchasing Organization . .	14	14	13	12	11

* Please note that system affiliate information for hospitals is derived from AHA membership. In years prior to 2003 the affiliation was derived from a question on the AHA Annual Survey of hospitals; therefore, non-responding hospitals were not included in the system affiliation counts. Years prior to 2003 have been updated to reflect this change, which now include affiliation for non-reporting hospitals.

TABLE 6

VERMONT

U.S. Registered Community Hospitals
(Nonfederal, short-term general and other special hospitals)

Utilization, Personnel, Revenue and Expenses, Community Health Indicators 2002–2006

	2006	2005	2004	2003	2002
TOTAL FACILITY (Includes Hospital and Nursing Home Units)					
Utilization - Inpatient					
Beds	1,313	1,358	1,473	1,506	1,576
Admissions	50,402	51,430	52,853	51,852	52,236
Inpatient Days	327,850	334,533	347,087	341,581	348,528
Average Length of Stay...........	6.5	6.5	6.6	6.6	6.7
Inpatient Surgeries..............	13,883	13,828	14,040	14,499	14,971
Births.........................	5,944	6,107	6,043	6,028	6,003
Utilization - Outpatient					
Emergency Outpatient Visits.......	260,429	256,116	261,642	251,346	230,643
Other Outpatient Visits...........	2,240,292	2,220,552	2,012,991	1,960,218	1,239,885
Total Outpatient Visits	2,500,721	2,476,668	2,274,633	2,211,564	1,470,528
Outpatient Surgeries	43,286	57,091	59,210	54,857	39,468
Personnel					
Full Time RNs	1,454	1,280	1,242	1,016	1,040
Full Time LPNs	223	219	161	219	216
Part Time RNs	1,286	1,326	1,262	1,619	1,770
Part Time LPNs	181	169	216	227	240
Total Full Time.................	8,781	8,264	7,761	7,224	7,981
Total Part Time	3,960	4,303	4,250	4,977	5,589
Revenue - Inpatient					
Gross Inpatient Revenue..........	$798,941,048	$715,536,841	$681,045,908	$669,226,956	$632,612,094
Revenue - Outpatient					
Gross Outpatient Revenue	$1,551,689,704	$1,385,916,565	$1,218,097,479	$1,056,083,809	$683,857,958
Revenue and Expenses - Totals					
(Includes Inpatient and Outpatient)					
Total Gross Revenue.............	$2,350,630,752	$2,101,453,406	$1,899,143,387	$1,725,310,765	$1,316,470,052
Deductions from Revenue.........	1,011,115,676	879,046,314	787,254,423	705,626,932	514,087,762
Net Patient Revenue	1,339,515,076	1,222,407,092	1,111,888,964	1,019,683,833	802,382,290
Other Operating Revenue	43,167,369	24,996,233	21,000,354	22,305,529	17,504,386
Other Nonoperating Revenue	61,745,217	26,468,077	17,165,067	10,299,848	260,503
Total Net Revenue...............	1,444,427,662	1,273,871,402	1,150,054,385	1,052,289,210	820,147,179
Total Expenses.................	1,332,522,993	1,217,413,378	1,103,050,959	1,012,039,974	812,757,084
HOSPITAL UNIT (Excludes Separate Nursing Home Units)					
Utilization - Inpatient					
Beds	1,053	1,090	1,205	1,258	1,325
Admissions	50,100	51,104	52,516	51,454	51,785
Inpatient Days	237,419	241,632	253,201	255,263	263,456
Average Length of Stay...........	4.7	4.7	4.8	5.0	5.1
Personnel					
Total Full Time.................	8,494	8,093	7,530	6,965	7,778
Total Part Time	3,791	4,181	4,108	4,765	5,469
Revenue and Expenses - Totals					
(Includes Inpatient and Outpatient)					
Total Net Revenue...............	$1,426,818,942	$1,255,847,385	$1,132,671,726	$1,034,057,663	$807,750,162
Total Expenses.................	1,315,948,812	1,199,376,861	1,085,829,448	994,881,487	798,095,694
COMMUNITY HEALTH INDICATORS PER 1000 POPULATION					
Total Population (in thousands)	624	622	621	619	616
Inpatient					
Beds	2.1	2.2	2.4	2.4	2.6
Admissions	80.8	82.6	85.1	83.8	84.8
Inpatient Days	525.5	537.5	559.1	552.2	565.6
Inpatient Surgeries..............	22.3	22.2	22.6	23.4	24.3
Births.........................	9.5	9.8	9.7	9.7	9.7
Outpatient					
Emergency Outpatient Visits.......	417.4	411.5	421.5	406.3	374.3
Other Outpatient Visits...........	3,590.7	3,567.8	3,242.6	3,168.7	2,012.0
Total Outpatient Visits	4,008.2	3,979.3	3,664.1	3,575.0	2,386.3
Outpatient Surgeries	69.4	91.7	95.4	88.7	64.0
Expense per Capita (per person)....	$2,135.8	$1,956.0	$1,776.8	$1,636.0	$1,318.9

TABLE 6

VIRGINIA

U.S. Registered Community Hospitals
(Nonfederal, short-term general and other special hospitals)

Overview 2002–2006

	2006	2005	2004	2003	2002
Total Community Hospitals in Virginia	88	87	88	84	86
Bed Size Category					
6-24	5	5	4	1	1
25-49	12	12	12	11	11
50-99	17	15	18	17	18
100-199	24	25	24	25	25
200-299	13	14	15	14	15
300-399	6	4	3	6	5
400-499	5	4	5	2	3
500 + ...	6	8	7	8	8
Location					
Hospitals Urban..........................	58	57	53	50	51
Hospitals Rural	30	30	35	34	35
Control					
State and Local Government...............	4	4	4	4	5
Not for Profit	64	62	64	63	67
Investor owned	20	21	20	17	14
Physician Models					
Independent Practice Association	11	11	9	12	8
Group Practice without Walls...............	10	9	7	7	1
Open Physician-Hospital Organization	9	10	12	14	20
Closed Physician-Hospital Organization	2	2	3	3	3
Management Service Organization	7	8	4	5	6
Integrated Salary Model....................	30	30	27	28	28
Equity Model	7	7	7	7	2
Foundation...............................	2	2	3	2	5
Insurance Products					
Health Maintenance Organization	21	22	22	22	26
Preferred Provider Organization.............	26	29	28	29	33
Indemnity Fee for Service	13	13	13	14	9
Managed Care Contracts					
Health Maintenance Organization	50	54	53	55	56
Preferred Provider Organization.............	56	61	60	63	64
Affiliations					
Hospitals in a System*....................	57	56	56	51	51
Hospitals in a Network....................	38	37	32	27	28
Hospitals in a Group Purchasing Organization..	61	70	63	67	66

* Please note that system affiliate information for hospitals is derived from AHA membership. In years prior to 2003 the affiliation was derived from a question on the AHA Annual Survey of hospitals; therefore, non-responding hospitals were not included in the system affiliation counts. Years prior to 2003 have been updated to reflect this change, which now include affiliation for non-reporting hospitals.

TABLE **6**

VIRGINIA

U.S. Registered Community Hospitals
(Nonfederal, short-term general and other special hospitals)

Utilization, Personnel, Revenue and Expenses, Community Health Indicators 2002–2006

	2006	2005	2004	2003	2002
TOTAL FACILITY (Includes Hospital and Nursing Home Units)					
Utilization - Inpatient					
Beds.........................	17,274	17,483	17,339	17,225	17,241
Admissions..................	778,680	780,063	770,482	758,258	746,686
Inpatient Days.................	4,416,114	4,500,420	4,468,361	4,367,997	4,278,445
Average Length of Stay...........	5.7	5.8	5.8	5.8	5.7
Inpatient Surgeries..............	233,922	239,260	236,905	233,220	236,774
Births.........................	98,948	96,713	94,851	92,014	90,401
Utilization - Outpatient					
Emergency Outpatient Visits.......	3,060,052	2,891,314	2,915,593	2,759,886	2,606,320
Other Outpatient Visits...........	10,592,692	10,407,953	9,033,065	8,431,492	8,183,177
Total Outpatient Visits...........	13,652,744	13,299,267	11,948,658	11,191,378	10,789,497
Outpatient Surgeries	473,915	498,917	484,775	489,438	503,094
Personnel					
Full Time RNs	21,187	20,788	19,372	18,335	18,038
Full Time LPNs	2,645	2,809	2,585	2,833	2,764
Part Time RNs.................	9,948	9,337	10,442	9,614	8,110
Part Time LPNs	793	783	929	939	844
Total Full Time.................	78,169	78,447	75,743	71,709	72,397
Total Part Time	26,965	25,534	27,658	26,516	23,323
Revenue - Inpatient					
Gross Inpatient Revenue..........	$19,234,761,450	$17,128,029,759	$15,465,159,071	$13,740,614,713	$12,167,189,859
Revenue - Outpatient					
Gross Outpatient Revenue	$13,231,876,352	$11,727,859,701	$9,538,948,095	$8,210,447,929	$7,232,253,089
Revenue and Expenses - Totals					
(Includes Inpatient and Outpatient)					
Total Gross Revenue.............	$32,466,637,802	$28,855,889,460	$25,004,107,166	$21,951,062,642	$19,399,442,948
Deductions from Revenue........	20,174,935,834	17,355,317,448	14,542,142,131	12,410,069,628	10,621,457,968
Net Patient Revenue	12,291,701,968	11,500,572,012	10,461,965,035	9,540,993,014	8,777,984,980
Other Operating Revenue	379,912,278	312,151,277	288,809,114	266,650,457	241,242,013
Other Nonoperating Revenue	245,713,096	180,752,253	187,888,489	185,982,334	-14,532,952
Total Net Revenue..............	12,917,327,342	11,993,475,542	10,938,662,638	9,993,625,805	9,004,694,041
Total Expenses.................	11,554,705,543	10,918,957,473	10,050,894,896	9,225,809,610	8,779,480,958
HOSPITAL UNIT (Excludes Separate Nursing Home Units)					
Utilization - Inpatient					
Beds.........................	16,411	16,453	16,158	15,890	15,938
Admissions..................	775,367	776,841	767,241	754,821	743,372
Inpatient Days.................	4,129,270	4,160,425	4,022,345	3,919,369	3,875,511
Average Length of Stay...........	5.3	5.4	5.2	5.2	5.2
Personnel					
Total Full Time.................	77,634	77,653	74,916	70,682	71,403
Total Part Time	26,744	25,226	27,424	26,126	23,004
Revenue and Expenses - Totals					
(Includes Inpatient and Outpatient)					
Total Net Revenue..............	$12,814,301,298	$11,935,132,273	$10,869,203,315	$9,930,690,590	$8,947,350,583
Total Expenses.................	11,498,207,599	10,867,011,952	9,993,659,840	9,167,578,607	8,727,817,754
COMMUNITY HEALTH INDICATORS PER 1000 POPULATION					
Total Population (in thousands)	7,643	7,564	7,472	7,376	7,286
Inpatient					
Beds	2.3	2.3	2.3	2.3	2.4
Admissions	101.9	103.1	103.1	102.8	102.5
Inpatient Days	577.8	595.0	598.0	592.2	587.2
Inpatient Surgeries.............	30.6	31.6	31.7	31.6	32.5
Births........................	12.9	12.8	12.7	12.5	12.4
Outpatient					
Emergency Outpatient Visits.......	400.4	382.2	390.2	374.2	357.7
Other Outpatient Visits...........	1,386.0	1,375.9	1,208.8	1,143.1	1,123.2
Total Outpatient Visits	1,786.3	1,758.2	1,599.0	1,517.3	1,480.9
Outpatient Surgeries	62.0	66.0	64.9	66.4	69.1
Expense per Capita (per person)....	$1,511.8	$1,443.5	$1,345.1	$1,250.8	$1,205.0

States

TABLE 6

WASHINGTON

U.S. Registered Community Hospitals
(Nonfederal, short-term general and other special hospitals)

Overview 2002–2006

	2006	2005	2004	2003	2002
Total Community Hospitals in Washington	88	86	85	85	86
Bed Size Category					
6-24	8	9	9	9	9
25-49	30	27	24	24	20
50-99	13	15	12	12	18
100-199	17	16	19	18	16
200-299	10	9	12	13	14
300-399	8	8	7	7	6
400-499	0	0	0	0	1
500 + ...	2	2	2	2	2
Location					
Hospitals Urban.........................	53	52	46	45	45
Hospitals Rural	35	34	39	40	41
Control					
State and Local Government................	41	40	39	39	40
Not for Profit	42	42	41	41	42
Investor owned	5	4	5	5	4
Physician Models					
Independent Practice Association	7	9	6	7	3
Group Practice without Walls...............	1	1	2	2	3
Open Physician-Hospital Organization	5	4	4	5	11
Closed Physician-Hospital Organization	2	5	4	4	1
Management Service Organization	4	5	5	5	6
Integrated Salary Model....................	35	42	34	37	36
Equity Model	0	0	0	0	0
Foundation...............................	1	3	1	1	0
Insurance Products					
Health Maintenance Organization	4	6	6	5	9
Preferred Provider Organization..............	8	11	8	8	12
Indemnity Fee for Service	0	2	2	3	3
Managed Care Contracts					
Health Maintenance Organization	31	37	34	40	41
Preferred Provider Organization..............	38	41	43	49	54
Affiliations					
Hospitals in a System*.....................	40	29	29	28	28
Hospitals in a Network	15	15	14	16	16
Hospitals in a Group Purchasing Organization..	54	58	42	64	62

* Please note that system affiliate information for hospitals is derived from AHA membership. In years prior to 2003 the affiliation was derived from a question on the AHA Annual Survey of hospitals; therefore, non-responding hospitals were not included in the system affiliation counts. Years prior to 2003 have been updated to reflect this change, which now include affiliation for non-reporting hospitals.

TABLE 6

WASHINGTON

U.S. Registered Community Hospitals
(Nonfederal, short-term general and other special hospitals)

Utilization, Personnel, Revenue and Expenses, Community Health Indicators 2002–2006

	2006	2005	2004	2003	2002
TOTAL FACILITY (Includes Hospital and Nursing Home Units)					
Utilization - Inpatient					
Beds	10,927	10,763	10,984	11,190	11,338
Admissions	556,700	543,329	528,145	515,939	518,562
Inpatient Days	2,486,577	2,481,368	2,464,033	2,477,079	2,486,925
Average Length of Stay...........	4.5	4.6	4.7	4.8	4.8
Inpatient Surgeries..............	161,357	172,394	172,224	172,130	162,809
Births......................	78,272	76,231	74,629	72,453	72,586
Utilization - Outpatient					
Emergency Outpatient Visits.......	2,147,309	2,150,665	2,070,588	2,030,209	1,936,458
Other Outpatient Visits...........	8,236,855	7,898,848	8,023,254	8,261,544	7,811,926
Total Outpatient Visits	10,384,164	10,049,513	10,093,842	10,291,753	9,748,384
Outpatient Surgeries	249,520	256,277	265,489	268,924	280,786
Personnel					
Full Time RNs	12,488	10,640	10,871	10,475	10,214
Full Time LPNs	954	804	842	913	1,060
Part Time RNs	11,236	11,885	12,266	12,041	11,477
Part Time LPNs	664	676	709	950	866
Total Full Time................	58,233	52,293	52,042	51,107	53,490
Total Part Time	33,984	34,010	35,860	35,276	32,880
Revenue - Inpatient					
Gross Inpatient Revenue..........	$13,933,139,987	$12,391,332,683	$11,175,038,171	$9,520,850,529	$8,210,414,712
Revenue - Outpatient					
Gross Outpatient Revenue	$10,552,552,309	$9,409,149,980	$8,233,809,398	$7,359,274,143	$6,583,605,589
Revenue and Expenses - Totals					
(Includes Inpatient and Outpatient)					
Total Gross Revenue.............	$24,485,692,296	$21,800,482,663	$19,408,847,569	$16,880,124,672	$14,794,020,301
Deductions from Revenue.........	14,099,862,736	12,092,084,642	10,469,471,708	8,552,487,105	7,178,544,115
Net Patient Revenue	10,385,829,560	9,708,398,021	8,939,375,861	8,327,637,567	7,615,476,186
Other Operating Revenue	515,593,853	501,680,129	532,612,476	469,719,678	473,047,880
Other Nonoperating Revenue	192,566,803	119,675,420	161,524,417	130,473,550	45,762,585
Total Net Revenue..............	11,093,990,216	10,329,753,570	9,633,512,754	8,927,830,795	8,134,286,651
Total Expenses................	10,650,112,282	9,877,966,089	9,016,549,152	8,358,507,505	7,830,121,368
HOSPITAL UNIT (Excludes Separate Nursing Home Units)					
Utilization - Inpatient					
Beds	10,679	10,433	10,498	10,475	10,494
Admissions	554,676	541,217	525,300	511,844	513,922
Inpatient Days	2,401,977	2,367,684	2,320,942	2,237,474	2,219,549
Average Length of Stay...........	4.3	4.4	4.4	4.4	4.3
Personnel					
Total Full Time................	57,925	52,000	51,635	50,508	52,927
Total Part Time	33,837	33,844	35,687	34,926	32,525
Revenue and Expenses - Totals					
(Includes Inpatient and Outpatient)					
Total Net Revenue..............	$11,062,106,616	$10,282,987,332	$9,591,633,736	$8,875,530,733	$8,082,984,927
Total Expenses................	10,623,552,352	9,848,163,539	8,979,129,740	8,315,286,786	7,788,632,966
COMMUNITY HEALTH INDICATORS PER 1000 POPULATION					
Total Population (in thousands)	6,396	6,292	6,206	6,130	6,070
Inpatient					
Beds	1.7	1.7	1.8	1.8	1.9
Admissions	87.0	86.4	85.1	84.2	85.4
Inpatient Days	388.8	394.4	397.1	404.1	409.7
Inpatient Surgeries..............	25.2	27.4	27.8	28.1	26.8
Births......................	12.2	12.1	12.0	11.8	12.0
Outpatient					
Emergency Outpatient Visits.......	335.7	341.8	333.7	331.2	319.0
Other Outpatient Visits...........	1,287.9	1,255.4	1,292.9	1,347.7	1,286.9
Total Outpatient Visits	1,623.6	1,597.2	1,626.6	1,678.8	1,605.9
Outpatient Surgeries	39.0	40.7	42.8	43.9	46.3
Expense per Capita (per person)....	$1,665.2	$1,569.9	$1,453.0	$1,363.5	$1,289.9

States

TABLE **6**

WEST VIRGINIA

U.S. Registered Community Hospitals
(Nonfederal, short-term general and other special hospitals)

Overview 2002–2006

	2006	2005	2004	2003	2002
Total Community Hospitals in West Virginia ...	56	57	57	57	57
Bed Size Category					
6-24	3	4	4	4	4
25-49	14	13	11	11	11
50-99	14	15	17	17	17
100-199	13	13	13	12	12
200-299	8	8	7	7	8
300-399	2	2	3	4	3
400-499	1	1	1	1	1
500 + ...	1	1	1	1	1
Location					
Hospitals Urban.........................	26	25	18	18	18
Hospitals Rural	30	32	39	39	39
Control					
State and Local Government................	10	10	10	10	10
Not for Profit	31	31	31	31	33
Investor owned	15	16	16	16	14
Physician Models					
Independent Practice Association	6	6	4	6	3
Group Practice without Walls................	2	2	1	2	1
Open Physician-Hospital Organization	15	16	15	15	16
Closed Physician-Hospital Organization	1	1	1	2	1
Management Service Organization	4	3	4	4	4
Integrated Salary Model....................	28	29	29	25	21
Equity Model	1	1	1	2	1
Foundation...............................	0	1	0	0	0
Insurance Products					
Health Maintenance Organization	6	8	8	5	6
Preferred Provider Organization..............	9	11	12	9	9
Indemnity Fee for Service	3	5	4	5	5
Managed Care Contracts					
Health Maintenance Organization	25	28	31	32	34
Preferred Provider Organization..............	37	40	44	45	48
Affiliations					
Hospitals in a System*.....................	24	25	25	23	24
Hospitals in a Network	24	25	27	28	30
Hospitals in a Group Purchasing Organization..	52	53	52	52	52

* Please note that system affiliate information for hospitals is derived from AHA membership. In years prior to 2003 the affiliation was derived from a question on the AHA Annual Survey of hospitals; therefore, non-responding hospitals were not included in the system affiliation counts. Years prior to 2003 have been updated to reflect this change, which now include affiliation for non-reporting hospitals.

TABLE **6**

WEST VIRGINIA

U.S. Registered Community Hospitals
(Nonfederal, short-term general and other special hospitals)

Utilization, Personnel, Revenue and Expenses, Community Health Indicators 2002–2006

	2006	2005	2004	2003	2002
TOTAL FACILITY (Includes Hospital and Nursing Home Units)					
Utilization - Inpatient					
Beds	7,197	7,243	7,412	7,779	7,821
Admissions	281,766	291,936	297,957	296,089	295,011
Inpatient Days	1,592,271	1,662,043	1,707,211	1,770,290	1,775,869
Average Length of Stay	5.7	5.7	5.7	6.0	6.0
Inpatient Surgeries	77,881	79,072	81,045	77,583	79,711
Births	21,137	20,817	21,164	21,302	20,659
Utilization - Outpatient					
Emergency Outpatient Visits	1,137,535	1,163,861	1,130,236	1,112,496	1,100,258
Other Outpatient Visits	5,074,611	4,951,884	4,915,115	4,644,732	4,585,150
Total Outpatient Visits	6,212,146	6,115,745	6,045,351	5,757,228	5,685,408
Outpatient Surgeries	213,317	207,093	209,671	200,952	201,288
Personnel					
Full Time RNs	7,271	7,298	7,111	6,459	6,836
Full Time LPNs	1,422	1,498	1,557	1,559	1,599
Part Time RNs	3,287	3,021	3,053	3,641	3,191
Part Time LPNs	481	465	490	514	532
Total Full Time	30,778	30,701	30,378	29,264	29,733
Total Part Time	10,013	9,906	9,794	9,749	9,691
Revenue - Inpatient					
Gross Inpatient Revenue	$4,197,327,290	$4,026,435,796	$4,044,864,251	$3,679,723,811	$3,247,995,766
Revenue - Outpatient					
Gross Outpatient Revenue	$3,747,433,060	$3,455,792,349	$3,060,476,434	$2,738,672,867	$2,395,425,269
Revenue and Expenses - Totals					
(Includes Inpatient and Outpatient)					
Total Gross Revenue	$7,944,760,350	$7,482,228,145	$7,105,340,685	$6,418,396,678	$5,643,421,035
Deductions from Revenue	4,125,056,133	3,830,700,396	3,631,517,398	3,177,374,702	2,606,272,014
Net Patient Revenue	3,819,704,217	3,651,527,749	3,473,823,287	3,241,021,976	3,037,149,021
Other Operating Revenue	126,071,335	116,366,406	105,961,591	99,592,313	87,401,673
Other Nonoperating Revenue	61,758,746	48,171,478	52,015,444	34,650,258	16,381,152
Total Net Revenue	4,007,534,298	3,816,065,633	3,631,800,322	3,375,264,547	3,140,931,846
Total Expenses	3,814,590,273	3,711,750,009	3,504,272,644	3,286,535,065	3,068,384,987
HOSPITAL UNIT (Excludes Separate Nursing Home Units)					
Utilization - Inpatient					
Beds	6,439	6,422	6,576	6,756	6,756
Admissions	275,550	285,425	291,135	288,258	286,752
Inpatient Days	1,350,098	1,396,933	1,433,988	1,439,093	1,435,794
Average Length of Stay	4.9	4.9	4.9	5.0	5.0
Personnel					
Total Full Time	30,217	30,096	29,662	28,411	28,849
Total Part Time	9,640	9,509	9,443	9,393	9,386
Revenue and Expenses - Totals					
(Includes Inpatient and Outpatient)					
Total Net Revenue	$3,947,204,453	$3,760,605,431	$3,573,095,326	$3,303,564,652	$3,073,370,762
Total Expenses	3,769,187,062	3,667,763,446	3,459,519,326	3,230,266,642	3,005,319,455
COMMUNITY HEALTH INDICATORS PER 1000 POPULATION					
Total Population (in thousands)	1,818	1,814	1,811	1,809	1,804
Inpatient					
Beds	4.0	4.0	4.1	4.3	4.3
Admissions	154.9	160.9	164.5	163.7	163.5
Inpatient Days	875.6	916.2	942.7	978.8	984.3
Inpatient Surgeries	42.8	43.6	44.8	42.9	44.2
Births	11.6	11.5	11.7	11.8	11.5
Outpatient					
Emergency Outpatient Visits	625.5	641.6	624.1	615.1	609.8
Other Outpatient Visits	2,790.6	2,729.7	2,714.2	2,568.1	2,541.5
Total Outpatient Visits	3,416.1	3,371.3	3,338.3	3,183.1	3,151.3
Outpatient Surgeries	117.3	114.2	115.8	111.1	111.6
Expense per Capita (per person)	$2,097.7	$2,046.1	$1,935.1	$1,817.1	$1,700.7

States

Overview 2002–2006

	2006	2005	2004	2003	2002
Total Community Hospitals in Wisconsin......	124	124	121	121	120
Bed Size Category					
6-24	11	12	10	8	8
25-49	31	26	27	26	29
50-99	27	31	27	30	27
100-199	37	35	36	35	36
200-299	10	12	13	14	14
300-399	5	5	4	4	4
400-499	2	2	3	3	1
500 + ...	1	1	1	1	1
Location					
Hospitals Urban...........................	67	67	57	57	55
Hospitals Rural	57	57	64	64	65
Control					
State and Local Government................	2	2	2	2	2
Not for Profit.............................	118	118	115	117	117
Investor owned	4	4	4	2	1
Physician Models					
Independent Practice Association	11	9	6	12	12
Group Practice without Walls................	1	1	3	11	9
Open Physician-Hospital Organization	4	4	4	8	8
Closed Physician-Hospital Organization	4	3	2	8	8
Management Service Organization	1	1	3	6	7
Integrated Salary Model....................	30	30	34	49	42
Equity Model	5	3	2	4	2
Foundation................................	2	3	3	3	2
Insurance Products					
Health Maintenance Organization	23	10	20	21	28
Preferred Provider Organization..............	25	9	20	21	21
Indemnity Fee for Service	9	3	5	8	5
Managed Care Contracts					
Health Maintenance Organization	111	108	105	113	102
Preferred Provider Organization..............	114	109	110	116	108
Affiliations					
Hospitals in a System*.....................	70	72	67	68	66
Hospitals in a Network.....................	42	40	42	46	41
Hospitals in a Group Purchasing Organization..	117	114	109	116	109

* Please note that system affiliate information for hospitals is derived from AHA membership. In years prior to 2003 the affiliation was derived from a question on the AHA Annual Survey of hospitals; therefore, non-responding hospitals were not included in the system affiliation counts. Years prior to 2003 have been updated to reflect this change, which now include affiliation for non-reporting hospitals.

States

TABLE **6**

WISCONSIN

U.S. Registered Community Hospitals
(Nonfederal, short-term general and other special hospitals)

Utilization, Personnel, Revenue and Expenses, Community Health Indicators 2002–2006

	2006	2005	2004	2003	2002
TOTAL FACILITY (Includes Hospital and Nursing Home Units)					
Utilization - Inpatient					
Beds	14,123	14,458	14,577	14,829	14,610
Admissions	609,108	611,669	598,542	588,466	579,830
Inpatient Days	3,210,210	3,302,565	3,335,415	3,355,918	3,396,381
Average Length of Stay.	5.3	5.4	5.6	5.7	5.9
Inpatient Surgeries	195,968	189,662	183,304	190,192	181,674
Births.	68,461	67,525	67,419	65,669	65,588
Utilization - Outpatient					
Emergency Outpatient Visits	2,091,172	1,965,535	1,861,206	1,813,690	1,833,344
Other Outpatient Visits.	10,420,878	10,760,999	9,957,806	10,001,511	9,778,893
Total Outpatient Visits	12,512,050	12,726,534	11,819,012	11,815,201	11,612,237
Outpatient Surgeries	449,460	537,342	418,490	416,065	388,879
Personnel					
Full Time RNs	12,971	12,197	11,027	10,729	10,225
Full Time LPNs	689	824	725	842	794
Part Time RNs	15,682	14,867	14,663	14,302	12,915
Part Time LPNs	1,094	1,152	1,105	1,010	1,125
Total Full Time	58,923	58,349	56,306	55,058	53,737
Total Part Time	49,217	48,137	47,844	44,896	42,826
Revenue - Inpatient					
Gross Inpatient Revenue.	$11,855,822,996	$11,202,143,456	$9,931,707,238	$8,686,033,584	$7,802,749,118
Revenue - Outpatient					
Gross Outpatient Revenue	$10,739,176,109	$9,561,512,469	$7,994,289,334	$7,135,965,468	$6,112,204,146
Revenue and Expenses - Totals					
(Includes Inpatient and Outpatient)					
Total Gross Revenue.	$22,594,999,105	$20,763,655,925	$17,925,996,572	$15,821,999,052	$13,914,953,264
Deductions from Revenue.	11,063,269,437	10,261,422,693	8,369,952,440	7,007,752,524	5,950,993,178
Net Patient Revenue	11,531,729,668	10,502,233,232	9,556,044,132	8,814,246,528	7,963,960,086
Other Operating Revenue	438,517,748	510,794,120	505,677,051	473,220,938	437,318,773
Other Nonoperating Revenue	227,736,515	161,419,465	197,222,441	89,274,796	92,711,281
Total Net Revenue.	12,197,983,931	11,174,446,817	10,258,943,624	9,376,742,262	8,493,990,140
Total Expenses.	11,210,657,463	10,255,161,431	9,417,648,940	8,797,685,529	7,917,744,877
HOSPITAL UNIT (Excludes Separate Nursing Home Units)					
Utilization - Inpatient					
Beds	12,196	12,387	12,516	12,634	12,413
Admissions	606,030	608,252	594,654	584,556	576,456
Inpatient Days	2,565,274	2,615,415	2,666,092	2,628,162	2,653,543
Average Length of Stay.	4.2	4.3	4.5	4.5	4.6
Personnel					
Total Full Time	58,161	57,472	53,258	54,308	53,066
Total Part Time	48,062	47,114	44,410	43,929	41,988
Revenue and Expenses - Totals					
(Includes Inpatient and Outpatient)					
Total Net Revenue.	$12,114,061,349	$11,078,760,380	$10,167,474,913	$9,306,678,467	$8,402,275,478
Total Expenses.	11,125,842,547	10,169,684,929	9,333,710,663	8,729,956,837	7,837,518,200
COMMUNITY HEALTH INDICATORS PER 1000 POPULATION					
Total Population (in thousands)	5,557	5,528	5,499	5,467	5,439
Inpatient					
Beds	2.5	2.6	2.7	2.7	2.7
Admissions	109.6	110.7	108.8	107.6	106.6
Inpatient Days	577.7	597.5	606.6	613.9	624.5
Inpatient Surgeries	35.3	34.3	33.3	34.8	33.4
Births.	12.3	12.2	12.3	12.0	12.1
Outpatient					
Emergency Outpatient Visits	376.3	355.6	338.5	331.8	337.1
Other Outpatient Visits.	1,875.4	1,946.8	1,810.9	1,829.5	1,798.1
Total Outpatient Visits	2,251.8	2,302.3	2,149.4	2,161.2	2,135.2
Outpatient Surgeries	80.9	97.2	76.1	76.1	71.5
Expense per Capita (per person). . . .	$2,017.6	$1,855.2	$1,712.7	$1,609.3	$1,455.9

States

TABLE 6

WYOMING

U.S. Registered Community Hospitals
(Nonfederal, short-term general and other special hospitals)

Overview 2002–2006

	2006	2005	2004	2003	2002
Total Community Hospitals in Wyoming.......	24	24	24	23	24
Bed Size Category					
6-24...	0	0	0	1	0
25-49..	10	10	9	8	9
50-99..	7	8	8	9	10
100-199...	4	3	4	4	4
200-299...	3	3	3	1	1
300-399...	0	0	0	0	0
400-499...	0	0	0	0	0
500 +...	0	0	0	0	0
Location					
Hospitals Urban................................	2	2	2	2	2
Hospitals Rural.................................	22	22	22	21	22
Control					
State and Local Government.................	17	17	17	15	16
Not for Profit...................................	4	4	4	5	5
Investor owned................................	3	3	3	3	3
Physician Models					
Independent Practice Association............	3	3	2	3	2
Group Practice without Walls.................	0	0	0	0	0
Open Physician-Hospital Organization........	1	1	2	2	2
Closed Physician-Hospital Organization.......	1	1	1	1	1
Management Service Organization............	1	1	1	2	1
Integrated Salary Model......................	11	10	9	9	7
Equity Model...................................	0	0	0	0	0
Foundation.....................................	0	0	0	0	0
Insurance Products					
Health Maintenance Organization............	1	1	0	1	1
Preferred Provider Organization..............	5	5	4	1	1
Indemnity Fee for Service....................	0	0	1	1	1
Managed Care Contracts					
Health Maintenance Organization............	3	3	3	4	3
Preferred Provider Organization..............	11	13	14	13	12
Affiliations					
Hospitals in a System*.......................	12	12	11	10	10
Hospitals in a Network.......................	4	4	4	4	2
Hospitals in a Group Purchasing Organization..	23	23	23	22	21

* Please note that system affiliate information for hospitals is derived from AHA membership. In years prior to 2003 the affiliation was derived from a question on the AHA Annual Survey of hospitals; therefore, non-responding hospitals were not included in the system affiliation counts. Years prior to 2003 have been updated to reflect this change, which now include affiliation for non-reporting hospitals.

TABLE **6**

WYOMING

U.S. Registered Community Hospitals
(Nonfederal, short-term general and other special hospitals)

Utilization, Personnel, Revenue and Expenses, Community Health Indicators 2002–2006

	2006	2005	2004	2003	2002
TOTAL FACILITY (Includes Hospital and Nursing Home Units)					
Utilization - Inpatient					
Beds	2,056	2,051	2,048	1,773	1,882
Admissions	52,586	51,200	50,509	52,612	49,201
Inpatient Days	421,089	421,352	394,422	342,260	370,143
Average Length of Stay.	8.0	8.2	7.8	6.5	7.5
Inpatient Surgeries.	14,128	13,175	14,626	13,178	13,393
Births.	6,824	6,603	6,220	6,048	5,945
Utilization - Outpatient					
Emergency Outpatient Visits	221,300	218,686	215,438	212,562	212,868
Other Outpatient Visits.	742,540	791,349	704,620	655,482	676,043
Total Outpatient Visits	963,840	1,010,035	920,058	868,044	888,911
Outpatient Surgeries	25,302	27,191	28,404	28,912	28,197
Personnel					
Full Time RNs	1,586	1,488	1,483	1,453	1,424
Full Time LPNs	160	173	176	177	185
Part Time RNs	457	370	400	443	426
Part Time LPNs	57	56	59	61	47
Total Full Time.	6,849	6,696	6,583	6,003	6,224
Total Part Time	1,989	1,776	1,716	1,666	1,798
Revenue - Inpatient					
Gross Inpatient Revenue.	$803,694,086	$734,933,760	$675,118,147	$591,634,445	$539,374,103
Revenue - Outpatient					
Gross Outpatient Revenue	$620,933,569	$561,095,096	$515,866,154	$478,863,281	$429,084,211
Revenue and Expenses - Totals					
(Includes Inpatient and Outpatient)					
Total Gross Revenue.	$1,424,627,655	$1,296,028,856	$1,190,984,301	$1,070,497,726	$968,458,314
Deductions from Revenue	606,943,644	534,882,813	487,084,081	429,180,139	371,291,521
Net Patient Revenue	817,684,011	761,146,043	703,900,220	641,317,587	597,166,793
Other Operating Revenue	46,089,909	40,147,046	34,461,766	32,237,152	28,889,946
Other Nonoperating Revenue	21,704,253	20,598,076	15,782,355	19,937,176	16,008,231
Total Net Revenue.	885,478,173	821,891,165	754,144,341	693,491,915	642,064,970
Total Expenses.	813,447,569	747,096,293	693,598,204	635,488,902	610,888,942
HOSPITAL UNIT (Excludes Separate Nursing Home Units)					
Utilization - Inpatient					
Beds	1,308	1,277	1,334	1,236	1,271
Admissions	51,024	49,554	49,081	51,509	47,931
Inpatient Days	180,631	178,182	197,165	172,278	178,227
Average Length of Stay.	3.5	3.6	4.0	3.3	3.7
Personnel					
Total Full Time.	6,291	6,120	5,757	5,592	5,750
Total Part Time	1,796	1,592	1,533	1,534	1,636
Revenue and Expenses - Totals					
(Includes Inpatient and Outpatient)					
Total Net Revenue.	$845,556,939	$779,859,233	$723,542,200	$669,886,380	$617,051,893
Total Expenses.	775,077,404	711,696,513	667,443,267	613,975,806	589,286,951
COMMUNITY HEALTH INDICATORS PER 1000 POPULATION					
Total Population (in thousands)	515	509	506	501	499
Inpatient					
Beds	4.0	4.0	4.1	3.5	3.8
Admissions	102.1	100.6	99.9	104.9	98.6
Inpatient Days	817.6	828.1	780.2	682.5	741.8
Inpatient Surgeries.	27.4	25.9	28.9	26.3	26.8
Births.	13.3	13.0	12.3	12.1	11.9
Outpatient					
Emergency Outpatient Visits	429.7	429.8	426.2	423.9	426.6
Other Outpatient Visits.	1,441.8	1,555.3	1,393.8	1,307.1	1,354.9
Total Outpatient Visits	1,871.5	1,985.1	1,820.0	1,730.9	1,781.5
Outpatient Surgeries	49.1	53.4	56.2	57.7	56.5
Expense per Capita (per person). . . .	$1,579.5	$1,468.4	$1,372.0	$1,267.2	$1,224.3

States

Table 7

Table		Page
7	Facilities and Services in the U. S. Census Divisions and States for 2006	154

The facilities and services presented in Table 7 are listed below in alphabetical order by major heading (where applicable).

Table 7

2006 Facilities and Services in the U.S. Census Divisions and States

These data include only hospital-based facilities and services as reported by responding hospitals in Section C of the 2006 AHA Annual Survey, beginning on page 197. All hospitals are represented with Community Hospitals listed separately under United States. No estimates have been made for nonresponding hospitals. Definitions of facilities and services are listed in the Glossary, page 187.

CLASSIFICATION	HOSPITALS REPORTING	GEN. MED. SURG. — ADULT (Number)	ADULT (Percent)	PEDIATRIC (Number)	PEDIATRIC (Percent)	OBSTETRICS INPATIENT CARE (Number)	OBST. (Percent)	NEONATAL INTERMEDIATE CARE (Number)	NEO. INT. (Percent)	NEONATAL (Number)	NEONATAL (Percent)	PEDIATRIC (Number)	PEDIATRIC (Percent)	INTENSIVE CARE — CARDIAC (Number)	CARDIAC (Percent)	MEDICAL SURGICAL (Number)	MED. SURG. (Percent)	OTHER (Number)	OTHER (Percent)
UNITED STATES	4,836	4,141	85.6	2,201	45.5	2,758	57.0	709	14.7	917	19.0	465	9.6	1,468	30.4	3,066	63.4	515	10.6
COMMUNITY HOSPITALS	4,120	3,870	93.9	2,139	51.9	2,714	65.9	694	16.8	904	21.9	453	11.0	1,413	34.3	2,933	71.2	488	11.8
CENSUS DIVISION 1, NEW ENGLAND	218	183	83.9	128	58.7	142	65.1	27	12.4	36	16.5	17	7.8	71	32.6	170	78.0	13	6.0
Connecticut	35	28	80.0	22	62.9	26	74.3	2	5.7	12	34.3	3	8.6	15	42.9	27	77.1	1	2.9
Maine	39	35	89.7	22	56.4	31	79.5	3	7.7	2	5.1	2	5.1	8	20.5	30	76.9	3	7.7
Massachusetts	84	67	79.8	49	58.3	43	51.2	15	17.9	15	17.9	7	8.3	33	39.3	63	75.0	7	8.3
New Hampshire	30	26	86.7	19	63.3	23	76.7	3	10.0	4	13.3	3	10.0	7	23.3	25	83.3	1	3.3
Rhode Island	13	12	92.3	7	53.8	7	53.8	2	15.4	2	15.4	1	7.7	3	23.1	11	84.6	1	7.7
Vermont	17	15	88.2	9	52.9	12	70.6	2	11.8	2	11.8	1	5.9	5	29.4	14	82.4	0	0.0
CENSUS DIVISION 2, MIDDLE ATLANTIC	410	352	85.9	212	51.7	251	61.2	98	23.9	100	24.4	48	11.7	176	42.9	316	77.1	41	10.0
New Jersey	71	58	81.7	46	64.8	48	67.6	39	54.9	20	28.2	13	18.3	38	53.5	58	81.7	6	8.5
New York	161	147	91.3	93	57.8	97	60.2	34	21.1	38	23.6	26	16.1	76	47.2	129	80.1	16	9.9
Pennsylvania	178	147	82.6	73	41.0	106	59.6	25	14.0	42	23.6	9	5.1	62	34.8	129	72.5	19	10.7
CENSUS DIVISION 3, SOUTH ATLANTIC	696	594	85.3	327	47.0	402	57.8	141	20.3	145	20.8	76	10.9	236	33.9	503	72.3	114	16.4
Delaware	9	6	66.7	3	33.3	4	44.4	1	11.1	3	33.3	2	22.2	6	66.7	6	66.7	2	22.2
District of Columbia	11	5	45.5	3	27.3	5	45.5	4	36.4	5	45.5	2	18.2	6	54.5	5	45.5	1	9.1
Florida	147	132	89.8	61	41.5	83	56.5	26	17.7	38	25.9	25	17.0	64	43.5	121	82.3	16	10.9
Georgia	129	110	85.3	53	41.1	71	55.0	31	24.0	26	20.2	7	5.4	36	27.9	84	65.1	19	14.7
Maryland	56	48	85.7	34	60.7	33	58.9	6	10.7	14	25.0	5	8.9	26	46.4	47	83.9	2	3.6
North Carolina	119	107	89.9	59	49.6	83	69.7	34	28.6	27	22.7	17	14.3	34	28.6	86	72.3	25	21.0
South Carolina	82	65	79.3	48	58.5	43	52.4	23	28.0	8	9.8	6	7.3	25	30.5	54	65.9	34	41.5
Virginia	76	64	84.2	37	48.7	50	65.8	14	18.4	20	26.3	8	10.5	24	31.6	62	81.6	12	15.8
West Virginia	67	57	85.1	29	43.3	30	44.8	2	3.0	2	6.0	4	6.0	19	28.4	38	56.7	3	4.5
CENSUS DIVISION 4, EAST NORTH CENTRAL	746	652	87.4	420	56.3	481	64.5	91	12.2	135	18.1	92	12.3	279	37.4	538	72.1	127	17.0
Illinois	170	156	91.8	108	63.5	108	63.5	38	22.4	34	20.0	26	15.3	53	31.2	129	75.9	15	8.8
Indiana	114	94	82.5	57	50.0	79	69.3	16	14.0	19	16.7	11	9.6	32	28.1	82	71.9	5	4.4
Michigan	152	131	86.2	77	50.7	91	59.9	13	8.6	27	17.8	13	8.6	53	34.9	101	66.4	15	9.9
Ohio	166	148	89.2	72	43.4	107	64.5	24	14.5	31	18.7	9	5.4	60	36.1	135	81.3	18	10.8
Wisconsin	144	123	85.4	106	73.6	96	66.7	0	0.0	24	16.7	33	22.9	81	56.3	91	63.2	74	51.4
CENSUS DIVISION 5, EAST SOUTH CENTRAL	375	333	88.8	175	46.7	186	49.6	67	17.9	64	17.1	40	10.7	124	33.1	218	58.1	42	11.2
Alabama	65	56	86.2	28	43.1	37	56.9	5	7.7	13	20.0	5	10.8	23	35.4	41	63.1	11	16.9
Kentucky	97	86	88.7	45	46.4	52	53.6	17	17.5	17	17.5	5	5.2	31	32.0	63	64.9	10	10.3
Mississippi	110	105	95.5	73	66.4	48	43.6	28	25.5	16	14.5	19	17.3	43	39.1	49	44.5	4	3.6
Tennessee	103	86	83.5	29	28.2	49	47.6	17	16.5	18	17.5	9	8.7	27	26.2	65	63.1	17	16.5
CENSUS DIVISION 6, WEST NORTH CENTRAL	706	640	90.7	319	45.2	389	55.1	73	10.3	82	11.6	47	6.7	157	22.2	361	51.1	45	6.4
Iowa	125	120	96.0	61	48.8	81	64.8	12	9.6	19	15.2	11	8.8	26	20.8	77	61.6	8	6.4
Kansas	154	138	89.6	49	31.8	69	44.8	11	7.1	11	7.1	5	3.2	11	7.1	53	34.4	2	1.3
Minnesota	109	102	93.6	67	61.5	85	78.0	12	11.0	16	14.7	13	11.9	34	31.2	68	62.4	12	11.0
Missouri	147	119	81.0	76	51.7	72	49.0	26	17.7	17	11.6	9	6.1	40	27.2	91	61.9	15	10.2
Nebraska	75	70	93.3	28	37.3	42	56.0	4	5.3	8	10.7	2	2.7	21	28.0	26	34.7	4	5.3
North Dakota	38	36	94.7	18	47.4	15	39.5	5	13.2	5	13.2	2	7.9	15	39.5	21	55.3	1	2.6
South Dakota	58	55	94.8	20	34.5	25	43.1	3	5.2	4	6.9	4	6.9	10	17.2	25	43.1	3	5.2
CENSUS DIVISION 7, WEST SOUTH CENTRAL	872	663	76.0	273	31.3	375	43.0	94	10.8	136	15.6	59	6.8	161	18.5	413	47.4	52	6.0
Arkansas	105	81	77.1	28	26.7	44	41.9	13	12.4	11	10.5	2	1.9	28	26.7	51	48.6	7	6.7
Louisiana	99	80	80.8	41	41.4	39	39.4	4	4.0	10	10.1	12	12.1	20	20.2	53	53.5	3	3.0
Oklahoma	124	107	86.3	28	22.6	54	43.5	6	4.8	10	8.1	5	4.0	21	16.9	47	37.9	4	3.0
Texas	544	395	72.6	176	32.4	238	43.8	71	13.1	95	17.5	40	7.4	92	16.9	262	48.2	38	7.0
CENSUS DIVISION 8, MOUNTAIN	341	298	87.4	141	41.3	208	61.0	58	17.0	65	19.1	35	10.3	85	24.9	195	57.2	33	9.7
Arizona	52	46	88.5	18	34.6	42	63.5	13	25.0	10	19.2	6	11.5	22	42.3	36	69.2	6	11.5
Colorado	64	58	90.6	31	48.4	42	65.6	10	15.6	20	31.3	6	9.4	15	23.4	43	67.2	6	9.4
Idaho	34	31	91.2	13	38.2	23	67.6	2	5.9	5	14.7	2	5.9	8	23.5	16	47.1	2	5.9
Montana	56	54	96.4	22	39.3	26	46.4	7	12.5	7	12.5	6	10.7	14	25.0	24	42.9	5	8.9
Nevada	33	22	66.7	8	24.2	14	42.4	4	12.1	6	18.2	4	12.1	6	18.2	16	48.5	5	15.2
New Mexico	38	29	76.3	19	50.0	22	57.9	6	15.8	3	7.9	3	7.9	6	15.8	19	50.0	4	10.5
Utah	36	32	88.9	20	55.6	28	77.8	12	33.3	13	36.1	4	11.1	13	36.1	21	58.3	3	8.3
Wyoming	28	26	92.9	10	35.7	20	71.4	4	14.3	1	3.6	2	7.1	1	3.6	20	71.4	2	7.1
CENSUS DIVISION 9, PACIFIC	472	426	90.3	206	43.6	324	68.6	60	12.7	154	32.6	51	10.8	179	37.9	352	74.6	48	10.2
Alaska	16	15	93.8	7	43.8	13	81.3	0	0.0	2	12.5	1	6.3	2	12.5	10	62.5	0	0.0
California	308	274	89.0	133	43.2	204	66.2	38	12.3	126	40.9	35	11.4	134	43.5	237	76.9	30	9.7
Hawaii	20	16	80.0	5	25.0	10	50.0	3	15.0	2	10.0	2	10.0	6	30.0	14	70.0	2	10.0
Oregon	60	58	96.7	28	46.7	52	86.7	8	13.3	9	15.0	5	8.3	18	30.0	50	83.3	5	8.3
Washington	68	63	92.6	33	48.5	45	66.2	11	16.2	15	22.1	8	11.8	19	27.9	41	60.3	12	17.6

Table 7 (Continued)

These data include only hospital-based facilities and services as reported by responding hospitals in Section C of the 2006 AHA Annual Survey, beginning on page 197. All hospitals are represented with Community Hospitals listed separately under United States. No estimates have been made for nonresponding hospitals. Definitions of facilities and services are listed in the Glossary, page 187.

CLASSIFICATION	HOSPITALS REPORTING	BURN CARE UNITS Number	Percent	LONG-TERM CARE ACUTE LONG-TERM CARE UNITS Number	Percent	SKILLED NURSING CARE UNITS Number	Percent	INTERMEDIATE CARE UNITS Number	Percent	OTHER LONG-TERM CARE UNITS Number	Percent	PSYCHIATRIC INPATIENT CARE UNITS Number	Percent	ALCOHOL/DRUG ABUSE OR DEPENDENCY INPATIENT CARE UNITS Number	Percent	OTHER SPECIAL CARE UNITS Number	Percent	PHYSICAL REHABILITATION INPATIENT CARE UNITS Number	Percent
UNITED STATES	4,836	204	4.2	380	7.9	1,436	29.7	469	9.7	324	6.7	1,675	34.6	510	10.5	735	15.2	1,457	30.1
COMMUNITY HOSPITALS	4,120	194	4.7	236	5.7	1,331	32.3	424	10.3	271	6.6	1,309	31.8	367	8.9	691	16.8	1,359	33.0
CENSUS DIVISION 1, NEW ENGLAND	218	11	5.0	13	6.0	52	23.9	25	11.5	10	4.6	114	52.3	26	11.9	23	10.6	51	23.4
Connecticut	35	1	2.9	1	2.9	2	5.7	2	5.7	0	0.0	26	74.3	7	20.0	7	20.0	13	37.1
Maine	39	2	5.1	2	5.1	11	28.2	7	17.9	3	7.7	13	33.3	6	15.4	2	5.1	8	20.5
Massachusetts	84	6	7.1	8	9.5	21	25.0	4	4.8	4	4.8	46	54.8	9	10.7	7	8.3	15	17.9
New Hampshire	30	1	3.3	1	3.3	11	36.7	9	30.0	1	3.3	14	46.7	1	3.3	5	16.7	7	23.3
Rhode Island	13	0	0.0	1	7.7	2	15.4	1	7.7	1	7.7	8	61.5	2	15.4	1	7.7	5	38.5
Vermont	17	1	5.9	0	0.0	5	29.4	2	11.8	1	5.9	7	41.2	1	5.9	1	5.9	3	17.6
CENSUS DIVISION 2, MIDDLE ATLANTIC	410	15	3.7	8	2.0	128	31.2	16	3.9	21	5.1	238	58.0	69	16.8	67	16.3	145	35.4
New Jersey	71	2	2.8	1	1.4	14	19.7	4	5.6	5	7.0	45	63.4	8	11.3	10	14.1	13	18.3
New York	161	7	4.3	3	1.9	57	35.4	7	4.3	12	7.5	97	60.2	44	27.3	26	16.1	61	37.9
Pennsylvania	178	6	3.4	4	2.2	57	32.0	5	2.8	4	2.2	96	53.9	17	9.6	31	17.4	71	39.9
CENSUS DIVISION 3, SOUTH ATLANTIC	696	28	4.0	79	11.4	214	30.7	66	9.5	58	8.3	254	36.5	81	11.6	131	18.8	211	30.3
Delaware	9	0	0.0	1	11.1	5	55.6	2	22.2	0	0.0	5	55.6	1	11.1	1	11.1	3	33.3
District of Columbia	11	2	18.2	3	27.3	5	45.5	1	9.1	2	18.2	7	63.6	2	18.2	1	9.1	3	27.3
Florida	147	5	3.4	6	4.1	20	13.6	6	4.1	2	1.4	48	32.7	14	9.5	38	25.9	36	24.5
Georgia	129	3	2.3	13	10.1	37	28.7	13	10.1	6	4.7	39	30.2	14	10.9	14	10.9	34	26.4
Maryland	56	1	1.8	4	7.1	16	28.6	2	3.6	3	5.4	34	60.7	6	10.7	14	25.0	14	25.0
North Carolina	119	8	6.7	10	8.4	47	39.5	15	12.6	7	5.9	48	40.3	16	13.4	31	26.1	31	26.1
South Carolina	82	2	2.4	36	43.9	37	45.1	11	13.4	31	37.8	24	29.3	14	17.1	16	19.5	54	65.9
Virginia	76	6	7.9	4	5.3	19	25.0	9	11.8	4	5.3	33	43.4	11	14.5	13	17.1	26	34.2
West Virginia	67	1	1.5	2	3.0	28	41.8	7	10.4	3	4.5	16	23.9	3	4.5	3	4.5	10	14.9
CENSUS DIVISION 4, EAST NORTH CENTRAL	746	43	5.8	61	8.2	219	29.4	77	10.3	55	7.4	295	39.5	116	15.5	194	26.0	274	36.7
Illinois	170	10	5.9	11	6.5	60	35.3	20	11.8	17	10.0	65	38.2	25	14.7	23	13.5	50	29.4
Indiana	114	5	4.4	12	10.5	34	29.8	14	12.3	8	7.0	42	36.8	13	11.4	17	14.9	39	34.2
Michigan	152	9	5.9	17	11.2	33	21.7	12	7.9	13	8.6	63	41.4	15	9.9	18	11.8	56	36.8
Ohio	166	7	4.2	7	4.2	59	35.5	10	6.0	12	7.2	78	47.0	21	12.7	25	15.1	60	36.1
Wisconsin	144	12	8.3	14	9.7	33	22.9	21	14.6	5	3.5	47	32.6	42	29.2	111	77.1	69	47.9
CENSUS DIVISION 5, EAST SOUTH CENTRAL	375	18	4.8	20	5.3	105	28.0	26	6.9	39	10.4	139	37.1	36	9.6	61	16.3	124	33.1
Alabama	65	5	7.7	2	3.1	10	15.4	5	7.7	4	6.2	27	41.5	4	6.2	10	15.4	17	26.2
Kentucky	97	6	6.2	10	10.3	33	34.0	9	9.3	8	8.2	31	32.0	8	8.2	15	15.5	26	26.8
Mississippi	110	2	1.8	0	0.0	31	28.2	0	0.0	23	20.9	44	40.0	15	13.6	18	16.4	51	46.4
Tennessee	103	5	4.9	8	7.8	31	30.1	12	11.7	4	3.9	37	35.9	9	8.7	18	17.5	30	29.1
CENSUS DIVISION 6, WEST NORTH CENTRAL	706	27	3.8	38	5.4	309	43.8	130	18.4	70	9.9	186	26.3	55	7.8	79	11.2	197	27.9
Iowa	125	6	4.8	6	4.8	66	52.8	40	32.0	15	12.0	41	32.8	15	12.0	12	9.6	28	22.4
Kansas	154	2	1.3	7	4.5	57	37.0	38	24.7	16	10.4	28	18.2	7	4.5	7	4.5	32	20.8
Minnesota	109	7	6.4	8	7.3	48	44.0	7	6.4	7	6.4	29	26.6	15	13.8	13	11.9	26	23.9
Missouri	147	8	5.4	9	6.1	51	34.7	17	11.6	11	7.5	61	41.5	18	12.2	34	23.1	80	54.4
Nebraska	75	3	4.0	3	4.0	36	48.0	15	20.0	10	13.3	11	14.7	3	4.0	7	9.3	13	17.3
North Dakota	38	0	0.0	0	0.0	20	52.6	4	10.5	2	5.3	9	23.7	2	5.3	2	5.3	9	23.7
South Dakota	58	1	1.7	5	8.6	31	53.4	9	15.5	9	15.5	7	12.1	1	1.7	4	6.9	9	15.5
CENSUS DIVISION 7, WEST SOUTH CENTRAL	872	23	2.6	106	12.2	130	14.9	37	4.2	20	2.3	207	23.7	54	6.2	85	9.7	241	27.6
Arkansas	105	3	2.9	9	8.6	25	23.8	9	8.6	3	2.9	36	34.3	5	4.8	5	4.8	32	30.5
Louisiana	99	3	3.0	12	12.1	18	18.2	5	5.1	3	3.0	37	37.4	6	6.1	6	6.1	31	31.3
Oklahoma	124	2	1.6	8	6.5	24	19.4	6	4.8	3	2.4	34	27.4	4	3.2	9	7.3	34	27.4
Texas	544	15	2.8	77	14.2	63	11.6	17	3.1	11	2.0	100	18.4	42	7.7	65	11.9	144	26.5
CENSUS DIVISION 8, MOUNTAIN	341	16	4.7	26	7.6	126	37.0	51	15.0	28	8.2	95	27.9	35	10.3	33	9.7	97	28.4
Arizona	52	2	3.8	4	7.7	5	9.6	6	11.5	2	3.8	19	36.5	3	5.8	4	7.7	19	36.5
Colorado	64	6	9.4	4	6.3	23	35.9	9	14.1	7	10.9	17	26.6	9	14.1	10	15.6	27	42.2
Idaho	34	0	0.0	0	0.0	14	41.2	4	11.8	0	0.0	9	26.5	1	2.9	1	2.9	5	14.7
Montana	56	2	3.6	8	14.3	42	75.0	9	16.1	10	17.9	8	19.6	5	8.9	7	12.5	11	19.6
Nevada	33	1	3.0	3	9.1	6	18.2	2	6.1	0	0.0	11	24.2	3	9.1	2	6.1	10	30.3
New Mexico	38	1	2.6	3	7.9	9	23.7	5	13.2	2	5.3	11	28.9	6	15.8	3	7.9	11	28.9
Utah	36	3	8.3	3	8.3	15	41.7	7	19.4	2	5.6	13	36.1	6	16.7	4	11.1	9	25.0
Wyoming	28	1	3.6	1	3.6	12	42.9	9	32.1	5	17.9	7	25.0	2	7.1	2	7.1	5	17.9
CENSUS DIVISION 9, PACIFIC	472	23	4.9	29	6.1	153	32.4	41	8.7	23	4.9	147	31.1	38	8.1	62	13.1	117	24.8
Alaska	16	1	6.3	0	0.0	7	43.8	5	31.3	1	6.3	7	43.8	2	12.5	1	6.3	2	12.5
California	308	15	4.9	22	7.1	113	36.7	17	5.5	15	4.9	94	30.5	24	7.8	36	11.7	76	24.7
Hawaii	20	1	5.0	1	5.0	9	45.0	5	25.0	1	5.0	7	35.0	0	0.0	3	15.0	1	5.0
Oregon	60	3	5.0	3	5.0	9	15.0	8	13.3	2	3.3	18	30.0	5	8.3	8	13.3	12	20.0
Washington	68	3	4.4	3	4.4	15	22.1	6	8.8	4	5.9	21	30.9	7	10.3	14	20.6	26	38.2

Table 7 (Continued)

These data include only hospital-based facilities and services as reported by responding hospitals in Section C of the 2006 AHA Annual Survey, beginning on page 197. All hospitals are represented with Community Hospitals listed separately under United States. No estimates have been made for nonresponding hospitals. Definitions of facilities and services are listed in the Glossary, page 187.

| | HOSPITALS REPORTING | ADULT DAY CARE PROGRAM | | AIRBORNE INFECTION ISOLATION ROOM | | ALCOHOL/DRUG ABUSE OR DEPENDENCY OUTPATIENT SERVICES | | ALZHEIMER CENTER | | AMBULANCE SERVICES | | AMBULATORY SURGERY CENTERS | | ARTHRITIS TREATMENT CENTER | | ASSISTED LIVING | | AUXILIARY | | BARIATRIC/WEIGHT CONTROL SERVICES | |
CLASSIFICATION		Number	Percent	Number	Percent	Number	Percent	Number	Percent	Number	Percent	Number	Percent	Number	Percent	Number	Percent	Number	Percent	Number	Percent
UNITED STATES	4,836	312	6.5	3,328	68.8	807	16.7	202	4.2	813	16.8	1,040	21.5	271	5.6	233	4.8	2,884	59.6	967	20.0
COMMUNITY HOSPITALS	4,120	278	6.7	3,014	73.2	617	15.0	170	4.1	775	18.8	980	23.8	255	6.2	216	5.2	2,798	67.9	906	22.0
CENSUS DIVISION 1, NEW ENGLAND	218	19	8.7	158	72.5	67	30.7	16	7.3	25	11.5	66	30.3	17	7.8	12	5.5	129	59.2	53	24.3
Connecticut	35	4	11.4	30	85.7	14	40.0	1	2.9	2	5.7	13	37.1	4	11.4	2	5.7	24	68.6	12	34.3
Maine	39	2	5.1	28	71.8	14	35.9	4	10.3	8	20.5	11	28.2	0	0.0	4	10.3	27	69.2	6	15.4
Massachusetts	84	6	7.1	55	65.5	29	34.5	9	10.7	7	8.3	21	25.0	9	10.7	2	2.4	40	47.6	22	26.2
New Hampshire	30	5	16.7	24	80.0	2	6.7	1	3.3	6	20.0	9	30.0	3	10.0	2	6.7	19	63.3	7	23.3
Rhode Island	13	0	0.0	6	46.2	4	30.8	0	0.0	1	7.7	6	46.2	0	0.0	1	7.7	7	53.8	3	23.1
Vermont	17	2	11.8	15	88.2	4	23.5	1	5.9	1	5.9	6	35.3	1	5.9	1	5.9	12	70.6	3	17.6
CENSUS DIVISION 2, MIDDLE ATLANTIC	410	45	11.0	294	71.7	113	27.6	25	6.1	72	17.6	133	32.4	46	11.2	18	4.4	278	67.8	131	32.0
New Jersey	71	8	11.3	57	80.3	25	35.2	6	8.5	15	21.1	15	21.1	7	9.9	4	5.6	56	78.9	27	38.0
New York	161	29	18.0	114	70.8	61	37.9	10	6.2	28	17.4	78	48.4	21	13.0	5	3.1	101	62.7	55	34.2
Pennsylvania	178	8	4.5	123	69.1	27	15.2	9	5.1	29	16.3	40	22.5	18	10.1	9	5.1	121	68.0	49	27.5
CENSUS DIVISION 3, SOUTH ATLANTIC	696	33	4.7	523	75.1	108	15.5	29	4.2	109	15.7	149	21.4	39	5.6	20	2.9	442	63.5	163	23.4
Delaware	9	2	22.2	5	55.6	1	11.1	1	11.1	1	11.1	2	22.2	1	11.1	0	0.0	4	44.4	3	33.3
District of Columbia	11	0	0.0	8	72.7	4	36.4	1	9.1	3	27.3	3	27.3	3	27.3	1	9.1	2	18.2	2	18.2
Florida	147	6	4.1	122	83.0	16	10.9	10	6.8	15	10.2	36	24.5	5	3.4	0	0.0	94	63.9	52	35.4
Georgia	129	5	3.9	88	68.2	21	16.3	4	3.1	29	22.5	27	20.9	3	2.3	7	5.4	84	65.1	22	17.1
Maryland	56	7	12.5	43	76.8	17	30.4	4	7.1	4	7.1	13	23.2	8	14.3	4	7.1	43	76.8	18	32.1
North Carolina	119	5	4.2	89	74.8	20	16.8	2	1.7	24	20.2	38	31.9	7	5.9	2	1.7	79	66.4	24	20.2
South Carolina	82	2	2.4	60	73.2	9	11.0	2	2.4	15	18.3	8	9.8	3	3.7	1	1.2	42	51.2	14	17.1
Virginia	76	4	5.3	63	82.9	12	15.8	5	6.6	13	17.1	16	21.1	5	6.6	5	6.6	57	75.0	20	26.3
West Virginia	67	2	3.0	45	67.2	8	11.9	0	0.0	5	7.5	6	9.0	4	6.0	0	0.0	37	55.2	8	11.9
CENSUS DIVISION 4, EAST NORTH CENTRAL	746	60	8.0	557	74.7	186	24.9	60	8.0	132	17.7	192	25.7	74	9.9	44	5.9	488	65.4	153	20.5
Illinois	170	20	11.8	133	78.2	46	27.1	10	5.9	28	16.5	38	22.4	19	11.2	7	4.1	116	68.2	42	24.7
Indiana	114	6	5.3	91	79.8	24	21.1	1	0.9	32	28.1	29	25.4	6	5.3	5	4.4	58	50.9	23	20.2
Michigan	152	11	7.2	115	75.7	32	21.1	8	5.3	22	14.5	40	26.3	10	6.6	10	6.6	109	71.7	43	28.3
Ohio	166	9	5.4	127	76.5	43	25.9	14	8.4	32	19.3	47	28.3	18	10.8	10	6.0	122	73.5	45	27.1
Wisconsin	144	14	9.7	91	63.2	41	28.5	27	18.8	18	12.5	38	26.4	21	14.6	10	6.9	83	57.6	0	0.0
CENSUS DIVISION 5, EAST SOUTH CENTRAL	375	8	2.1	210	56.0	46	12.3	3	0.8	50	13.3	54	14.4	10	2.7	6	1.6	158	42.1	56	14.9
Alabama	65	2	3.1	36	55.4	6	9.2	2	3.1	8	12.3	13	20.0	3	4.6	3	4.6	34	52.3	20	30.8
Kentucky	97	4	4.1	75	77.3	15	15.5	1	1.0	14	14.4	17	17.5	3	3.1	1	1.0	63	64.9	16	16.5
Mississippi	110	1	0.9	24	21.8	12	10.9	0	0.0	10	9.1	8	7.3	0	0.0	0	0.0	16	14.5	3	2.7
Tennessee	103	1	1.0	75	72.8	13	12.6	0	0.0	18	17.5	16	15.5	4	3.9	2	1.9	45	43.7	17	16.5
CENSUS DIVISION 6, WEST NORTH CENTRAL	706	69	9.8	431	61.0	99	14.0	36	5.1	194	27.5	114	16.1	30	4.2	81	11.5	478	67.7	106	15.0
Iowa	125	9	7.2	63	50.4	25	20.0	7	5.6	56	44.8	28	22.4	5	4.0	11	8.8	110	88.0	19	15.2
Kansas	154	14	9.1	91	59.1	7	4.5	3	1.9	23	14.9	14	9.1	5	3.2	13	8.4	83	53.9	14	9.1
Minnesota	109	21	19.3	70	64.2	23	21.1	11	10.1	43	39.4	22	20.2	4	3.7	19	17.4	76	69.7	28	25.7
Missouri	147	5	3.4	112	76.2	27	18.4	7	4.8	33	22.4	25	17.0	12	8.2	3	2.0	102	69.4	19	12.9
Nebraska	75	8	10.7	42	56.0	7	9.3	3	4.0	16	21.3	11	14.7	1	1.3	12	16.0	46	61.3	11	14.7
North Dakota	38	4	10.5	27	71.1	5	13.2	0	0.0	10	26.3	6	15.8	1	2.6	4	10.5	28	73.7	9	23.7
South Dakota	58	8	13.8	26	44.8	5	8.6	5	8.6	13	22.4	8	13.8	2	3.4	19	32.8	33	56.9	6	10.3
CENSUS DIVISION 7, WEST SOUTH CENTRAL	872	16	1.8	607	69.6	62	7.1	9	1.0	120	13.8	123	14.1	18	2.1	23	2.6	438	50.2	133	15.3
Arkansas	105	3	2.9	79	75.2	6	5.7	4	3.8	15	14.3	20	19.0	2	1.9	1	1.0	69	65.7	9	8.6
Louisiana	99	6	6.1	58	58.6	7	7.1	3	3.0	11	11.1	24	24.2	3	3.0	1	1.0	45	45.5	14	14.1
Oklahoma	124	2	1.6	80	64.5	8	6.5	1	0.8	20	16.1	13	10.5	1	0.8	4	3.2	61	49.2	11	8.9
Texas	544	5	0.9	390	71.7	41	7.5	1	0.2	74	13.6	66	12.1	12	2.2	17	3.1	263	48.3	99	18.2
CENSUS DIVISION 8, MOUNTAIN	341	32	9.4	225	66.0	60	17.6	12	3.5	68	19.9	79	23.2	13	3.8	19	5.6	197	57.8	53	15.5
Arizona	52	1	1.9	43	82.7	10	19.2	3	5.8	2	3.8	15	28.8	1	1.9	1	1.9	33	63.5	12	23.1
Colorado	64	4	6.3	46	71.9	13	20.3	2	3.1	15	23.4	14	21.9	5	7.8	3	4.7	38	59.4	19	29.7
Idaho	34	6	17.6	20	58.8	5	14.7	0	0.0	7	20.6	9	26.5	2	5.9	1	2.9	25	73.5	5	14.7
Montana	56	16	28.6	31	55.4	4	7.1	4	7.1	16	28.6	10	17.9	1	1.8	11	19.6	30	53.6	3	5.4
Nevada	33	1	3.0	20	60.6	6	18.2	0	0.0	4	12.1	6	18.2	2	6.1	1	3.0	14	42.4	6	18.2
New Mexico	38	1	2.6	20	52.6	9	23.7	0	0.0	8	21.1	9	23.7	2	5.3	0	0.0	19	50.0	1	2.6
Utah	36	2	5.6	28	77.8	7	19.4	0	0.0	6	16.7	11	30.6	0	0.0	0	0.0	18	50.0	4	11.1
Wyoming	28	1	3.6	17	60.7	6	21.4	3	10.7	10	35.7	5	17.9	0	0.0	2	7.1	20	71.4	3	10.7
CENSUS DIVISION 9, PACIFIC	472	30	6.4	323	68.4	66	14.0	12	2.5	43	9.1	130	27.5	24	5.1	10	2.1	276	58.5	119	25.2
Alaska	16	1	6.3	10	62.5	5	31.3	1	6.3	3	18.8	4	25.0	0	0.0	1	6.3	7	43.8	4	25.0
California	308	20	6.5	208	67.5	42	13.6	7	2.3	24	7.8	83	26.9	14	4.5	3	1.0	181	58.8	80	26.0
Hawaii	20	2	10.0	15	75.0	3	15.0	0	0.0	1	5.0	6	30.0	1	5.0	0	0.0	5	25.0	5	25.0
Oregon	60	4	6.7	52	86.7	7	11.7	2	3.3	7	11.7	16	26.7	4	6.7	2	3.3	44	73.3	16	26.7
Washington	68	3	4.4	38	55.9	9	13.2	2	2.9	8	11.8	21	30.9	5	7.4	4	5.9	39	57.4	14	20.6

Table 7 (Continued)

These data include only hospital-based facilities and services as reported by responding hospitals in Section C of the 2006 AHA Annual Survey, beginning on page 199. All hospitals are represented with Community Hospitals listed separately under United States. No estimates have been made for nonresponding hospitals. Definitions of facilities and services are listed in the Glossary, page 211.

CARDIOLOGY AND CARDIAC SERVICES

CLASSIFICATION	HOSPITALS REPORTING	BIRTHING/LDR/LDRP ROOM Number	Percent	BREAST CANCER SCREENING Number	Percent	ADULT DIAGNOSTIC/INVASIVE CATHETERIZATION Number	Percent	PEDIATRIC DIAGNOSTIC/INVASIVE CATHETERIZATION Number	Percent	ADULT INTERVENTIONAL CARDIAC CATHETERIZATION Number	Percent	PEDIATRIC INTERVENTIONAL CARDIAC CATHETERIZATION Number	Percent	ADULT CARDIAC SURGERY Number	Percent	PEDIATRIC CARDIAC SURGERY Number	Percent	CARDIAC REHABILITATION Number	Percent
UNITED STATES	4,836	2,718	56.2	3,367	69.6	1,728	35.7	226	4.7	1,356	28.0	200	4.1	1,072	22.2	193	4.0	2,408	49.8
COMMUNITY HOSPITALS	4,120	2,682	65.1	3,283	79.7	1,655	40.2	221	5.4	1,294	31.4	196	4.8	1,030	25.0	189	4.6	2,340	56.8
CENSUS DIVISION 1, NEW ENGLAND	218	144	66.1	169	77.5	89	40.8	12	5.5	57	26.1	11	5.0	42	19.3	11	5.0	142	65.1
Connecticut	35	26	74.3	26	74.3	19	54.3	3	8.6	16	45.7	3	8.6	13	37.1	3	8.6	23	65.7
Maine	39	31	79.5	34	87.2	11	28.2	1	2.6	5	12.8	1	2.6	4	10.3	1	2.6	28	71.8
Massachusetts	84	46	54.8	62	73.8	36	42.9	4	4.8	22	26.2	4	4.8	16	19.0	4	4.8	49	58.3
New Hampshire	30	23	76.7	24	80.0	13	43.3	2	6.7	9	30.0	1	3.3	5	16.7	1	3.3	22	73.3
Rhode Island	13	6	46.2	10	76.9	6	46.2	1	7.7	3	23.1	1	7.7	2	15.4	1	7.7	7	53.8
Vermont	17	12	70.6	13	76.5	4	23.5	1	5.9	2	11.8	1	5.9	2	11.8	1	5.9	13	76.5
CENSUS DIVISION 2, MIDDLE ATLANTIC	410	243	59.3	323	78.8	192	46.8	25	6.1	139	33.9	22	5.4	101	24.6	23	5.6	243	59.3
New Jersey	71	45	63.4	55	77.5	49	69.0	5	7.0	35	49.3	5	7.0	16	22.5	5	7.0	46	64.8
New York	161	97	60.2	130	80.7	59	36.6	13	8.1	40	24.8	11	6.8	29	18.0	12	7.5	79	49.1
Pennsylvania	178	101	56.7	138	77.5	84	47.2	7	3.9	64	36.0	6	3.4	56	31.5	6	3.4	118	66.3
CENSUS DIVISION 3, SOUTH ATLANTIC	696	396	56.9	524	75.3	335	48.1	30	4.3	212	30.5	28	4.0	160	23.0	28	4.0	348	50.0
Delaware	9	5	55.6	5	55.6	5	55.6	0	0.0	4	44.4	0	0.0	3	33.3	0	0.0	5	55.6
District of Columbia	11	5	45.5	5	45.5	6	54.5	1	9.1	6	54.5	1	9.1	3	27.3	1	9.1	5	45.5
Florida	147	79	53.7	113	76.9	93	63.3	10	6.8	63	42.9	8	5.4	58	39.5	10	6.8	70	47.6
Georgia	129	70	54.3	97	75.2	49	38.0	3	2.3	30	23.3	3	2.3	20	15.5	3	2.3	52	40.3
Maryland	56	33	58.9	41	73.2	35	62.5	4	7.1	23	41.1	3	5.4	10	17.9	2	3.6	33	58.9
North Carolina	119	83	69.7	95	79.8	58	48.7	5	4.2	31	26.1	6	5.0	24	20.2	5	4.2	66	55.5
South Carolina	82	42	51.2	56	68.3	32	39.0	1	1.2	17	20.7	1	1.2	18	22.0	1	1.2	35	42.7
Virginia	76	49	64.5	62	81.6	36	47.4	5	6.6	29	38.2	5	6.6	18	23.7	5	6.6	50	65.8
West Virginia	67	30	44.8	50	74.6	21	31.3	1	1.5	9	13.4	1	1.5	6	9.0	1	1.5	32	47.8
CENSUS DIVISION 4, EAST NORTH CENTRAL	746	478	64.1	593	79.5	269	36.1	37	5.0	217	29.1	34	4.6	179	24.0	30	4.0	499	66.9
Illinois	170	105	61.8	149	87.6	81	47.6	10	5.9	73	42.9	10	5.9	57	33.5	8	4.7	117	68.8
Indiana	114	79	69.3	87	76.3	44	38.6	4	3.5	35	30.7	2	1.8	28	24.6	4	3.5	77	67.5
Michigan	152	90	59.2	121	79.6	57	37.5	5	3.3	42	27.6	5	3.3	35	23.0	5	3.3	83	54.6
Ohio	166	107	64.5	131	78.9	86	51.8	11	6.6	66	39.8	10	6.0	58	34.9	9	5.4	115	69.3
Wisconsin	144	97	67.4	105	72.9	1	0.7	7	4.9	1	0.7	7	4.9	1	0.7	4	2.8	107	74.3
CENSUS DIVISION 5, EAST SOUTH CENTRAL	375	178	47.5	263	70.1	133	35.5	11	2.9	108	28.8	9	2.4	87	23.2	9	2.4	134	35.7
Alabama	65	36	55.4	44	67.7	31	47.7	2	3.1	23	35.4	2	3.1	23	35.4	2	3.1	31	47.7
Kentucky	97	50	51.5	81	83.5	40	41.2	2	2.1	29	29.9	2	2.1	23	23.7	2	2.1	46	47.4
Mississippi	110	44	40.0	62	56.4	25	22.7	2	1.8	24	21.8	1	0.9	17	15.5	1	0.9	15	13.6
Tennessee	103	48	46.6	76	73.8	37	35.9	5	4.9	32	31.1	4	3.9	24	23.3	4	3.9	42	40.8
CENSUS DIVISION 6, WEST NORTH CENTRAL	706	405	57.4	487	69.0	142	20.1	16	2.3	132	18.7	13	1.8	97	13.7	15	2.1	473	67.0
Iowa	125	82	65.6	112	89.6	22	17.6	2	1.6	23	18.4	2	1.6	12	9.6	2	1.6	106	84.8
Kansas	154	73	47.4	78	50.6	22	14.3	1	0.6	20	13.0	0	0.0	16	10.4	0	0.0	70	45.5
Minnesota	109	86	78.9	88	80.7	15	13.8	3	2.8	14	12.8	3	2.8	14	12.8	3	2.8	84	77.1
Missouri	147	72	49.0	102	69.4	55	37.4	5	3.4	49	33.3	4	2.7	35	23.8	6	4.1	87	59.2
Nebraska	75	51	68.0	53	70.7	15	20.0	2	2.7	14	18.7	1	1.3	10	13.3	1	1.3	55	73.3
North Dakota	38	18	47.4	22	57.9	6	15.8	2	5.3	6	15.8	1	2.6	6	15.8	2	5.3	30	78.9
South Dakota	58	23	39.7	32	55.2	7	12.1	2	3.4	6	10.3	2	3.4	4	6.9	1	1.7	41	70.7
CENSUS DIVISION 7, WEST SOUTH CENTRAL	872	364	41.7	432	49.5	255	29.2	29	3.3	211	24.2	24	2.8	182	20.9	25	2.9	267	30.6
Arkansas	105	44	41.9	61	58.1	28	26.7	1	1.0	25	23.8	1	1.0	20	19.0	1	1.0	36	34.3
Louisiana	99	36	36.4	57	57.6	35	35.4	6	6.1	31	31.3	5	5.1	23	23.2	2	2.0	26	26.3
Oklahoma	124	54	43.5	60	48.4	30	24.2	3	2.4	24	19.4	2	1.6	19	15.3	3	2.4	26	21.0
Texas	544	230	42.3	254	46.7	162	29.8	19	3.5	131	24.1	16	2.9	120	22.1	19	3.5	179	32.9
CENSUS DIVISION 8, MOUNTAIN	341	203	59.5	233	68.3	116	34.0	20	5.9	106	31.1	20	5.9	75	22.0	15	4.4	132	38.7
Arizona	52	30	57.7	33	63.5	32	61.5	4	5.8	30	57.7	4	7.7	23	44.2	3	5.8	29	55.8
Colorado	64	43	67.2	51	79.7	26	40.6	4	6.3	26	40.6	4	6.3	17	26.6	3	4.7	35	54.7
Idaho	34	23	67.6	19	55.9	8	23.5	2	5.9	7	20.6	2	5.9	5	14.7	1	2.9	8	23.5
Montana	56	26	46.4	37	66.1	10	17.9	2	3.6	8	14.3	2	3.6	5	8.9	1	1.8	25	44.6
Nevada	33	12	36.4	17	51.5	12	36.4	4	12.1	10	30.3	3	9.1	7	21.2	2	6.1	6	18.2
New Mexico	38	21	55.3	24	63.2	11	28.9	2	5.3	10	26.3	2	5.3	7	18.4	1	2.6	7	18.4
Utah	36	29	80.6	31	86.1	15	41.7	3	8.3	12	33.3	3	8.3	9	25.0	4	11.1	12	33.3
Wyoming	28	19	67.9	21	75.0	2	7.1	0	0.0	3	10.7	0	0.0	2	7.1	0	0.0	10	35.7
CENSUS DIVISION 9, PACIFIC	472	307	65.0	343	72.7	197	41.7	46	9.7	174	36.9	39	8.3	149	31.6	37	7.8	170	36.0
Alaska	16	11	68.8	13	81.3	2	12.5	1	6.3	1	6.3	1	6.3	1	6.3	0	0.0	5	31.3
California	308	191	62.0	210	68.2	138	44.8	31	10.1	125	40.6	27	8.8	114	37.0	25	8.1	113	36.7
Hawaii	20	10	50.0	13	65.0	8	40.0	3	15.0	7	35.0	2	10.0	6	30.0	1	5.0	6	30.0
Oregon	60	50	83.3	53	88.3	21	35.0	5	8.3	15	25.0	4	6.7	12	20.0	4	6.7	22	36.7
Washington	68	45	66.2	54	79.4	28	41.2	6	8.8	26	38.2	5	7.4	16	23.5	7	10.3	24	35.3

AHA Hospital Statistics © 2008 Health Forum LLC, an affiliate of the American Hospital Association   157

Table 7 (Continued)

These data include only hospital-based facilities and services as reported by responding hospitals in Section C of the 2006 AHA Annual Survey, beginning on page 197. All hospitals are represented with Community Hospitals listed separately under United States. No estimates have been made for nonresponding hospitals. Definitions of facilities and services are listed in the Glossary, page 187.

CLASSIFICATION	HOSPITALS REPORTING	CASE MANAGEMENT Number	Percent	CHAPLAINCY/PASTORAL CARE SERVICES Number	Percent	CHEMOTHERAPY Number	Percent	CHILDREN WELLNESS PROGRAM Number	Percent	CHIROPRACTIC SERVICES Number	Percent	COMMUNITY OUTREACH Number	Percent	COMPLEMENTARY MEDICINE SERVICES Number	Percent	CRISIS PREVENTION Number	Percent	DENTAL SERVICES Number	Percent
UNITED STATES	4,836	3,940	81.5	3,076	63.6	2,456	50.8	913	18.9	120	2.5	3,165	65.4	914	18.9	1,021	21.1	1,113	23.0
COMMUNITY HOSPITALS	4,120	3,482	84.5	2,785	67.6	2,352	57.1	879	21.3	91	2.2	2,932	71.2	864	21.0	880	21.4	932	22.6
CENSUS DIVISION 1, NEW ENGLAND	218	199	91.3	164	75.2	154	70.6	69	31.7	13	6.0	179	82.1	83	38.1	75	34.4	67	30.7
Connecticut	35	31	88.6	29	82.9	26	74.3	13	37.1	3	8.6	29	82.9	13	37.1	21	60.0	16	45.7
Maine	39	37	94.9	24	61.5	29	74.4	10	25.6	1	2.6	32	82.1	11	28.2	7	17.9	9	23.1
Massachusetts	84	78	92.9	65	77.4	57	67.9	23	27.4	6	7.1	70	83.3	35	41.7	28	33.3	20	23.8
New Hampshire	30	28	93.3	22	73.3	21	70.0	13	43.3	1	3.3	25	83.3	14	46.7	12	40.0	14	46.7
Rhode Island	13	11	84.6	11	84.6	11	84.6	4	30.8	0	0.0	9	69.2	2	15.4	4	30.8	5	38.5
Vermont	17	14	82.4	13	76.5	10	58.8	6	35.3	2	11.8	14	82.4	8	47.1	3	17.6	3	17.6
CENSUS DIVISION 2, MIDDLE ATLANTIC	410	366	89.3	320	78.0	272	66.3	142	34.6	19	4.6	328	80.0	128	31.2	158	38.5	174	42.4
New Jersey	71	63	88.7	63	88.7	55	77.5	33	46.5	5	7.0	63	88.7	25	35.2	39	54.9	31	43.7
New York	161	148	91.9	126	78.3	107	66.5	54	33.5	10	6.2	132	82.0	58	36.0	68	42.2	73	45.3
Pennsylvania	178	155	87.1	131	73.6	110	61.8	55	30.9	4	2.2	133	74.7	45	25.3	51	28.7	70	39.3
CENSUS DIVISION 3, SOUTH ATLANTIC	696	605	86.9	529	76.0	386	55.5	133	19.1	12	1.7	501	72.0	125	18.0	148	21.3	171	24.6
Delaware	9	8	88.9	7	77.8	6	66.7	4	44.4	0	0.0	6	66.7	3	33.3	4	44.4	3	33.3
District of Columbia	11	10	90.9	9	81.8	6	54.5	2	18.2	0	0.0	7	63.6	3	27.3	3	27.3	4	36.4
Florida	147	135	91.8	111	75.5	95	64.6	20	13.6	4	2.7	96	65.3	27	18.4	26	17.7	21	14.3
Georgia	129	113	87.6	91	70.5	60	46.5	14	10.9	3	2.3	90	69.8	12	9.3	25	19.4	32	24.8
Maryland	56	49	87.5	49	87.5	40	71.4	18	32.1	1	1.8	47	83.9	22	39.3	23	41.1	15	26.8
North Carolina	119	107	89.9	99	83.2	72	60.5	24	20.2	3	2.5	90	75.6	17	14.3	20	16.8	31	26.1
South Carolina	82	65	79.3	54	65.9	31	37.8	22	26.8	0	0.0	65	79.3	3	3.7	5	6.1	17	20.7
Virginia	76	68	89.5	64	84.2	50	65.8	14	18.4	1	1.3	59	77.6	27	35.5	29	38.2	29	38.2
West Virginia	67	50	74.6	45	67.2	26	38.8	15	22.4	0	0.0	41	61.2	11	16.4	13	19.4	19	28.4
CENSUS DIVISION 4, EAST NORTH CENTRAL	746	628	84.2	521	69.8	445	59.7	184	24.7	29	3.9	534	71.6	214	28.7	212	28.4	200	26.8
Illinois	170	148	87.1	139	81.8	112	65.9	50	29.4	8	4.7	127	74.7	44	25.9	56	32.9	49	28.8
Indiana	114	100	87.7	82	71.9	69	60.5	29	25.4	1	0.9	83	72.8	27	23.7	22	19.3	26	22.8
Michigan	152	124	81.6	111	73.0	90	59.2	39	25.7	6	3.9	115	75.7	52	34.2	54	35.5	45	29.6
Ohio	166	151	91.0	123	74.1	111	66.9	43	25.9	10	6.0	132	79.5	43	25.9	44	26.5	56	33.7
Wisconsin	144	105	72.9	66	45.8	63	43.8	23	16.0	4	2.8	77	53.5	48	33.3	36	25.0	24	16.7
CENSUS DIVISION 5, EAST SOUTH CENTRAL	375	300	80.0	207	55.2	127	33.9	33	8.8	2	0.5	225	60.0	29	7.7	46	12.3	76	20.3
Alabama	65	58	89.2	39	60.0	30	46.2	5	7.7	1	1.5	36	55.4	3	4.6	8	12.3	6	9.2
Kentucky	97	87	89.7	79	81.4	46	47.4	17	17.5	1	1.0	64	66.0	19	19.6	16	16.5	23	23.7
Mississippi	110	62	56.4	19	17.3	11	10.0	3	2.7	0	0.0	61	55.5	2	1.8	5	4.5	33	30.0
Tennessee	103	93	90.3	70	68.0	40	38.8	8	7.8	0	0.0	64	62.1	5	4.9	17	16.5	14	13.6
CENSUS DIVISION 6, WEST NORTH CENTRAL	706	460	65.2	375	53.1	378	53.5	113	16.0	15	2.1	428	60.6	123	17.4	121	17.1	133	18.8
Iowa	125	96	76.8	60	48.0	87	69.6	26	20.8	2	1.6	93	74.4	37	29.6	26	20.8	24	19.2
Kansas	154	79	51.3	74	48.1	46	29.9	14	9.1	0	0.0	53	34.4	10	6.5	9	5.8	20	13.0
Minnesota	109	70	64.2	59	54.1	74	67.9	20	18.3	6	5.5	84	77.1	32	29.4	25	22.9	15	13.8
Missouri	147	123	83.7	107	72.8	69	46.9	24	16.3	6	4.1	97	66.0	28	19.0	38	25.9	50	34.0
Nebraska	75	42	56.0	33	44.0	45	60.0	13	17.3	0	0.0	46	61.3	5	6.7	13	17.3	11	14.7
North Dakota	38	17	44.7	24	63.2	26	68.4	9	23.7	0	0.0	20	52.6	7	18.4	5	13.2	3	7.9
South Dakota	58	33	56.9	18	31.0	31	53.4	7	12.1	1	1.7	35	60.3	4	6.9	5	8.6	10	17.2
CENSUS DIVISION 7, WEST SOUTH CENTRAL	872	713	81.8	435	49.9	257	29.5	95	10.9	4	0.5	404	46.3	59	6.8	79	9.1	141	16.2
Arkansas	105	90	85.7	57	54.3	34	32.4	6	5.7	0	0.0	61	58.1	7	6.7	12	11.4	18	17.1
Louisiana	99	84	84.8	45	45.5	38	38.4	20	20.2	0	0.0	52	52.5	11	11.1	18	18.2	20	20.2
Oklahoma	124	92	74.2	62	50.0	31	25.0	8	6.5	2	1.6	50	40.3	5	4.0	5	4.0	20	16.1
Texas	544	447	82.2	271	49.8	154	28.3	61	11.2	2	0.4	241	44.3	36	6.6	44	8.1	83	15.3
CENSUS DIVISION 8, MOUNTAIN	341	276	80.9	194	56.9	172	50.4	56	16.4	9	2.6	220	64.5	62	18.2	82	24.0	67	19.6
Arizona	52	50	96.2	45	86.5	31	59.6	12	23.1	1	1.9	33	63.5	14	26.9	16	30.8	15	28.8
Colorado	64	54	84.4	47	73.4	42	65.6	10	15.6	3	4.7	47	73.4	23	35.9	14	21.9	13	20.3
Idaho	34	24	70.6	19	55.9	17	50.0	6	17.6	2	5.9	25	73.5	6	17.6	5	14.7	9	26.5
Montana	56	29	51.8	21	37.5	21	37.5	11	19.6	1	1.8	34	60.7	7	12.5	10	17.9	5	8.9
Nevada	33	32	97.0	16	48.5	13	39.4	3	9.1	0	0.0	17	51.5	1	3.0	5	15.2	1	3.0
New Mexico	38	33	86.8	21	55.3	13	34.2	6	15.8	1	2.6	25	65.8	3	7.9	8	21.1	9	23.7
Utah	36	31	86.1	13	36.1	20	55.6	5	13.9	1	2.8	25	69.4	5	13.9	18	50.0	9	25.0
Wyoming	28	23	82.1	12	42.9	15	53.6	3	10.7	0	0.0	14	50.0	3	10.7	6	21.4	6	21.4
CENSUS DIVISION 9, PACIFIC	472	393	83.3	331	70.1	265	56.1	88	18.6	17	3.6	346	73.3	91	19.3	100	21.2	84	17.8
Alaska	16	11	68.8	9	56.3	10	62.5	3	18.8	1	6.3	10	62.5	2	12.5	6	37.5	4	25.0
California	308	266	86.4	216	70.1	171	55.5	60	19.5	14	4.5	234	76.0	56	18.2	59	19.2	62	20.1
Hawaii	20	16	80.0	10	50.0	13	65.0	2	10.0	1	5.0	12	60.0	5	25.0	4	20.0	4	20.0
Oregon	60	49	81.7	48	80.0	35	58.3	11	18.3	1	1.7	47	78.3	14	23.3	10	16.7	7	11.7
Washington	68	51	75.0	48	70.6	36	52.9	12	17.6	0	0.0	43	63.2	14	20.6	21	30.9	7	10.3

Table 7 (Continued)

These data include only hospital-based facilities and services as reported by responding hospitals in Section C of the 2006 AHA Annual Survey, beginning on page 197. All hospitals are represented with Community Hospitals listed separately under United States. No estimates have been made for nonresponding hospitals. Definitions of facilities and services are listed in the Glossary, page 187.

RADIOLOGY, DIAGNOSTIC

CLASSIFICATION	HOSPITALS REPORTING	CT SCANNER Number	CT SCANNER Percent	DIAGNOSTIC RADIOISOTOPE FACILITY Number	Percent	ELECTRON BEAM COMPUTED TOMOGRAPHY (EBCT) Number	Percent	FULL-FIELD DIGITAL MAMMOGRAPHY (FFDM) Number	Percent	MAGNETIC RESONANCE IMAGING (MRI) Number	Percent	MULTI-SLICE SPIRAL COMPUTED TOMOGRAPHY (<64 SLICE CT) Number	Percent	MULTI-SLICE SPIRAL COMPUTED TOMOGRAPHY (64+ SLICE CT) Number	Percent	POSITRON EMISSION TOMOGRAPHY (PET) Number	Percent	POSITRON EMISSION TOMOGRAPHY/CT (PET/CT) Number	Percent	SINGLE PHOTON EMISSION COMPUTERIZED TOMOGRAPHY (SPECT) Number	Percent	ULTRASOUND Number	Percent
UNITED STATES	4,896	3,926	81.2	2,665	55.1	306	6.3	836	17.3	2,822	58.4	2,544	52.6	929	19.2	689	14.2	661	13.7	1,743	36.0	3,861	79.8
COMMUNITY HOSPITALS	4,120	3,711	90.1	2,570	62.4	291	7.1	811	19.7	2,693	65.4	2,438	59.2	885	21.5	671	16.3	644	15.6	1,695	41.1	3,653	88.7
CENSUS DIVISION 1. NEW ENGLAND	218	183	83.9	152	69.7	11	5.0	48	22.0	128	58.7	127	58.3	63	28.9	53	24.3	46	21.1	113	51.8	183	83.9
Connecticut	35	28	80.0	26	74.3	6	17.1	10	28.6	26	74.3	21	60.0	12	34.3	16	45.7	18	51.4	24	68.6	28	80.0
Maine	39	35	89.7	30	76.9	0	0.0	10	25.6	20	51.3	19	48.7	11	28.2	4	10.3	2	5.1	20	51.3	33	84.6
Massachusetts	84	68	81.0	57	67.9	2	2.4	15	17.9	47	56.0	52	61.9	22	26.2	18	21.4	13	15.5	40	47.6	70	83.3
New Hampshire	30	27	90.0	18	60.0	1	3.3	6	20.0	17	56.7	19	63.3	10	33.3	9	30.0	7	23.3	14	46.7	27	90.0
Rhode Island	13	11	84.6	9	69.2	1	7.7	4	30.8	10	76.9	7	53.8	3	23.1	2	15.4	2	15.4	8	61.5	11	84.6
Vermont	17	14	82.4	12	70.6	1	5.9	3	17.6	8	47.1	9	52.9	5	29.4	4	23.5	4	23.5	7	41.2	14	82.4
CENSUS DIVISION 2. MIDDLE ATLANTIC	410	347	84.6	291	71.0	51	12.4	114	27.8	267	65.1	250	61.0	109	26.6	96	23.4	81	19.8	222	54.1	351	85.6
New Jersey	71	58	81.7	52	73.2	15	21.1	25	35.2	47	66.2	46	64.8	22	31.0	19	26.8	20	28.2	44	62.0	58	81.7
New York	161	142	88.2	117	72.7	18	11.2	51	31.7	98	60.9	94	58.4	45	28.0	35	21.7	29	18.0	74	46.0	144	89.4
Pennsylvania	178	147	82.6	122	68.5	18	10.1	38	21.3	122	68.5	110	61.8	42	23.6	42	23.6	32	18.0	104	58.4	149	83.7
CENSUS DIVISION 3. SOUTH ATLANTIC	696	581	83.5	461	66.2	57	8.2	124	17.8	470	67.5	433	62.2	147	21.1	131	18.8	122	17.5	317	45.5	583	83.8
Delaware	9	6	66.7	5	55.6	2	22.2	1	11.1	5	55.6	5	55.6	2	22.2	3	33.3	2	22.2	6	44.4	6	66.7
District of Columbia	11	6	54.5	6	54.5	0	0.0	4	36.4	6	54.5	6	54.5	2	18.2	2	18.2	2	18.2	5	45.5	7	63.6
Florida	147	130	88.4	113	76.9	26	17.7	38	25.9	118	80.3	105	71.4	36	24.5	40	27.2	36	24.5	70	47.6	132	89.8
Georgia	129	109	84.5	80	62.0	4	3.1	25	19.4	88	68.2	72	55.8	22	17.1	17	13.2	21	16.3	50	38.8	109	84.5
Maryland	56	48	85.7	41	73.2	3	5.4	9	16.1	37	66.1	37	66.1	16	28.6	13	23.2	11	19.6	34	60.7	47	83.9
North Carolina	119	103	86.6	73	61.3	10	8.4	15	12.6	78	65.5	78	65.5	33	27.7	22	18.5	20	16.8	52	43.7	103	86.6
South Carolina	82	61	74.4	51	62.2	4	4.9	7	8.5	44	53.7	40	48.8	7	8.5	9	11.0	6	7.3	25	30.5	61	74.4
Virginia	76	64	84.2	55	72.4	6	7.9	18	23.7	60	78.9	54	71.1	19	25.0	16	21.1	18	23.7	49	64.5	66	86.8
West Virginia	67	54	80.6	37	55.2	2	3.0	7	10.4	34	50.7	36	53.7	10	14.9	9	13.4	6	9.0	28	41.8	52	77.6
CENSUS DIVISION 4. EAST NORTH CENTRAL	746	647	86.7	487	65.3	58	7.8	146	19.6	468	62.7	451	60.5	186	24.9	142	19.0	154	20.6	359	48.1	632	84.7
Illinois	170	157	92.4	117	68.8	11	6.5	33	19.4	98	57.6	112	65.9	45	26.5	26	15.3	29	17.1	78	45.9	152	89.4
Indiana	114	94	82.5	68	59.6	6	5.3	29	25.4	82	71.9	65	57.0	31	27.2	17	14.9	19	16.7	40	35.1	94	82.5
Michigan	152	129	84.9	102	67.1	10	6.6	27	17.8	83	54.6	91	59.9	39	25.7	27	17.8	33	21.7	82	53.9	129	84.9
Ohio	166	153	92.2	127	76.5	17	10.2	33	19.9	129	77.7	115	69.3	43	25.9	45	27.1	43	25.9	102	61.4	150	90.4
Wisconsin	144	114	79.2	73	50.7	14	9.7	24	16.7	76	52.8	68	47.2	28	19.4	27	18.8	30	20.8	57	39.6	107	74.3
CENSUS DIVISION 5. EAST SOUTH CENTRAL	375	306	81.6	199	53.1	13	3.5	61	16.3	225	60.0	154	41.1	69	18.4	49	13.1	43	11.5	127	33.9	306	81.6
Alabama	65	56	86.2	40	61.5	1	1.5	16	24.6	43	66.2	32	49.2	13	20.0	10	15.4	10	15.4	26	40.0	54	83.1
Kentucky	97	86	88.7	55	56.7	6	6.2	21	21.6	61	62.9	49	50.5	23	23.7	12	12.4	13	13.4	33	34.0	87	89.7
Mississippi	110	80	72.7	51	46.4	4	3.6	8	7.3	48	43.6	17	15.5	11	10.0	13	11.8	8	7.3	32	29.1	84	76.4
Tennessee	103	84	81.6	53	51.5	2	1.9	16	15.5	73	70.9	56	54.4	22	21.4	14	13.6	12	11.7	36	35.0	81	78.6
CENSUS DIVISION 6. WEST NORTH CENTRAL	706	562	79.6	276	39.1	17	2.4	80	11.3	354	50.1	343	48.6	77	10.9	66	9.3	74	10.5	178	25.2	525	74.4
Iowa	125	113	90.4	52	41.6	3	2.4	18	14.4	63	50.4	78	62.4	12	9.6	10	8.0	13	10.4	39	31.2	108	86.4
Kansas	154	109	70.8	52	33.8	1	0.6	6	3.9	56	36.4	51	33.1	12	7.8	5	3.2	5	3.2	27	17.5	92	59.7
Minnesota	109	95	87.2	43	39.4	5	4.6	17	15.6	57	52.3	67	61.5	15	13.8	8	7.3	12	11.0	24	22.0	86	78.9
Missouri	147	119	81.0	76	51.7	3	2.0	21	14.3	108	73.5	81	55.1	15	10.2	23	15.6	20	13.6	55	37.4	116	78.9
Nebraska	75	62	82.7	25	33.3	2	2.7	11	14.7	33	44.0	32	42.7	12	16.0	9	12.0	15	20.0	17	22.7	56	74.7
North Dakota	38	29	76.3	12	31.6	3	7.9	3	7.9	18	47.4	19	50.0	3	7.9	6	15.8	6	15.8	7	18.4	26	68.4
South Dakota	58	35	60.3	16	27.6	0	0.0	4	6.9	19	32.8	15	25.9	8	13.8	5	8.6	3	5.2	9	15.5	41	70.7
CENSUS DIVISION 7. WEST SOUTH CENTRAL	872	620	71.1	353	40.5	36	4.1	101	11.6	418	47.9	363	41.6	131	15.0	50	5.7	52	6.0	176	20.2	594	68.1
Arkansas	105	79	75.2	37	35.2	5	4.8	6	5.7	55	52.4	51	48.6	12	11.4	4	3.8	3	2.9	18	17.1	76	72.4
Louisiana	99	70	70.7	46	46.5	6	6.1	21	21.2	44	44.4	45	45.5	23	23.2	6	6.1	9	9.1	23	23.2	74	74.7
Oklahoma	124	90	72.6	43	34.7	4	3.2	19	15.3	56	45.2	39	31.5	20	16.1	11	8.9	8	6.5	20	16.1	89	71.8
Texas	544	381	70.0	227	41.7	21	3.9	55	10.1	263	48.3	228	41.9	76	14.0	29	5.3	32	5.9	115	21.1	355	65.3
CENSUS DIVISION 8. MOUNTAIN	341	274	80.4	158	46.3	21	6.2	51	15.0	205	60.1	173	50.7	64	18.8	29	8.5	25	7.3	84	24.6	270	79.2
Arizona	52	45	86.5	32	61.5	4	7.7	8	15.4	38	73.1	32	61.5	18	34.6	8	15.4	6	11.5	25	48.1	44	84.6
Colorado	64	55	85.9	34	53.1	5	7.8	9	14.1	45	70.3	39	60.9	11	17.2	9	14.1	7	10.9	19	29.7	56	87.5
Idaho	34	30	88.2	11	32.4	0	0.0	4	11.8	20	58.8	20	58.8	4	11.8	2	5.9	1	2.9	5	14.7	30	88.2
Montana	56	39	69.6	19	33.9	2	3.6	7	12.5	19	33.9	21	37.5	6	10.7	1	1.8	1	1.8	9	16.1	39	69.6
Nevada	33	22	66.7	13	39.4	1	3.0	7	21.2	20	60.6	14	42.4	6	18.2	2	6.1	2	6.1	7	21.2	21	63.6
New Mexico	38	28	73.7	15	39.5	2	5.3	2	5.3	19	50.0	20	52.6	4	10.5	2	5.3	2	5.3	7	18.4	27	71.1
Utah	36	31	86.1	20	55.6	3	8.3	11	30.6	27	75.0	15	41.7	11	30.6	5	13.9	6	16.7	7	19.4	29	80.6
Wyoming	28	24	85.7	14	50.0	4	14.3	3	10.7	17	60.7	12	42.9	4	14.3	0	0.0	0	0.0	5	17.9	24	85.7
CENSUS DIVISION 9. PACIFIC	472	406	86.0	288	61.0	42	8.9	111	23.5	287	60.8	250	53.0	83	17.6	73	15.5	64	13.6	167	35.4	417	88.3
Alaska	16	14	87.5	5	31.3	0	0.0	4	25.0	9	56.3	4	25.0	4	25.0	0	0.0	0	0.0	2	12.5	15	93.8
California	308	262	85.1	195	63.3	30	9.7	67	21.8	191	62.0	154	50.0	53	17.2	50	16.2	44	14.3	114	37.0	269	87.3
Hawaii	20	14	70.0	12	60.0	1	5.0	4	20.0	12	60.0	8	40.0	0	0.0	2	10.0	2	10.0	5	25.0	15	75.0
Oregon	60	58	96.7	38	63.3	3	5.0	21	35.0	36	60.0	45	75.0	13	21.7	7	11.7	5	8.3	25	41.7	58	96.7
Washington	68	58	85.3	38	55.9	8	11.8	15	22.1	39	57.4	39	57.4	13	16.2	14	20.6	13	19.1	21	30.9	60	88.2

Table 7 (Continued)

These data include only hospital-based facilities and services as reported by responding hospitals in Section C of the 2006 AHA Annual Survey, beginning on page 197. All hospitals are represented with Community Hospitals listed separately under United States. No estimates have been made for nonresponding hospitals. Definitions of facilities and services are listed in the Glossary, page 187.

CLASSIFICATION	HOSPITALS REPORTING	ENABLING SERVICES		ENROLLMENT ASSISTANCE SERVICES		EXTRACORPOREAL SHOCK WAVE LITHOTRIPTER (ESWL)		EMERGENCY SERVICES				TRAUMA CENTER (CERTIFIED)		FITNESS CENTER		REPRODUCTIVE HEALTH			
								EMERGENCY DEPARTMENT		FREESTANDING/ SATELLITE EMERGENCY DEPARTMENT						FERTILITY CLINIC		GENETIC TESTING/ COUNSELING	
		Number	Percent	Number	Percent	Number	Percent	Number	Percent	Number	Percent	Number	Percent	Number	Percent	Number	Percent	Number	Percent
UNITED STATES	4,836	1,052	21.8	2,019	41.7	1,089	22.5	4,061	84.0	189	3.9	1,469	30.4	1,348	27.9	300	6.2	492	10.2
COMMUNITY HOSPITALS	4,120	965	23.4	1,860	45.1	1,055	25.6	3,833	93.0	179	4.3	1,436	34.9	1,253	30.4	290	7.0	481	11.7
CENSUS DIVISION 1, NEW ENGLAND	218	70	32.1	143	65.6	93	42.7	180	82.6	14	6.4	71	32.6	59	27.1	32	14.7	37	17.0
Connecticut	35	14	40.0	21	60.0	17	48.6	28	80.0	6	17.1	14	40.0	16	45.7	5	14.3	9	25.7
Maine	39	8	20.5	23	59.0	18	46.2	35	89.7	1	2.6	10	25.6	12	30.8	5	12.8	4	10.3
Massachusetts	84	28	33.3	63	75.0	30	35.7	63	75.0	4	4.8	25	29.8	11	13.1	11	13.1	18	21.4
New Hampshire	30	13	43.3	22	73.3	15	50.0	27	90.0	3	10.0	14	46.7	12	40.0	6	20.0	4	13.3
Rhode Island	13	2	15.4	6	46.2	8	61.5	12	92.3	0	0.0	3	23.1	3	23.1	2	15.4	1	7.7
Vermont	17	5	29.4	8	47.1	5	29.4	15	88.2	0	0.0	5	29.4	5	29.4	3	17.6	1	5.9
CENSUS DIVISION 2, MIDDLE ATLANTIC	410	142	34.6	235	57.3	126	30.7	343	83.7	12	2.9	88	21.5	125	30.5	53	12.9	92	22.4
New Jersey	71	36	50.7	46	64.8	20	28.2	57	80.3	2	2.8	13	18.3	22	31.0	9	12.7	23	32.4
New York	161	50	31.1	91	56.5	47	29.2	137	85.1	6	3.7	44	27.3	42	26.1	27	16.8	39	24.2
Pennsylvania	178	56	31.5	98	55.1	59	33.1	149	83.7	4	2.2	31	17.4	61	34.3	17	9.6	30	16.9
CENSUS DIVISION 3, SOUTH ATLANTIC	696	184	26.4	338	48.6	199	28.6	580	83.3	22	3.2	149	21.4	211	30.3	40	5.7	81	11.6
Delaware	9	3	33.3	4	44.4	4	44.4	6	66.7	1	11.1	4	44.4	4	44.4	0	0.0	1	11.1
District of Columbia	11	3	27.3	5	45.5	2	18.2	6	54.5	1	9.1	4	36.4	3	27.3	2	18.2	4	36.4
Florida	147	34	23.1	67	45.6	50	34.0	130	88.4	3	2.0	24	16.3	59	40.1	7	4.8	25	17.0
Georgia	129	35	27.1	66	51.2	37	28.7	106	82.2	2	1.6	20	15.5	29	22.5	5	3.9	9	7.0
Maryland	56	25	44.6	37	66.1	23	41.1	47	83.9	2	3.6	12	21.4	13	23.2	7	12.5	18	32.1
North Carolina	119	31	26.1	54	45.4	20	16.8	104	87.4	3	2.5	19	16.0	37	31.1	9	7.6	10	8.4
South Carolina	82	8	9.8	26	31.7	17	20.7	60	73.2	3	3.7	22	26.8	23	28.0	3	3.7	5	6.1
Virginia	76	31	40.8	51	67.1	29	38.2	65	85.5	6	7.9	16	21.1	21	27.6	4	5.3	5	6.6
West Virginia	67	14	20.9	28	41.8	17	25.4	56	83.6	1	1.5	28	41.8	22	32.8	3	4.5	6	6.0
CENSUS DIVISION 4, EAST NORTH CENTRAL	746	226	30.3	364	48.8	183	24.5	647	86.7	56	7.5	252	33.8	251	33.6	60	8.0	99	13.3
Illinois	170	44	25.9	88	51.8	29	17.1	158	92.9	11	6.5	65	38.2	53	31.2	16	9.4	28	16.5
Indiana	114	24	21.1	58	50.9	28	24.6	91	79.8	3	2.6	19	16.7	33	28.9	5	4.4	11	9.6
Michigan	152	59	38.8	84	55.3	44	28.9	127	83.6	11	7.2	43	28.3	49	32.2	18	11.8	19	12.5
Ohio	166	56	33.7	85	51.2	49	29.5	150	90.4	19	11.4	47	28.3	60	36.1	17	10.2	26	15.7
Wisconsin	144	43	29.9	49	34.0	33	22.9	121	84.0	12	8.3	78	54.2	56	38.9	4	2.8	15	10.4
CENSUS DIVISION 5, EAST SOUTH CENTRAL	375	45	12.0	98	26.1	92	24.5	314	83.7	19	5.1	122	32.5	107	28.5	16	4.3	13	3.5
Alabama	65	11	16.9	21	32.3	20	30.8	57	87.7	0	0.0	20	30.8	21	32.3	2	3.1	3	4.6
Kentucky	97	14	14.4	43	44.3	22	22.7	86	88.7	4	4.1	21	21.6	26	26.8	7	7.2	4	4.1
Mississippi	110	1	0.9	5	5.5	19	17.3	87	79.1	14	12.7	68	61.8	32	29.1	5	4.5	1	0.9
Tennessee	103	19	18.4	28	27.2	31	30.1	84	81.6	1	1.0	13	12.6	28	27.2	2	1.9	5	4.9
CENSUS DIVISION 6, WEST NORTH CENTRAL	706	136	19.3	237	33.6	90	12.7	624	88.4	22	3.1	214	30.3	237	33.6	30	4.2	45	6.4
Iowa	125	32	25.6	52	41.6	12	9.6	119	95.2	1	0.8	84	67.2	53	42.4	8	6.4	7	5.6
Kansas	154	16	10.4	31	20.1	19	12.3	128	83.1	2	1.3	12	7.8	42	27.3	2	1.3	5	3.2
Minnesota	109	18	16.5	38	34.9	13	11.9	101	92.7	4	3.7	31	28.4	30	27.5	6	5.5	10	9.2
Missouri	147	44	29.9	64	43.5	28	19.0	121	82.3	9	6.1	29	19.7	50	34.0	8	5.4	18	12.2
Nebraska	75	10	13.3	18	24.0	9	12.0	67	89.3	3	4.0	25	33.3	28	37.3	3	4.0	2	2.7
North Dakota	38	10	26.3	21	55.3	4	10.5	36	94.7	3	7.9	23	60.5	16	42.1	1	2.6	1	2.6
South Dakota	58	6	10.3	13	22.4	5	8.6	52	89.7	0	0.0	10	17.2	18	31.0	0	0.0	2	3.4
CENSUS DIVISION 7, WEST SOUTH CENTRAL	872	93	10.7	262	30.0	145	16.6	670	76.8	19	2.2	290	33.3	180	20.6	26	3.0	44	5.0
Arkansas	105	7	6.7	33	31.4	17	16.2	81	77.1	3	2.9	16	15.2	21	20.0	1	1.0	3	2.9
Louisiana	99	7	7.1	32	32.3	9	9.1	70	70.7	3	3.0	15	15.2	17	17.2	4	4.0	6	6.1
Oklahoma	124	5	4.0	18	14.5	17	13.7	109	87.9	3	2.4	42	33.9	21	16.9	4	3.2	6	4.8
Texas	544	74	13.6	179	32.9	102	18.8	410	75.4	10	1.8	217	39.9	121	22.2	17	3.1	29	5.3
CENSUS DIVISION 8, MOUNTAIN	341	60	17.6	139	40.8	67	19.6	290	85.0	15	4.4	123	36.1	81	23.8	15	4.4	21	6.2
Arizona	52	11	21.2	25	48.1	18	34.6	44	84.6	1	1.9	17	32.7	12	23.1	3	5.8	5	9.6
Colorado	64	15	23.4	29	45.3	11	17.2	56	87.5	7	10.9	47	73.4	24	37.5	5	7.8	7	10.9
Idaho	34	6	17.6	12	35.3	7	20.6	30	88.2	0	0.0	7	20.6	8	23.5	0	0.0	2	5.9
Montana	56	6	10.7	26	46.4	7	12.5	52	92.9	1	1.8	12	21.4	10	17.9	1	1.8	2	3.6
Nevada	33	4	12.1	7	21.2	3	9.1	21	63.6	3	9.1	5	15.2	3	9.1	0	0.0	0	0.0
New Mexico	38	6	15.8	17	44.7	10	26.3	30	78.9	1	2.6	6	15.8	8	21.1	1	2.6	1	2.6
Utah	36	11	30.6	16	44.4	5	13.9	32	88.9	0	0.0	11	30.6	12	33.3	5	13.9	3	8.3
Wyoming	28	1	3.6	7	25.0	6	21.4	25	89.3	2	7.1	18	64.3	4	14.3	0	0.0	1	3.6
CENSUS DIVISION 9, PACIFIC	472	96	20.3	203	43.0	94	19.9	413	87.5	10	2.1	160	33.9	97	20.6	28	5.9	60	12.7
Alaska	16	1	6.3	6	37.5	2	12.5	16	100.0	0	0.0	2	12.5	2	12.5	1	6.3	3	18.8
California	308	58	18.8	135	43.8	64	20.8	259	84.1	7	2.3	60	19.5	58	18.8	20	6.5	44	14.3
Hawaii	20	3	15.0	6	30.0	4	20.0	16	80.0	0	0.0	4	20.0	2	10.0	1	5.0	1	5.0
Oregon	60	19	31.7	37	61.7	11	18.3	58	96.7	0	0.0	42	70.0	19	31.7	3	5.0	3	5.0
Washington	68	15	22.1	19	27.9	13	19.1	64	94.1	3	4.4	52	76.5	16	23.5	3	4.4	9	13.2

Table 7 (Continued)

These data include only hospital-based facilities and services as reported by responding hospitals in Section C of the 2006 AHA Annual Survey, beginning on page 197. All hospitals are represented with Community Hospitals listed separately under United States. No estimates have been made for nonresponding hospitals. Definitions of facilities and services are listed in the Glossary, page 187.

Facilities and Services

CLASSIFICATION	HOSPITALS REPORTING	GERIATRIC SERVICES Number	Percent	HEALTH FAIR Number	Percent	HEALTH INFORMATION CENTER Number	Percent	HEALTH SCREENINGS Number	Percent	HEMODIALYSIS Number	Percent	HIV/AIDS SERVICES Number	Percent	HOME HEALTH SERVICES Number	Percent	IMAGE-GUIDED RADIATION THERAPY (IGRT) Number	Percent	INTENSITY-MODULATED RADIATION THERAPY (IMRT) Number	Percent	SHAPED BEAM RADIATION SYSTEM Number	Percent
UNITED STATES	4,836	1,865	38.6	3,420	70.7	2,203	45.6	3,500	72.4	1,367	28.3	1,203	24.9	1,618	33.5	487	10.1	946	19.6	772	16.0
COMMUNITY HOSPITALS	4,120	1,670	40.5	3,220	78.2	2,035	49.4	3,281	79.6	1,270	30.8	1,094	26.6	1,550	37.6	476	11.6	923	22.4	752	18.3
CENSUS DIVISION 1, NEW ENGLAND	218	112	51.4	164	75.2	140	64.2	187	85.8	75	34.4	102	46.8	51	23.4	19	8.7	55	25.2	42	19.3
Connecticut	35	20	57.1	25	71.4	25	71.4	27	77.1	16	45.7	22	62.9	10	28.6	6	17.1	17	48.6	11	31.4
Maine	39	16	41.0	30	76.9	18	46.2	35	89.7	6	15.4	13	33.3	9	23.1	1	2.6	5	12.8	4	10.3
Massachusetts	84	42	50.0	60	71.4	56	66.7	69	82.1	34	40.5	39	46.4	22	26.2	8	9.5	23	27.4	20	23.8
New Hampshire	30	16	53.3	28	93.3	19	63.3	27	90.0	9	30.0	16	53.3	6	20.0	2	6.7	6	20.0	5	16.7
Rhode Island	13	10	76.9	10	76.9	11	84.6	12	92.3	8	61.5	6	46.2	3	23.1	1	7.7	1	7.7	0	0.0
Vermont	17	8	47.1	11	64.7	11	64.7	17	100.0	2	11.8	6	35.3	1	5.9	1	5.9	3	17.6	2	11.8
CENSUS DIVISION 2, MIDDLE ATLANTIC	410	230	56.1	323	78.8	226	55.1	333	81.2	185	45.1	182	44.4	126	30.7	76	18.5	145	35.4	119	29.0
New Jersey	71	48	67.6	57	80.3	46	64.8	57	80.3	46	64.8	40	56.3	21	29.6	17	23.9	38	53.5	35	49.3
New York	161	92	57.1	129	80.1	90	55.9	129	80.1	88	54.7	73	45.3	36	22.4	30	18.6	50	31.1	37	23.0
Pennsylvania	178	90	50.6	137	77.0	90	50.6	147	82.6	51	28.7	69	38.8	69	38.8	29	16.3	57	32.0	47	26.4
CENSUS DIVISION 3, SOUTH ATLANTIC	696	282	40.5	553	79.5	357	51.3	551	79.2	267	38.4	225	32.3	200	28.7	81	11.6	166	23.9	135	19.4
Delaware	9	6	66.7	5	55.6	4	44.4	5	55.6	4	44.4	4	44.4	5	55.6	1	11.1	4	44.4	4	44.4
District of Columbia	11	6	54.5	8	72.7	6	54.5	6	54.5	6	54.5	5	45.5	2	18.2	2	18.2	3	27.3	3	27.3
Florida	147	61	41.5	109	74.1	75	51.0	113	76.9	70	47.6	51	34.7	35	23.8	23	15.6	38	25.9	34	23.1
Georgia	129	41	31.8	99	76.7	60	46.5	101	78.3	43	33.3	35	27.1	22	17.1	6	4.7	20	15.5	19	14.7
Maryland	56	31	55.4	48	85.7	40	71.4	49	87.5	34	60.7	24	42.9	13	23.2	11	19.6	19	33.9	15	26.8
North Carolina	119	47	39.5	97	81.5	62	52.1	97	81.5	38	31.9	30	25.2	45	37.8	15	12.6	33	27.7	25	21.0
South Carolina	82	39	47.6	64	78.0	35	42.7	62	75.6	25	30.5	31	37.8	18	22.0	5	6.1	14	17.1	9	11.0
Virginia	76	30	39.5	66	86.8	48	63.2	64	84.2	35	46.1	32	42.1	33	43.4	14	18.4	27	35.5	20	26.3
West Virginia	67	21	31.3	57	85.1	27	40.3	54	80.6	12	17.9	13	19.4	27	40.3	4	6.0	8	11.9	6	9.0
CENSUS DIVISION 4, EAST NORTH CENTRAL	748	384	51.5	552	74.0	474	63.5	591	79.2	221	29.6	194	26.0	278	37.3	97	13.0	193	25.9	153	20.5
Illinois	170	85	50.0	136	80.0	92	54.1	145	85.3	51	30.0	56	32.9	72	42.4	19	11.2	51	30.0	40	23.5
Indiana	114	45	39.5	86	75.4	60	52.6	90	78.9	24	21.1	23	20.2	46	40.4	22	19.3	33	28.9	22	19.3
Michigan	152	72	47.4	110	72.4	85	55.9	123	80.9	51	33.6	52	34.2	60	39.5	18	11.8	34	22.4	30	19.7
Ohio	166	74	44.6	144	86.7	101	60.8	150	90.4	63	38.0	55	33.1	72	43.4	20	12.0	43	25.9	37	22.3
Wisconsin	144	108	75.0	76	52.8	136	94.4	83	57.6	32	22.2	8	5.6	28	19.4	18	12.5	32	22.2	24	16.7
CENSUS DIVISION 5, EAST SOUTH CENTRAL	375	102	27.2	230	61.3	109	29.1	221	58.9	68	18.1	78	20.8	119	31.7	26	6.9	58	15.5	40	10.7
Alabama	65	16	24.6	51	78.5	27	41.5	46	70.8	19	29.2	14	21.5	24	36.9	4	6.2	11	16.9	7	10.8
Kentucky	97	29	29.9	86	88.7	52	53.6	83	85.6	19	19.6	16	16.5	43	44.3	6	6.2	15	15.5	10	10.3
Mississippi	110	19	17.3	22	20.0	8	7.3	19	17.3	0	0.0	29	26.4	18	16.4	8	7.3	7	6.4	5	4.5
Tennessee	103	38	36.9	71	68.9	22	21.4	73	70.9	30	29.1	19	18.4	34	33.0	8	7.8	25	24.3	18	17.5
CENSUS DIVISION 6, WEST NORTH CENTRAL	706	262	37.1	490	69.4	269	38.1	525	74.4	133	18.8	127	18.0	330	46.7	48	6.8	96	13.6	83	11.8
Iowa	125	57	45.6	101	80.8	62	49.6	117	93.6	28	22.4	28	22.4	71	56.8	8	6.4	13	10.4	11	8.8
Kansas	154	43	27.9	82	53.2	31	20.1	75	48.7	11	7.1	19	12.3	58	37.7	5	3.2	15	9.7	14	9.1
Minnesota	109	50	45.9	75	68.8	43	39.4	85	78.0	15	13.8	18	16.5	56	51.4	10	9.2	16	14.7	11	10.1
Missouri	147	59	40.1	112	76.2	77	52.4	118	80.3	45	30.6	42	28.6	60	40.8	11	7.5	27	18.4	26	17.7
Nebraska	75	18	24.0	58	77.3	24	32.0	52	69.3	14	18.7	7	9.3	39	52.0	7	9.3	12	16.0	11	14.7
North Dakota	38	17	44.7	24	63.2	14	36.8	28	73.7	9	23.7	4	10.5	17	44.7	4	10.5	6	15.8	5	13.2
South Dakota	58	18	31.0	38	65.5	18	31.0	50	86.2	11	19.0	9	15.5	29	50.0	3	5.2	7	12.1	5	8.6
CENSUS DIVISION 7, WEST SOUTH CENTRAL	872	246	28.2	540	61.9	256	29.4	513	58.8	173	19.8	114	13.1	236	27.1	41	4.7	60	6.9	61	7.0
Arkansas	105	30	28.6	74	70.5	29	27.6	77	73.3	18	17.1	17	16.2	54	51.4	6	5.7	5	4.8	5	4.8
Louisiana	99	30	30.3	62	62.6	32	32.3	60	60.6	24	24.2	17	17.2	13	13.1	6	6.1	11	11.1	9	9.1
Oklahoma	124	24	19.4	68	54.8	37	29.8	61	49.2	21	16.9	11	8.9	50	40.3	8	6.5	0	0.0	15	12.1
Texas	544	162	29.8	336	61.8	158	29.0	315	57.9	110	20.2	69	12.7	119	21.9	21	3.9	44	8.1	32	5.9
CENSUS DIVISION 8, MOUNTAIN	341	105	30.8	239	70.1	138	40.5	241	70.7	87	25.5	63	18.5	117	34.3	32	9.4	62	18.2	50	14.7
Arizona	52	13	25.0	32	61.5	26	50.0	35	67.3	28	53.8	14	26.9	13	25.0	7	13.5	12	23.1	10	19.2
Colorado	64	21	32.8	44	68.8	29	45.3	46	71.9	18	28.1	17	26.6	22	34.4	7	10.9	17	26.6	11	17.2
Idaho	34	10	29.4	25	73.5	15	44.1	26	76.5	5	14.7	4	11.8	13	38.2	4	11.8	6	17.6	5	14.7
Montana	56	24	42.9	47	83.9	19	33.9	46	82.1	6	10.7	10	17.9	24	42.9	3	5.4	5	8.9	5	8.9
Nevada	33	6	18.2	18	54.5	9	27.3	17	51.5	5	15.2	6	18.2	9	27.3	3	9.1	2	6.1	2	6.1
New Mexico	38	6	15.8	23	60.5	10	26.3	23	60.5	8	21.1	4	10.5	12	31.6	1	2.6	7	18.4	4	10.5
Utah	36	14	38.9	30	83.3	22	61.1	29	80.6	10	27.8	6	16.7	13	36.1	4	11.1	7	19.4	7	19.4
Wyoming	28	11	39.3	20	71.4	8	28.6	19	67.9	7	25.0	2	7.1	11	39.3	3	10.7	5	17.9	4	14.3
CENSUS DIVISION 9, PACIFIC	472	142	30.1	329	69.7	234	49.6	338	71.6	158	33.5	118	25.0	161	34.1	67	14.2	111	23.5	89	18.9
Alaska	16	5	31.3	13	81.3	6	37.5	12	75.0	2	12.5	5	31.3	10	62.5	1	6.3	2	12.5	1	6.3
California	308	94	30.5	216	70.1	154	50.0	214	69.5	115	37.3	83	26.9	92	29.9	42	13.6	72	23.4	61	19.8
Hawaii	20	6	30.0	9	45.0	5	25.0	13	65.0	8	40.0	5	25.0	4	20.0	4	20.0	5	25.0	2	10.0
Oregon	60	20	33.3	46	76.7	37	61.7	54	90.0	16	26.7	12	20.0	36	60.0	10	16.7	15	25.0	12	20.0
Washington	68	17	25.0	45	66.2	32	47.1	45	66.2	17	25.0	13	19.1	19	27.9	10	14.7	17	25.0	13	19.1

AHA Hospital Statistics © 2008 Health Forum LLC, an affiliate of the American Hospital Association 161

Table 7 (Continued)

These data include only hospital-based facilities and services as reported by responding hospitals in Section C of the 2006 AHA Annual Survey, beginning on page 197. All hospitals are represented with Community Hospitals listed separately under United States. No estimates have been made for nonresponding hospitals. Definitions of facilities and services are listed in the Glossary, page 187.

CLASSIFICATION	HOSPITALS REPORTING	MEALS ON WHEELS		NEUROLOGICAL SERVICES		NUTRITION PROGRAMS CENTER		OCCUPATIONAL HEALTH SERVICES		ONCOLOGY SERVICES		ORTHOPEDIC SERVICES		FREESTANDING OUTPATIENT CARE CENTER		HOSPITAL-BASED OUTPATIENT CARE CENTER SERVICES		OUTPATIENT SURGERY	
		Number	Percent	Number	Percent	Number	Percent	Number	Percent	Number	Percent	Number	Percent	Number	Percent	Number	Percent	Number	Percent
UNITED STATES	4,836	531	11.0	2,122	43.9	3,534	73.1	3,041	62.9	2,488	51.4	3,176	65.7	1,294	26.8	3,484	72.0	3,936	81.4
COMMUNITY HOSPITALS	4,120	523	12.7	1,969	47.8	3,193	77.5	2,801	68.0	2,389	58.0	2,974	72.2	1,180	28.6	3,236	78.5	3,722	90.3
CENSUS DIVISION 1, NEW ENGLAND	218	14	6.4	139	63.8	201	92.2	171	78.4	167	76.6	178	81.7	85	39.0	185	84.9	184	84.4
Connecticut	35	5	14.3	29	82.9	31	88.6	25	71.4	26	74.3	28	80.0	17	48.6	30	85.7	28	80.0
Maine	39	4	10.3	18	46.2	37	94.9	26	66.7	32	82.1	35	89.7	16	41.0	30	76.9	35	89.7
Massachusetts	84	3	3.6	57	67.9	76	90.5	69	82.1	65	77.4	66	78.6	32	38.1	73	86.9	67	79.8
New Hampshire	30	1	3.3	16	53.3	30	100.0	27	90.0	23	76.7	26	86.7	12	40.0	27	90.0	27	90.0
Rhode Island	13	1	7.7	11	84.6	11	84.6	10	76.9	11	84.6	10	76.9	4	30.8	11	84.6	12	92.3
Vermont	17	0	0.0	8	47.1	16	94.1	14	82.4	10	58.8	13	76.5	4	23.5	14	82.4	15	88.2
CENSUS DIVISION 2, MIDDLE ATLANTIC	410	49	12.0	278	67.8	348	84.9	308	75.1	282	68.8	340	82.9	197	48.0	330	80.5	348	84.9
New Jersey	71	15	21.1	53	74.6	60	84.5	47	66.2	54	76.1	56	78.9	28	39.4	60	84.5	58	81.7
New York	161	18	11.2	112	69.6	134	83.2	121	75.2	108	67.1	137	85.1	92	57.1	135	83.9	143	88.8
Pennsylvania	178	16	9.0	113	63.5	154	86.5	140	78.7	120	67.4	147	82.6	77	43.3	135	75.8	147	82.6
CENSUS DIVISION 3, SOUTH ATLANTIC	696	38	5.5	374	53.7	555	79.7	462	66.4	396	56.9	522	75.0	220	31.6	519	74.6	576	82.8
Delaware	9	0	0.0	5	55.6	6	66.7	4	44.4	5	55.6	7	66.7	4	44.4	5	55.6	6	66.7
District of Columbia	11	1	9.1	7	63.6	9	81.8	7	63.6	6	54.5	7	63.6	4	36.4	7	63.6	6	54.5
Florida	147	2	1.4	102	69.4	119	81.0	103	70.1	106	72.1	121	82.3	46	31.8	113	76.9	131	89.1
Georgia	129	3	2.3	57	44.2	101	78.3	80	62.0	57	44.2	88	68.2	41	31.8	86	66.7	104	80.6
Maryland	56	3	5.4	42	75.0	47	83.9	43	76.8	42	75.0	49	87.5	24	42.9	45	80.4	48	85.7
North Carolina	119	11	9.2	57	47.9	99	83.2	87	73.1	72	60.5	96	80.7	35	29.4	91	76.5	108	90.8
South Carolina	82	5	6.1	32	39.0	63	76.8	50	61.0	30	36.6	58	70.7	25	30.5	61	74.4	59	72.0
Virginia	76	9	11.8	45	59.2	63	82.9	56	73.7	51	67.1	60	78.9	26	34.2	59	77.6	64	84.2
West Virginia	67	4	6.0	27	40.3	48	71.6	32	47.8	27	40.3	37	55.2	15	22.4	52	77.6	50	74.6
CENSUS DIVISION 4, EAST NORTH CENTRAL	746	160	21.4	377	50.5	618	82.8	529	70.9	491	65.8	549	73.6	260	34.9	602	80.7	652	87.4
Illinois	170	35	20.6	99	58.2	135	79.4	113	66.5	117	68.8	131	77.1	55	32.4	142	83.5	157	92.4
Indiana	114	33	28.9	52	45.6	93	81.6	80	70.2	73	64.0	83	72.8	35	30.7	80	70.2	92	80.7
Michigan	152	13	8.6	82	53.9	128	84.2	118	77.6	93	61.2	117	77.0	60	39.5	121	79.6	130	85.5
Ohio	166	36	21.7	95	57.2	143	86.1	129	77.7	121	72.9	144	86.7	63	38.0	141	84.9	153	92.2
Wisconsin	144	43	29.9	49	34.0	119	82.6	89	61.8	87	60.4	74	51.4	47	32.6	118	81.9	120	83.3
CENSUS DIVISION 5, EAST SOUTH CENTRAL	375	12	3.2	131	34.9	220	58.7	195	52.0	147	39.2	189	50.4	67	17.9	200	53.3	284	75.7
Alabama	65	4	6.2	29	44.6	38	58.5	35	53.8	28	43.1	41	63.1	11	16.9	48	73.8	54	83.1
Kentucky	97	5	5.2	47	48.5	73	75.3	62	63.9	46	47.4	69	71.1	29	29.9	68	70.1	82	84.5
Mississippi	110	1	0.9	16	14.5	37	33.6	33	30.0	30	27.3	19	17.3	6	5.5	20	18.2	66	60.0
Tennessee	103	2	1.9	39	37.9	72	69.9	65	63.1	43	41.7	60	58.3	21	20.4	64	62.1	82	79.6
CENSUS DIVISION 6, WEST NORTH CENTRAL	706	156	22.1	191	27.1	478	67.7	439	62.2	318	45.0	375	53.1	96	13.6	520	73.7	606	85.8
Iowa	125	46	36.8	31	24.8	109	87.2	88	70.4	75	60.0	80	64.0	14	11.2	111	88.8	118	94.4
Kansas	154	36	23.4	26	16.9	76	49.4	78	50.6	44	28.6	60	39.0	13	8.4	94	61.0	123	79.9
Minnesota	109	31	28.4	29	26.6	80	73.4	79	72.5	55	50.5	67	61.5	17	15.6	86	78.9	101	92.7
Missouri	147	19	12.9	73	49.7	110	74.8	102	69.4	75	51.0	97	66.0	36	24.5	115	78.2	115	78.2
Nebraska	75	10	13.3	17	22.7	48	64.0	38	50.7	38	50.7	42	56.0	8	10.7	53	70.7	70	93.3
North Dakota	38	4	10.5	7	18.4	25	65.8	23	60.5	23	60.5	11	28.9	3	7.9	23	60.5	33	86.8
South Dakota	58	10	17.2	8	13.8	30	51.7	31	53.4	16	27.6	18	31.0	5	8.6	38	65.5	46	79.3
CENSUS DIVISION 7, WEST SOUTH CENTRAL	872	46	5.3	275	31.5	529	60.7	419	48.1	264	30.3	449	51.5	144	16.5	539	61.8	601	68.9
Arkansas	105	7	6.7	30	28.6	64	61.0	44	41.9	34	32.4	54	51.4	16	15.2	76	72.4	77	73.3
Louisiana	99	3	3.0	28	28.3	63	63.6	46	46.5	37	37.4	46	46.5	21	21.2	54	54.5	70	70.7
Oklahoma	124	18	14.5	29	23.4	54	43.5	54	43.5	29	23.4	64	51.6	9	7.3	63	50.8	95	76.6
Texas	544	18	3.3	188	34.6	348	64.0	275	50.6	164	30.1	285	52.4	98	18.0	346	63.6	359	66.0
CENSUS DIVISION 8, MOUNTAIN	341	25	7.3	128	37.5	235	68.9	203	59.5	148	43.4	221	64.8	79	23.2	230	67.4	270	79.2
Arizona	52	7	13.5	33	63.5	46	88.5	35	67.3	30	57.7	41	78.8	18	34.6	38	73.1	45	86.5
Colorado	64	5	7.8	34	53.1	50	78.1	46	71.9	39	60.9	49	76.6	25	39.1	51	79.7	57	89.1
Idaho	34	1	2.9	8	23.5	21	61.8	20	58.8	22	29.4	22	64.7	7	20.6	23	67.6	29	85.3
Montana	53	9	16.1	14	25.0	33	58.9	30	53.6	17	30.4	25	44.6	5	8.9	40	71.4	35	62.5
Nevada	33	0	0.0	11	33.3	17	51.5	18	54.5	12	36.4	20	60.6	9	27.3	16	48.5	21	63.6
New Mexico	38	1	2.6	9	23.7	22	57.9	17	44.7	15	36.8	18	47.4	5	13.2	26	68.4	27	71.1
Utah	36	1	2.8	14	38.9	26	72.2	22	61.1	15	41.7	24	66.7	9	25.0	20	55.6	32	88.9
Wyoming	28	1	3.6	5	17.9	20	71.4	15	53.6	11	39.3	22	78.6	1	3.6	16	57.1	24	85.7
CENSUS DIVISION 9, PACIFIC	472	31	6.6	229	48.5	350	74.2	315	66.7	275	58.3	353	74.8	146	30.9	359	76.1	415	87.9
Alaska	16	0	0.0	4	25.0	13	81.3	10	62.5	9	56.3	10	62.5	2	12.5	12	75.0	14	87.5
California	308	23	7.5	159	51.6	215	69.8	205	66.6	184	59.7	229	74.4	98	31.8	224	72.7	268	87.0
Hawaii	20	1	5.0	9	45.0	15	75.0	17	85.0	11	55.0	14	70.0	4	20.0	16	80.0	16	70.0
Oregon	60	2	3.3	25	41.7	56	93.3	38	63.3	31	51.7	48	80.0	21	35.0	50	83.3	57	95.0
Washington	68	5	7.4	32	47.1	51	75.0	45	66.2	40	58.8	52	76.5	21	30.9	57	83.8	62	91.2

TABLE 8

U.S. CENSUS DIVISION 2, MIDDLE ATLANTIC

U.S. Community Hospitals
(Nonfederal, short-term general and other special hospitals)

2006 Utilization, Personnel and Finances

FULL-TIME EQUIVALENT PERSONNEL					FULL-TIME EQUIV. TRAINEES			EXPENSES						
								LABOR				TOTAL		
Physicians and Dentists	Registered Nurses	Licensed Practical Nurses	Other Salaried Personnel	Total Personnel	Medical and Dental Residents	Other Trainees	Total Trainees	Payroll (in thousands)	Employee Benefits (in thousands)	Total (in thousands)	Percent of Total	Amount (in thousands)	Adjusted per Admission	Adjusted per Inpatient Day
82,249	1,138,633	112,897	2,419,268	4,343,480	85,320	7,428	92,748	$225,892,043	$57,781,527	$283,673,571	51.4	$551,835,328	$8,970.31	$1,612.23
9,876	143,037	32,484	356,147	641,178	1,422	280	1,702	27,189,409	7,290,060	34,479,464	53.5	64,488,354	5,979.83	914.81
72,373	995,596	80,413	2,063,121	3,702,302	83,898	7,148	91,046	198,702,635	50,491,466	249,194,107	51.1	487,346,974	9,605.99	1,793.12
18,049	175,212	14,140	393,778	692,250	24,085	1,066	25,151	38,851,348	10,184,222	49,035,580	53.7	91,387,151	10,226.65	1,647.50
1,226	11,046	2,558	29,243	51,414	416	24	440	2,214,467	597,793	2,812,263	53.4	5,264,329	6,266.08	841.17
16,823	164,166	11,582	364,535	640,836	23,669	1,042	24,711	36,636,881	9,586,429	46,223,317	53.7	86,122,822	10,637.64	1,750.04
2,206	31,754	1,638	70,820	120,034	2,576	69	2,645	6,987,248	1,717,436	8,704,687	54.9	15,863,979	10,030.03	1,909.68
2,206	31,754	1,638	70,820	120,034	2,576	69	2,645	6,987,248	1,717,436	8,704,687	54.9	15,863,979	10,030.03	1,909.68
9	380	43	1,220	1,869	20	0	20	77,633	19,742	97,375	53.2	183,179	9,314.48	2,122.14
60	1,330	80	2,565	4,721	41	0	41	302,041	95,689	397,730	58.7	677,801	10,049.98	1,945.75
476	4,707	275	11,772	18,790	272	11	283	776,149	185,716	961,865	50.9	1,889,264	8,878.25	1,802.95
386	7,022	439	14,656	25,779	512	19	531	1,595,634	397,841	1,993,475	53.6	3,720,678	9,741.52	1,827.51
510	6,547	196	15,633	26,036	440	7	447	1,654,744	393,818	2,048,563	55.6	3,682,183	10,150.55	2,098.07
645	9,095	332	18,789	32,132	1,198	16	1,214	1,999,315	477,414	2,476,730	56.8	4,362,292	11,094.53	1,909.29
0	246	5	523	885	0	6	6	42,062	15,606	57,668	56.3	102,414	7,263.92	1,614.04
115	1,831	123	4,099	7,180	91	10	101	399,186	92,417	491,604	53.5	918,619	10,206.65	1,881.56
2	451	123	1,355	2,187	0	0	0	114,823	33,491	148,314	56.9	260,759	8,438.00	1,604.45
3	145	22	208	455	2	0	2	25,661	5,702	31,363	47.0	66,789	7,548.48	1,927.03
10,211	83,470	7,101	197,705	342,252	14,339	408	14,747	20,876,562	5,592,476	26,469,040	55.4	47,808,815	11,543.27	1,601.58
557	4,435	1,180	13,683	22,970	87	3	90	1,038,703	261,704	1,300,406	58.2	2,235,760	6,501.06	675.96
9,654	79,035	5,921	184,022	319,282	14,252	405	14,657	19,837,859	5,330,772	25,168,634	55.2	45,573,055	11,999.87	1,716.92
265	3,715	361	8,548	14,847	225	13	238	664,780	148,270	813,051	51.1	1,589,871	8,424.63	1,361.14
102	888	86	2,510	4,090	77	0	77	198,001	63,827	261,828	51.9	504,751	7,523.95	1,338.85
455	4,899	340	11,566	19,888	510	54	564	990,467	271,177	1,261,644	52.5	2,404,541	9,786.25	1,032.90
70	600	62	1,351	2,364	8	2	10	106,588	31,201	137,789	57.4	239,994	6,740.65	901.05
71	493	224	1,634	2,816	0	0	0	113,777	23,108	136,885	59.7	229,471	7,413.76	1,255.03
3	239	6	466	870	0	0	0	38,893	15,806	54,699	52.6	103,893	6,329.14	1,261.85
3	378	61	926	1,510	6	0	6	75,722	16,014	91,737	53.5	171,491	7,153.49	1,242.69
1,277	12,331	705	25,107	44,170	1,601	33	1,634	3,151,109	861,679	4,012,789	57.7	6,953,452	11,765.99	1,803.34
6,466	44,484	2,769	108,236	185,251	10,754	275	11,029	12,381,014	3,323,987	15,705,000	55.1	28,480,555	13,832.09	1,992.22
69	2,200	135	4,059	7,491	24	4	28	422,551	118,510	541,061	55.6	972,800	8,588.18	1,537.64
659	4,800	610	10,468	19,646	585	10	595	905,237	233,031	1,138,266	55.3	2,059,507	9,459.78	1,155.50
142	2,786	315	6,299	11,045	423	14	437	562,213	166,642	728,857	53.9	1,351,078	10,086.13	1,565.14
72	1,222	247	2,852	5,294	39	0	39	227,507	57,520	285,028	55.7	511,652	6,876.40	896.20
5,632	59,988	5,401	125,253	229,964	7,170	589	7,759	10,987,538	2,874,310	13,861,853	50.0	27,714,357	8,626.16	1,600.87
669	6,611	1,378	15,560	28,444	329	21	350	1,175,765	336,089	1,511,857	49.9	3,028,569	6,103.23	1,026.35
4,963	53,377	4,023	109,693	201,520	6,841	568	7,409	9,811,774	2,538,221	12,349,996	50.0	24,685,788	9,087.01	1,718.92
383	3,956	204	6,451	13,690	354	44	398	612,895	165,861	778,756	49.1	1,585,656	9,194.34	1,704.76
31	815	108	1,511	2,805	17	0	17	131,248	38,761	170,010	50.8	334,636	6,751.05	1,400.00
112	1,608	107	2,570	5,038	103	7	110	212,351	75,043	287,394	51.5	558,199	8,247.13	1,622.35
590	3,029	333	7,256	12,744	613	224	837	567,041	151,337	718,378	53.3	1,348,570	10,278.66	1,866.71
33	1,008	124	2,697	4,373	81	2	83	165,087	45,832	210,919	48.3	436,490	7,651.54	1,442.62
127	1,581	225	3,874	7,096	56	2	58	356,584	115,314	471,898	54.5	865,875	9,495.80	1,882.77
8	210	73	840	1,225	0	3	3	48,469	16,676	65,146	48.1	135,491	8,045.80	1,649.66
2,242	20,555	987	40,356	75,315	3,871	225	4,096	4,329,712	1,049,478	5,379,189	51.0	10,538,594	10,434.52	1,982.17
1,011	14,076	648	29,300	52,407	1,397	53	1,450	2,219,207	539,273	2,758,482	46.3	5,954,427	8,462.49	1,589.73
156	1,364	241	3,203	5,859	80	2	82	260,711	74,735	335,445	52.8	635,772	9,100.14	1,641.57
177	2,302	484	5,349	9,356	76	1	77	384,646	106,295	490,942	49.0	1,002,597	6,673.92	1,237.32
2	308	51	636	1,206	0	0	0	56,937	14,982	71,919	52.7	136,511	5,309.42	1,414.27
12	621	105	1,289	2,377	28	5	33	102,966	31,518	134,484	55.4	242,852	6,897.64	909.92
52	1,204	234	2,775	5,108	158	0	158	252,272	75,503	327,775	51.6	635,396	7,674.05	1,698.05
27	740	99	1,586	2,921	7	0	7	111,647	37,612	149,259	54.3	274,723	5,162.80	968.98

MSAs

TABLE 8

U.S. CENSUS DIVISION 3, SOUTH ATLANTIC

U.S. Community Hospitals
(Nonfederal, short-term general and other special hospitals)

2006 Utilization, Personnel and Finances

MSAs

CLASSIFICATION	Hospitals	Beds	Admissions	Inpatient Days	Adjusted Patient Days	Average Daily Census	Adjusted Average Daily Census	Average Stay (days)	Surgical Operations	NEWBORNS Bassinets	NEWBORNS Births	OUTPATIENT VISITS Emergency	OUTPATIENT VISITS Total
UNITED STATES	4,927	802,658	35,377,659	196,366,512	342,281,133	538,496	938,580	5.6	27,330,824	57,832	4,075,193	118,374,029	599,553,025
Nonmetropolitan	2,001	145,328	4,662,402	30,375,652	70,493,783	83,319	193,322	6.5	4,130,326	11,655	481,086	22,555,781	112,987,297
Metropolitan	2,926	657,330	30,715,257	165,990,860	271,787,350	455,177	745,258	5.4	23,200,498	46,177	3,594,107	95,818,248	486,565,728
CENSUS DIVISION 3, SOUTH ATLANTIC	741	153,115	6,862,970	38,694,981	65,016,483	106,079	178,283	5.6	5,303,318	10,077	754,948	23,813,876	90,169,850
Nonmetropolitan	245	25,769	889,863	5,874,493	12,197,133	16,088	33,416	6.6	738,050	1,850	83,420	4,517,505	15,816,887
Metropolitan	496	127,346	5,973,107	32,820,488	52,819,350	89,991	144,867	5.5	4,565,268	8,227	671,528	19,296,371	74,352,963
Delaware	6	2,138	105,164	669,392	1,103,514	1,834	3,024	6.4	94,474	98	12,361	382,935	1,839,908
Nonmetropolitan	2	439	15,181	133,920	264,658	367	725	8.8	10,876	28	1,858	73,181	468,138
Metropolitan	4	1,699	89,983	535,472	838,856	1,467	2,299	6.0	83,598	70	10,503	309,754	1,371,770
Dover	1	335	18,431	99,842	176,661	274	484	5.4	17,274	20	2,336	65,773	408,464
Wilmington	3	1,364	71,552	435,630	662,195	1,193	1,815	6.1	66,324	50	8,167	243,981	963,306
District of Columbia	11	3,601	139,515	979,850	1,407,189	2,685	3,855	7.0	100,161	201	14,120	396,343	1,608,964
Metropolitan	11	3,601	139,515	979,850	1,407,189	2,685	3,855	7.0	100,161	201	14,120	396,343	1,608,964
Washington-Arlington-Alexandria	11	3,601	139,515	979,850	1,407,189	2,685	3,855	7.0	100,161	201	14,120	396,343	1,608,964
Florida	203	51,423	2,373,712	12,432,951	18,820,423	34,118	51,645	5.2	1,456,328	2,672	225,049	7,165,036	22,759,029
Nonmetropolitan	30	2,051	98,506	434,583	816,680	1,191	2,239	4.4	66,317	91	5,175	464,793	1,301,373
Metropolitan	173	49,372	2,275,206	11,998,368	18,003,743	32,927	49,406	5.3	1,390,011	2,581	219,874	6,700,243	21,457,656
Cape Coral-Fort Myers	5	1,736	77,310	388,574	596,624	1,120	1,714	5.0	48,561	123	8,676	210,561	1,008,905
Deltona-Daytona Beach-Ormond Beach	5	1,300	64,462	303,655	465,618	832	1,276	4.7	35,211	56	4,371	269,543	562,664
Fort Lauderdale-Pompano Beach-Deerfield Beach	18	5,429	245,112	1,284,009	1,942,736	3,518	5,323	5.2	130,246	268	25,162	808,383	2,125,552
Fort Walton Beach-Crestview-Destin	3	422	20,459	102,697	147,961	281	405	5.0	14,942	48	2,217	73,253	191,848
Gainesville	3	1,168	60,475	343,645	477,549	941	1,309	5.7	49,903	45	5,856	126,526	870,908
Jacksonville	12	3,236	161,659	884,556	1,373,164	2,423	3,763	5.5	129,626	252	16,021	536,517	1,532,078
Lakeland	4	1,475	69,290	330,179	469,318	905	1,286	4.8	36,837	52	6,800	262,506	588,333
Miami-Miami Beach-Kendall	26	8,101	331,149	2,046,298	2,938,984	5,607	8,053	6.2	183,638	285	29,749	841,151	2,878,713
Naples-Marco Island	2	618	36,642	167,356	224,536	459	615	4.6	14,167	36	4,370	124,046	325,496
Ocala	2	614	37,041	171,289	240,102	469	658	4.6	23,667	26	2,265	144,330	238,199
Orlando-Kissimmee	10	5,016	265,064	1,345,869	2,014,962	3,688	5,520	5.1	159,822	381	31,132	798,980	2,135,984
Palm Bay-Melbourne-Titusville	6	1,341	64,741	323,628	531,728	886	1,457	5.0	34,459	83	5,346	189,403	877,567
Panama City-Lynn Haven	3	597	30,430	141,015	227,192	387	622	4.6	20,308	28	3,061	98,749	309,998
Pensacola-Ferry Pass-Brent	6	1,524	59,659	302,752	513,515	830	1,407	5.1	50,838	68	5,982	229,680	911,101
Port St. Lucie-Fort Pierce	3	835	42,588	202,681	304,133	556	833	4.8	22,032	66	4,540	96,212	210,447
Punta Gorda	3	638	26,133	128,683	191,535	353	525	4.9	25,709	10	1,216	77,594	227,667
Sarasota-Bradenton-Venice	7	2,049	78,569	411,799	606,581	1,128	1,662	5.2	48,926	64	6,144	270,876	889,136
Tallahassee	3	745	35,245	178,254	298,660	488	818	5.1	25,399	56	5,131	118,182	472,175
Tampa-St. Petersburg-Clearwater	34	8,448	368,930	1,932,161	2,903,736	5,293	7,956	5.2	231,855	435	34,460	916,825	3,544,333
Vero Beach	3	484	21,068	118,460	185,444	324	507	5.6	10,210	22	1,337	58,919	219,377
West Palm Beach-Boca Raton-Boynton Beach	15	3,596	179,180	890,808	1,349,665	2,439	3,697	5.0	93,655	177	16,038	448,007	1,337,175
Georgia	147	24,772	956,395	6,221,330	11,141,312	17,041	30,521	6.5	777,713	1,963	140,741	3,629,453	13,782,727
Nonmetropolitan	64	6,833	157,024	1,613,712	3,353,257	4,418	9,187	10.3	136,553	407	19,086	842,584	2,884,356
Metropolitan	83	17,939	799,371	4,607,618	7,788,055	12,623	21,334	5.8	641,160	1,556	121,655	2,786,869	10,898,371
Albany	3	634	24,913	144,340	301,193	395	825	5.8	19,389	44	3,052	90,924	829,428
Athens-Clarke County	2	503	27,108	118,327	213,945	324	586	4.4	26,241	29	3,796	96,062	372,416
Atlanta-Sandy Springs-Marietta	42	9,620	447,508	2,642,865	4,297,288	7,238	11,772	5.9	328,994	887	78,532	1,561,024	5,376,025
Augusta-Richmond County	7	1,473	62,034	331,693	552,462	909	1,513	5.3	59,616	136	7,315	208,475	1,125,627
Brunswick	1	229	10,174	59,117	97,893	162	268	5.8	6,780	30	1,278	32,441	146,250
Chattanooga	2	307	6,467	71,643	150,142	196	411	11.1	9,400	15	889	33,082	186,000
Columbus	5	1,067	37,166	227,453	395,135	624	1,083	6.1	28,500	31	4,219	138,089	356,490
Dalton	2	290	12,299	47,435	81,347	130	223	3.9	9,009	39	2,414	58,859	222,652
Gainesville	1	418	24,194	118,067	183,242	323	502	4.9	12,511	40	3,225	58,092	334,628
Hinesville-Fort Stewart	1	91	2,276	25,203	60,482	69	166	11.1	2,377	8	474	10,100	50,533
Macon	5	908	42,988	241,020	382,520	661	1,047	5.6	42,125	96	4,307	108,265	557,941
Rome	2	534	25,170	120,858	217,925	331	597	4.8	21,196	30	2,553	101,788	293,001
Savannah	4	1,162	45,139	296,440	524,468	813	1,437	6.6	40,916	71	5,503	167,545	556,956
Valdosta	4	478	18,525	106,085	203,884	291	559	5.7	15,712	66	2,336	56,035	248,485
Warner Robins	2	225	13,410	57,072	126,129	157	345	4.3	18,394	34	1,762	66,088	241,939

TABLE 8

U.S. CENSUS DIVISION 3, SOUTH ATLANTIC

U.S. Community Hospitals
(Nonfederal, short-term general and other special hospitals)

2006 Utilization, Personnel and Finances

FULL-TIME EQUIVALENT PERSONNEL					FULL-TIME EQUIV. TRAINEES			EXPENSES						
								LABOR				TOTAL		
Physicians and Dentists	Registered Nurses	Licensed Practical Nurses	Other Salaried Personnel	Total Personnel	Medical and Dental Residents	Other Trainees	Total Trainees	Payroll (in thousands)	Employee Benefits (in thousands)	Total (in thousands)	Percent of Total	Amount (in thousands)	Adjusted per Admission	Adjusted per Inpatient Day
82,249	1,138,633	112,897	2,419,268	4,343,480	85,320	7,428	92,748	$225,892,043	$57,781,527	$283,673,571	51.4	$551,835,328	$8,970.31	$1,612.23
9,876	143,037	32,484	356,147	641,178	1,422	280	1,702	27,189,409	7,290,060	34,479,464	53.5	64,488,354	5,979.83	914.81
72,373	995,596	80,413	2,063,121	3,702,302	83,898	7,148	91,046	198,702,635	50,491,466	249,194,107	51.1	487,346,974	9,605.99	1,793.12
8,882	220,056	20,612	424,301	790,163	12,159	969	13,128	39,024,015	9,516,836	48,540,859	50.0	97,065,907	8,457.72	1,492.94
1,075	26,127	5,614	56,951	107,873	151	15	166	4,413,927	1,186,381	5,600,310	52.4	10,683,185	5,801.89	875.88
7,807	193,929	14,998	367,350	682,290	12,008	954	12,962	34,610,088	8,330,455	42,940,549	49.7	86,382,722	8,965.25	1,635.44
255	4,048	275	8,909	15,285	258	2	260	804,887	244,533	1,049,419	58.2	1,802,837	10,559.58	1,633.72
10	598	50	1,140	2,112	0	0	0	101,326	35,433	136,759	53.9	253,844	8,471.64	959.14
245	3,450	225	7,769	13,173	258	2	260	703,561	209,100	912,660	58.9	1,548,993	11,004.03	1,846.55
11	733	81	1,363	2,561	0	0	0	117,960	37,821	155,780	55.4	281,047	8,617.89	1,590.88
234	2,717	144	6,406	10,612	258	2	260	585,601	171,279	756,880	59.7	1,267,946	11,723.53	1,914.76
1,080	5,197	404	12,592	21,850	1,256	79	1,335	1,343,767	262,808	1,606,575	53.6	2,998,369	14,753.65	2,130.75
1,080	5,197	404	12,592	21,850	1,256	79	1,335	1,343,767	262,808	1,606,575	53.6	2,998,369	14,753.65	2,130.75
1,080	5,197	404	12,592	21,850	1,256	79	1,335	1,343,767	262,808	1,606,575	53.6	2,998,369	14,753.65	2,130.75
1,882	68,728	5,866	126,847	237,236	2,544	290	2,834	11,912,213	2,849,753	14,761,969	49.2	30,009,186	8,294.11	1,594.50
92	2,284	481	4,935	9,279	5	0	5	394,536	96,383	490,917	49.6	989,273	5,412.76	1,211.34
1,790	66,444	5,385	121,912	227,957	2,539	290	2,829	11,517,677	2,753,370	14,271,052	49.2	29,019,912	8,447.41	1,611.88
146	1,709	249	5,034	7,914	9	2	11	409,092	77,448	486,541	56.1	866,529	7,276.81	1,452.39
59	1,788	185	3,740	6,578	43	0	43	317,721	75,392	393,113	51.6	762,144	7,651.51	1,636.84
235	6,802	474	10,189	20,728	104	3	107	1,203,805	252,570	1,456,374	52.5	2,776,250	7,424.08	1,429.04
7	495	69	779	1,590	10	1	11	67,352	14,652	82,005	46.3	177,104	5,930.53	1,196.96
21	1,905	96	3,864	6,610	22	3	25	362,395	90,918	453,313	47.7	950,180	11,222.95	1,989.70
18	5,246	186	9,198	17,323	36	32	68	808,246	251,701	1,059,947	48.4	2,191,400	8,615.55	1,595.88
26	1,860	318	3,741	7,108	0	42	42	310,332	64,083	374,415	52.4	715,128	7,228.85	1,523.76
396	10,930	781	19,887	37,070	1,350	139	1,489	2,072,062	477,837	2,549,901	48.2	5,287,780	10,947.65	1,799.19
4	997	88	2,344	3,729	0	0	0	211,155	42,006	253,162	61.1	414,657	8,459.45	1,846.73
1	975	33	1,601	3,115	0	0	0	141,865	34,981	176,847	45.4	389,826	7,506.17	1,623.58
239	8,501	592	17,525	31,974	318	6	324	1,432,590	376,268	1,808,857	47.8	3,785,378	9,624.63	1,878.64
3	1,701	98	3,035	6,091	0	35	35	354,690	81,773	436,463	50.7	861,325	7,918.70	1,619.86
5	498	147	1,587	2,498	0	0	0	119,836	31,285	151,121	55.7	271,315	5,436.74	1,194.21
27	2,055	108	3,017	5,811	0	0	0	258,061	59,465	317,525	42.3	750,198	7,415.29	1,460.91
6	1,004	50	1,760	3,268	0	0	0	182,948	53,838	236,785	52.8	448,243	6,903.16	1,473.84
7	719	113	1,129	2,300	11	1	12	111,786	25,675	137,461	45.5	302,065	7,741.89	1,577.08
27	2,433	281	4,368	7,962	32	1	33	342,623	86,752	429,376	50.1	857,323	7,408.53	1,413.37
54	1,038	140	1,958	3,764	31	0	31	175,102	34,816	209,918	49.1	427,845	7,251.24	1,432.55
420	10,997	924	19,432	37,010	509	24	533	1,840,814	436,565	2,277,379	48.2	4,726,243	8,502.40	1,627.64
26	588	74	1,081	2,132	2	0	2	93,254	23,050	116,303	52.0	223,715	6,778.62	1,206.37
63	4,203	379	6,643	13,382	62	1	63	701,949	162,296	864,246	47.1	1,835,263	6,790.63	1,359.79
873	31,815	4,578	64,376	119,220	1,126	71	1,197	5,631,234	1,383,469	7,014,704	50.7	13,846,913	8,205.40	1,242.84
210	4,679	1,721	11,218	21,770	37	2	39	836,859	212,821	1,049,679	53.1	1,977,613	5,837.37	589.76
663	27,136	2,857	53,158	97,450	1,089	69	1,158	4,794,375	1,170,648	5,965,025	50.3	11,869,300	8,800.22	1,524.04
76	785	193	2,548	4,045	18	0	18	158,755	47,029	205,784	45.2	455,734	8,821.45	1,513.10
22	873	52	2,114	3,299	6	0	6	173,938	45,831	219,768	59.0	372,307	7,598.41	1,740.20
368	15,746	1,305	27,525	53,439	259	62	321	2,700,030	630,808	3,330,839	49.9	6,676,252	9,087.66	1,553.60
12	2,344	308	4,381	7,959	442	0	442	385,372	108,402	493,773	51.2	964,398	9,271.81	1,745.64
24	291	44	663	1,192	35	0	35	55,727	14,628	70,356	50.1	140,454	8,337.01	1,434.77
6	211	77	666	1,139	0	0	0	41,075	10,379	51,454	55.6	92,530	6,844.94	616.28
34	844	180	2,118	3,930	39	0	39	182,111	48,196	230,308	48.4	476,035	7,368.28	1,204.74
3	289	70	816	1,257	0	0	0	76,652	19,510	96,162	52.8	182,046	8,570.90	2,237.89
42	648	44	1,448	2,499	65	7	72	107,960	27,660	135,620	50.6	267,904	7,134.79	1,462.02
5	81	22	226	399	1	0	1	13,256	3,641	16,897	55.9	30,230	5,534.59	499.82
4	1,674	117	3,595	5,646	96	0	96	289,782	83,918	373,699	51.1	730,875	10,680.31	1,910.68
53	745	168	1,680	2,892	20	0	20	137,601	27,260	164,862	49.5	332,982	7,420.70	1,527.96
4	1,714	114	3,540	6,363	108	0	108	315,101	69,590	384,691	49.2	770,453	10,645.58	1,469.02
8	590	115	1,210	2,269	0	0	0	97,335	17,171	114,506	49.6	230,681	6,619.44	1,131.43
2	301	48	628	1,122	0	0	0	59,682	16,624	76,306	52.1	146,421	4,933.49	1,160.88

Table continues

MSAs

TABLE 8

U.S. CENSUS DIVISION 3, SOUTH ATLANTIC CONTINUED

U.S. Community Hospitals
(Nonfederal, short-term general and other special hospitals)

2006 Utilization, Personnel and Finances

CLASSIFICATION	Hospitals	Beds	Admissions	Inpatient Days	Adjusted Patient Days	Average Daily Census	Adjusted Average Daily Census	Average Stay (days)	Surgical Operations	NEWBORNS Bassinets	NEWBORNS Births	OUTPATIENT VISITS Emergency	OUTPATIENT VISITS Total
Maryland	50	11,479	690,371	3,167,502	4,875,206	8,677	13,358	4.6	541,711	871	69,138	2,299,181	7,007,817
Nonmetropolitan	6	418	31,294	113,334	216,386	311	593	3.6	30,187	51	2,660	152,570	535,494
Metropolitan	44	11,061	659,077	3,054,168	4,658,820	8,366	12,765	4.6	511,524	820	66,478	2,146,611	6,472,323
Baltimore-Towson	23	6,996	416,178	1,968,523	2,958,721	5,392	8,106	4.7	334,045	424	35,496	1,244,517	3,919,481
Bethesda-Gaithersburg-Frederick	7	1,509	105,525	428,956	673,488	1,175	1,846	4.1	67,245	202	18,621	331,541	894,096
Cumberland	2	403	17,974	109,142	194,582	299	533	6.1	11,426	12	981	55,025	291,263
Hagerstown-Martinsburg	1	296	15,981	69,414	119,593	190	328	4.3	8,879	41	1,881	68,268	202,363
Salisbury	3	514	24,404	121,601	184,729	333	506	5.0	19,915	28	2,055	74,304	498,947
Washington-Arlington-Alexandria	7	1,221	70,869	330,496	482,704	906	1,323	4.7	62,916	101	6,786	339,107	522,989
Wilmington	1	122	8,146	26,036	45,003	71	123	3.2	7,098	12	658	33,849	143,184
North Carolina	114	23,441	1,015,594	6,131,924	11,546,885	16,795	31,631	6.0	855,583	1,617	120,778	3,849,736	17,212,819
Nonmetropolitan	58	6,846	274,824	1,642,553	3,479,753	4,498	9,530	6.0	217,489	611	28,526	1,373,808	4,777,608
Metropolitan	56	16,595	740,770	4,489,371	8,067,132	12,297	22,101	6.1	638,094	1,006	92,252	2,475,928	12,435,211
Asheville	5	1,351	58,139	343,530	622,187	941	1,704	5.9	57,644	58	5,165	167,925	1,040,635
Burlington	1	210	10,343	45,977	110,571	126	303	4.4	9,134	20	1,261	49,983	134,249
Charlotte-Gastonia-Concord	13	3,365	166,288	904,133	1,661,231	2,476	4,549	5.4	129,325	286	24,987	625,451	3,293,791
Durham	5	1,890	88,065	550,365	975,888	1,507	2,674	6.2	83,613	69	8,790	204,077	2,180,002
Fayetteville	1	581	30,001	177,688	293,542	487	804	5.9	24,171	48	4,156	93,294	497,570
Goldsboro	1	267	13,398	66,129	121,949	181	334	4.9	12,405	30	1,507	46,195	143,082
Greensboro-High Point	4	2,016	74,976	545,621	1,046,593	1,494	2,867	7.3	54,409	123	9,493	288,828	1,069,262
Greenville	1	761	34,588	217,804	301,046	597	825	6.3	30,161	42	3,766	78,565	276,405
Hickory-Lenoir-Morganton	5	1,072	33,962	253,148	505,367	694	1,385	7.5	27,434	51	3,218	128,627	608,969
Jacksonville	1	133	5,710	33,433	63,348	92	174	5.9	3,122	23	1,607	44,496	153,497
Raleigh-Cary	6	1,749	88,015	480,299	920,923	1,316	2,524	5.5	99,262	116	15,264	327,785	1,614,330
Rocky Mount	3	472	19,016	104,479	178,054	286	487	5.5	12,720	31	1,766	75,483	254,192
Wilmington	4	885	38,930	227,888	434,236	624	1,191	5.9	35,573	52	4,260	149,642	454,552
Winston-Salem	6	1,843	79,339	538,877	832,197	1,476	2,280	6.8	59,121	57	7,012	195,577	714,675
South Carolina	66	11,790	521,773	3,083,647	5,059,865	8,444	13,864	5.9	478,313	790	52,676	1,893,605	6,093,696
Nonmetropolitan	25	3,135	110,747	704,781	1,320,853	1,929	3,621	6.4	94,871	257	11,466	537,588	1,078,477
Metropolitan	41	8,655	411,026	2,378,866	3,739,012	6,515	10,243	5.8	383,442	533	41,210	1,356,017	5,015,219
Anderson	2	350	16,046	100,378	151,428	275	415	6.3	9,434	0	0	67,664	476,085
Augusta-Richmond County	2	245	12,326	59,377	94,994	162	261	4.8	10,564	18	1,235	52,691	187,102
Charleston-North Charleston	7	1,629	84,889	458,271	732,040	1,254	2,006	5.4	79,779	127	9,796	267,863	1,315,178
Charlotte-Gastonia-Concord	2	300	17,208	86,178	120,744	236	331	5.0	18,842	32	2,351	43,514	69,853
Columbia	7	2,012	94,647	547,370	829,035	1,500	2,271	5.8	66,055	115	9,636	222,533	926,943
Florence	6	961	49,450	277,347	399,406	760	1,093	5.6	52,428	40	2,821	145,487	223,175
Greenville	9	1,532	64,070	417,954	666,383	1,144	1,825	6.5	69,519	70	6,818	237,900	828,860
Myrtle Beach-Conway-North Myrtle Beach	3	658	27,494	171,958	299,741	471	821	6.3	22,819	54	2,949	145,833	387,851
Spartanburg	2	710	35,338	186,455	290,277	511	795	5.3	37,457	57	4,072	120,458	463,289
Sumter	1	258	9,558	73,578	154,964	202	425	7.7	16,545	20	1,532	52,074	136,883
Virginia	88	17,274	778,680	4,416,114	7,749,713	12,098	21,237	5.7	707,837	1,398	98,948	3,060,052	13,652,744
Nonmetropolitan	30	3,156	100,149	608,034	1,193,557	1,665	3,272	6.1	94,512	205	7,576	537,432	2,203,693
Metropolitan	58	14,118	678,531	3,808,080	6,556,156	10,433	17,965	5.6	613,325	1,193	91,372	2,522,620	11,449,051
Blacksburg-Christiansburg-Radford	4	315	16,022	66,607	128,315	183	352	4.2	17,280	37	1,502	68,012	191,426
Charlottesville	3	771	39,798	214,684	388,632	589	1,064	5.4	69,905	45	3,507	91,556	1,864,301
Danville	1	186	13,117	65,485	101,727	179	279	5.0	8,717	20	1,112	35,150	147,657
Harrisonburg	1	244	13,199	53,465	120,976	146	331	4.1	19,331	28	1,783	64,584	474,817
Kingsport-Bristol-Bristol	1	135	5,055	18,593	44,477	51	122	3.7	8,558	12	668	30,642	104,540
Lynchburg	2	655	27,498	302,613	482,198	829	1,321	11.0	16,472	48	2,545	76,505	86,628
Richmond	13	3,576	144,300	861,352	1,370,617	2,360	3,757	6.0	130,255	197	16,478	541,436	1,769,816
Roanoke	3	1,281	53,587	330,303	489,948	905	1,343	6.2	45,233	73	4,631	268,178	1,168,684
Virginia Beach-Norfolk-Newport News	15	3,155	156,770	885,754	1,673,481	2,427	4,585	5.7	140,144	324	19,290	682,903	3,380,005
Washington-Arlington-Alexandria	14	3,389	184,664	905,407	1,588,175	2,480	4,352	4.9	147,281	385	37,460	595,616	1,963,203
Winchester	1	411	24,521	103,817	167,610	284	459	4.2	10,149	24	2,396	68,038	297,974
West Virginia	56	7,197	281,766	1,592,271	3,312,376	4,387	9,148	5.7	291,198	467	21,137	1,137,535	6,212,146
Nonmetropolitan	30	2,891	102,138	623,576	1,551,989	1,709	4,249	6.1	87,245	200	7,073	535,549	2,567,748
Metropolitan	26	4,306	179,628	968,695	1,760,387	2,678	4,899	5.4	203,953	267	14,064	601,986	3,644,398
Charleston	7	1,238	51,490	280,016	510,490	793	1,473	5.4	82,739	62	4,111	145,521	896,901
Cumberland	1	25	1,086	3,429	11,714	9	32	3.2	1,585	0	0	13,555	44,596
Hagerstown-Martinsburg	2	200	7,599	43,758	98,683	120	270	5.8	9,053	21	964	41,589	199,906
Huntington-Ashland	3	686	37,306	178,544	302,543	489	829	4.8	24,382	55	3,013	113,519	553,962
Morgantown	4	762	32,113	200,059	290,619	548	797	6.2	32,330	14	2,201	77,491	712,757
Parkersburg-Marietta-Vienna	3	496	19,091	101,776	187,134	278	513	5.3	21,004	50	1,650	74,806	370,689
Washington-Arlington-Alexandria	1	45	2,085	9,573	31,707	26	87	4.6	1,814	10	265	19,579	65,281
Weirton-Steubenville	1	238	7,342	31,135	70,751	85	194	4.2	6,756	21	370	34,936	112,488
Wheeling	3	572	21,047	108,374	223,332	297	612	5.1	23,991	34	1,490	74,625	656,691
Winchester	1	44	469	12,031	33,414	33	92	25.7	299	0	0	6,365	31,127

MSAs

TABLE 8 U.S. CENSUS DIVISION 3, SOUTH ATLANTIC CONTINUED

U.S. Community Hospitals
(Nonfederal, short-term general and other special hospitals)

2006 Utilization, Personnel and Finances

Physicians and Dentists	Registered Nurses	Licensed Practical Nurses	Other Salaried Personnel	Total Personnel	Medical and Dental Residents	Other Trainees	Total Trainees	Payroll (in thousands)	Employee Benefits (in thousands)	Total (in thousands)	Percent of Total	Amount (in thousands)	Adjusted per Admission	Adjusted per Inpatient Day
1,823	19,194	710	41,846	74,202	1,289	114	1,403	3,923,370	918,033	4,841,404	49.4	9,794,446	9,133.52	2,009.03
39	857	46	1,901	3,408	1	7	8	150,598	40,660	191,258	54.5	351,143	5,908.42	1,622.76
1,784	18,337	664	39,945	70,794	1,288	107	1,395	3,772,772	877,373	4,650,146	49.2	9,443,303	9,322.74	2,026.97
1,681	12,631	353	27,804	49,185	1,233	105	1,338	2,573,632	605,266	3,178,896	48.5	6,557,529	10,363.59	2,216.34
23	2,303	43	4,906	8,433	0	0	0	527,262	112,068	639,330	49.6	1,287,686	7,856.25	1,911.97
23	538	28	1,077	1,942	0	0	0	86,028	27,218	113,246	52.0	217,717	6,762.45	1,118.90
5	411	32	971	1,677	0	0	0	83,977	22,456	106,433	56.8	187,440	6,807.59	1,567.32
24	647	82	1,364	2,625	0	0	0	131,179	31,808	162,987	48.3	337,315	9,190.63	1,826.00
26	1,647	106	3,368	6,145	55	2	57	335,329	69,861	405,191	52.4	773,044	7,308.87	1,601.49
2	160	20	455	787	0	0	0	35,366	8,697	44,063	53.4	82,572	5,864.47	1,834.80
1,097	38,386	2,372	73,527	136,886	2,284	237	2,521	6,582,526	1,619,328	8,201,852	52.2	15,721,864	8,239.94	1,361.57
209	8,651	1,004	18,108	33,959	15	1	16	1,410,693	377,087	1,787,777	53.5	3,342,544	5,794.43	960.57
888	29,735	1,368	55,419	102,927	2,269	236	2,505	5,171,833	1,242,241	6,414,075	51.8	12,379,319	9,299.71	1,534.54
80	2,451	146	5,247	8,826	0	5	5	396,417	97,571	493,988	54.0	915,632	8,999.11	1,471.64
1	310	11	964	1,413	0	0	0	59,395	14,005	73,400	48.6	151,167	6,077.32	1,367.15
333	6,523	197	11,472	21,880	227	15	242	1,161,205	270,166	1,431,372	48.6	2,946,008	9,384.79	1,773.39
17	4,424	79	7,126	14,121	984	133	1,117	814,148	173,187	987,336	51.3	1,924,410	12,548.73	1,971.96
82	975	205	2,380	4,281	0	0	0	219,329	50,625	269,953	57.4	470,292	9,488.96	1,602.13
0	324	24	894	1,411	0	0	0	66,238	17,789	84,027	56.3	149,154	6,036.91	1,223.09
179	2,737	177	5,455	10,130	53	4	57	451,822	146,485	598,306	57.0	1,050,362	7,329.66	1,003.60
0	1,282	36	3,330	5,255	330	3	333	253,842	72,058	325,900	49.6	656,862	13,739.86	2,181.93
74	1,341	90	2,520	4,634	13	3	16	217,351	50,605	267,955	52.1	514,332	7,574.07	1,017.74
0	290	20	522	939	0	0	0	36,703	8,137	44,840	52.7	85,078	7,863.74	1,343.02
108	3,847	143	5,423	11,607	0	0	0	615,054	127,531	742,585	53.8	1,379,217	8,126.52	1,497.65
4	588	25	1,238	2,249	0	0	0	102,600	27,922	130,522	54.9	237,945	7,230.19	1,336.37
6	1,399	49	2,647	4,973	62	0	62	230,953	61,303	292,256	49.5	590,070	8,510.54	1,358.87
4	3,244	166	6,201	11,208	600	73	673	546,777	124,858	671,635	51.3	1,308,791	10,799.05	1,572.69
676	17,611	1,704	30,253	60,545	1,076	0	1,076	2,774,963	723,651	3,498,619	46.5	7,522,996	8,884.84	1,486.80
118	3,254	557	6,776	12,765	28	0	28	551,042	153,416	704,461	49.1	1,434,445	7,161.77	1,086.00
558	14,357	1,147	23,477	47,780	1,048	0	1,048	2,223,921	570,236	2,794,158	45.9	6,088,551	9,418.72	1,628.39
37	435	40	1,578	2,401	29	0	29	133,874	34,244	168,118	51.8	324,294	13,106.47	2,141.57
0	277	42	402	899	0	0	0	44,362	8,937	53,299	40.4	131,991	6,568.67	1,389.46
4	3,379	196	4,096	9,694	557	0	557	533,622	127,453	661,075	44.2	1,496,102	10,962.95	2,043.74
0	587	27	701	1,568	0	0	0	71,014	16,911	87,925	38.2	229,946	9,402.84	1,904.41
21	3,172	261	5,396	11,041	226	0	226	519,742	125,685	645,428	47.0	1,373,689	9,618.39	1,656.97
19	1,467	221	2,793	5,387	21	0	21	172,554	47,355	219,909	47.0	467,988	6,264.82	1,171.71
300	2,580	90	3,540	7,680	162	0	162	349,812	99,808	449,620	43.5	1,032,430	10,037.62	1,549.30
8	831	125	1,229	2,702	0	0	0	121,824	32,023	153,848	49.5	310,782	6,874.19	1,036.84
169	1,331	123	2,938	5,177	53	0	53	218,595	60,145	278,740	49.8	560,160	10,193.26	1,929.74
0	298	22	804	1,231	0	0	0	58,521	17,674	76,196	47.3	161,169	8,006.42	1,040.04
727	26,159	3,039	46,939	89,682	1,815	157	1,972	4,559,794	1,068,076	5,627,871	48.7	11,554,706	8,299.95	1,490.98
169	3,168	876	6,738	12,872	39	2	41	497,739	124,229	621,969	51.4	1,211,226	5,744.06	1,014.80
558	22,991	2,163	40,201	76,810	1,776	155	1,931	4,062,055	943,847	5,005,902	48.4	10,343,479	8,756.19	1,577.67
14	476	76	918	1,710	4	0	4	81,944	20,216	102,160	49.6	205,770	6,622.99	1,603.63
39	2,002	164	3,608	6,512	722	18	740	362,127	89,858	451,985	47.6	949,280	12,649.81	2,442.62
0	197	37	578	960	0	0	0	63,594	14,130	77,724	47.0	165,517	8,123.14	1,627.07
28	440	74	904	1,737	0	0	0	86,547	20,798	107,344	53.7	199,793	6,689.65	1,651.51
10	187	48	278	674	0	0	0	23,004	6,846	29,850	47.9	62,273	5,149.96	1,400.12
44	948	56	848	2,230	15	0	15	147,540	37,828	185,368	50.8	364,930	8,459.60	756.81
64	5,541	607	7,860	16,667	678	103	781	849,230	200,540	1,049,771	47.9	2,193,275	9,533.86	1,600.21
126	1,856	134	3,387	6,340	192	13	205	334,421	81,224	415,644	48.7	853,426	10,504.61	1,741.87
55	4,980	566	9,766	18,281	65	4	69	933,763	205,720	1,139,484	47.9	2,381,032	8,022.29	1,422.80
167	5,395	315	10,071	18,481	100	17	117	1,059,718	235,972	1,295,689	49.2	2,632,307	8,174.69	1,657.44
11	969	86	1,983	3,218	0	0	0	120,168	30,716	150,883	44.9	335,877	8,484.09	2,003.92
469	8,918	1,664	19,012	35,257	511	19	530	1,491,260	447,185	1,938,446	50.8	3,814,590	6,602.52	1,151.62
228	2,636	879	6,135	11,708	26	3	29	471,134	146,353	617,490	55.0	1,123,096	4,633.87	723.65
241	6,282	785	12,877	23,549	485	16	501	1,020,126	300,832	1,320,956	49.1	2,691,494	8,025.18	1,528.92
84	2,119	202	3,550	7,034	139	0	139	305,432	81,119	386,551	47.1	821,095	8,451.83	1,608.45
0	35	7	92	178	0	0	0	5,936	1,315	7,251	49.3	14,712	3,965.40	1,255.90
3	266	32	632	1,067	0	0	0	45,142	12,569	57,710	55.6	103,857	6,391.97	1,052.43
26	1,026	139	2,309	3,917	0	0	0	179,264	73,425	252,690	52.1	485,448	7,510.60	1,604.56
31	1,264	136	2,763	4,932	296	14	310	220,641	60,596	281,236	46.8	601,364	12,240.01	2,069.25
6	507	109	1,286	2,171	0	0	0	89,785	25,098	114,882	45.6	252,034	6,964.57	1,346.81
5	67	13	128	295	0	0	0	14,961	3,881	18,842	57.7	32,663	4,729.60	1,030.14
0	238	30	452	846	0	0	0	35,968	10,519	46,486	54.5	85,326	5,114.23	1,206.00
77	742	108	1,615	2,994	50	2	52	119,561	31,521	151,082	53.0	285,150	6,566.34	1,276.80
0	18	9	50	115	0	0	0	3,436	790	4,226	42.9	9,846	7,556.62	294.68

MSAs

TABLE 8

U.S. CENSUS DIVISION 4, EAST NORTH CENTRAL

U.S. Community Hospitals
(Nonfederal, short-term general and other special hospitals)

2006 Utilization, Personnel and Finances

CLASSIFICATION	Hospitals	Beds	Admissions	Inpatient Days	Adjusted Patient Days	Average Daily Census	Adjusted Average Daily Census	Average Stay (days)	Surgical Operations	NEWBORNS Bassinets	NEWBORNS Births	OUTPATIENT VISITS Emergency	OUTPATIENT VISITS Total
UNITED STATES	4,927	802,658	35,377,659	196,366,512	342,281,133	538,496	938,580	5.6	27,330,824	57,832	4,075,193	118,374,029	599,553,025
Nonmetropolitan	2,001	145,328	4,662,402	30,375,652	70,493,783	83,319	193,322	6.5	4,130,326	11,655	481,086	22,555,781	112,987,297
Metropolitan	2,926	657,330	30,715,257	165,990,860	271,787,350	455,177	745,258	5.4	23,200,498	46,177	3,594,107	95,818,248	486,565,728
CENSUS DIVISION 4, EAST NORTH CENTRAL.	741	125,144	5,666,562	29,071,025	56,341,325	79,664	154,355	5.1	4,731,006	10,131	596,871	20,042,357	119,408,746
Nonmetropolitan	273	19,997	722,979	4,041,090	11,566,374	11,074	31,689	5.6	720,659	1,982	77,742	3,862,797	22,773,474
Metropolitan	468	105,147	4,943,583	25,029,935	44,774,951	68,590	122,666	5.1	4,010,347	8,149	519,129	16,179,560	96,635,272
Illinois	190	34,178	1,583,620	8,072,145	14,368,661	22,117	39,361	5.1	1,137,100	2,682	170,858	5,079,148	29,564,619
Nonmetropolitan	64	4,556	166,508	906,737	2,239,462	2,484	6,134	5.4	139,299	344	13,866	857,237	4,429,404
Metropolitan	126	29,622	1,417,112	7,165,408	12,129,199	19,633	33,227	5.1	997,801	2,338	156,992	4,221,911	25,135,215
Bloomington-Normal	2	368	16,353	66,500	117,107	183	321	4.1	13,414	33	2,479	62,196	447,423
Champaign-Urbana	4	554	27,075	128,484	247,355	352	677	4.7	20,950	47	3,421	98,013	477,345
Chicago-Naperville-Joliet	78	21,130	1,038,127	5,256,003	8,560,972	14,400	23,452	5.1	657,791	1,630	117,078	2,905,842	17,053,693
Danville	2	290	9,443	56,197	103,576	154	284	6.0	5,260	26	893	42,217	256,938
Davenport-Moline-Rock Island . . .	5	569	25,806	126,836	289,731	348	794	4.9	20,632	85	2,598	90,986	454,915
Decatur	2	535	20,827	112,187	197,756	307	541	5.4	17,806	36	1,785	90,714	436,509
Kankakee-Bradley	2	417	20,980	95,388	173,791	262	476	4.5	16,831	33	1,713	60,324	513,546
Lake County-Kenosha County . . .	5	820	52,317	224,058	407,713	615	1,117	4.3	38,915	115	6,370	164,234	1,146,567
Peoria	6	1,245	55,520	308,868	580,315	845	1,590	5.6	76,443	73	4,936	177,861	1,551,052
Rockford	5	911	43,501	217,391	359,328	596	984	5.0	31,178	68	5,116	147,215	798,747
Springfield	2	960	41,924	210,321	341,158	576	935	5.0	42,392	48	3,541	114,081	760,470
St. Louis	13	1,823	65,239	363,175	750,397	995	2,056	5.6	56,189	144	7,062	268,228	1,238,010
Indiana.	114	18,076	726,020	3,801,325	7,439,256	10,417	20,382	5.2	645,893	1,678	85,960	2,704,727	16,520,457
Nonmetropolitan	40	2,475	94,135	404,527	1,220,027	1,108	3,342	4.3	104,181	294	12,358	596,711	3,443,021
Metropolitan	74	15,601	631,885	3,396,798	6,219,229	9,309	17,040	5.4	541,712	1,384	73,602	2,108,016	13,077,436
Anderson	2	231	8,956	57,125	159,426	157	437	6.4	13,126	10	445	42,038	399,818
Bloomington	2	283	15,437	66,912	132,925	184	364	4.3	13,644	24	2,215	63,668	716,440
Cincinnati-Middletown	1	97	4,898	20,131	48,007	55	132	4.1	6,715	11	588	17,626	143,897
Columbus	1	235	9,517	42,339	87,829	116	241	4.4	12,097	20	1,408	35,870	199,695
Elkhart-Goshen	2	405	18,654	83,285	161,503	229	443	4.5	13,310	53	3,185	82,911	565,545
Evansville	6	1,194	43,517	250,937	448,070	690	1,228	5.8	24,038	63	4,927	138,262	675,393
Fort Wayne	7	1,677	61,883	358,728	602,162	981	1,650	5.8	51,062	148	7,421	183,926	826,011
Gary	10	2,479	103,685	550,296	958,065	1,507	2,623	5.3	63,439	258	9,875	313,841	1,609,754
Indianapolis	20	5,220	206,025	1,183,026	2,146,270	3,243	5,880	5.7	193,086	457	25,679	661,666	5,157,198
Kokomo	4	390	13,617	84,173	200,977	230	550	6.2	14,790	40	1,575	90,663	419,790
Lafayette	1	451	18,010	86,509	134,263	237	368	4.8	12,851	24	2,579	52,334	301,463
Louisville	6	644	29,849	130,285	273,807	357	750	4.4	30,884	42	2,800	113,065	574,230
Michigan City-La Porte	2	395	13,765	76,265	165,094	209	452	5.5	11,813	35	1,433	48,616	213,974
Muncie	1	386	17,060	94,099	178,472	258	489	5.5	14,621	24	1,623	57,212	340,782
South Bend-Mishawaka	3	878	40,418	186,726	285,659	511	784	4.6	30,714	107	5,344	113,163	405,345
Terre Haute	6	636	26,594	125,962	236,700	345	649	4.7	35,522	68	2,505	93,155	528,101
Michigan.	142	25,945	1,205,481	6,245,033	12,874,982	17,116	35,274	5.2	1,105,179	1,826	123,600	4,326,912	28,125,103
Nonmetropolitan	58	4,383	159,541	912,516	3,156,763	2,503	8,649	5.7	180,048	404	16,588	783,052	6,111,181
Metropolitan	84	21,562	1,045,940	5,332,517	9,718,219	14,613	26,625	5.1	925,131	1,422	107,012	3,543,860	22,013,922
Ann Arbor	5	1,489	80,619	412,664	756,147	1,130	2,073	5.1	91,878	70	7,149	202,126	2,902,832
Battle Creek	3	386	16,054	67,260	165,681	184	454	4.2	11,477	24	1,762	69,143	287,901
Bay City.	1	320	16,906	76,877	124,517	211	341	4.5	11,328	24	980	39,471	337,976
Detroit-Livonia-Dearborn.	18	5,617	275,173	1,416,777	2,479,565	3,883	6,794	5.1	204,991	320	26,265	1,049,174	4,603,304
Flint	3	1,257	71,105	318,120	524,292	872	1,436	4.5	46,063	89	6,393	222,019	1,830,043
Grand Rapids-Wyoming	8	2,248	92,641	518,685	898,973	1,422	2,463	5.6	88,165	159	12,884	293,899	1,625,072
Holland-Grand Haven	3	272	11,415	47,185	106,204	129	291	4.1	8,737	49	2,187	93,927	502,060
Jackson.	2	441	17,689	87,234	182,604	239	500	4.9	19,363	24	1,908	54,502	383,939
Kalamazoo-Portage.	4	911	45,979	244,616	438,664	671	1,202	5.3	33,353	70	5,054	147,427	1,030,573
Lansing-East Lansing	5	996	51,555	242,452	483,762	665	1,325	4.7	44,042	62	5,944	186,009	1,150,810
Monroe	1	173	8,770	37,313	91,372	102	250	4.3	9,962	13	914	41,159	208,282
Muskegon-Norton Shores	2	411	20,114	82,811	221,028	227	606	4.1	30,677	38	2,415	104,471	655,366
Niles-Benton Harbor	2	719	16,772	168,223	304,316	461	834	10.0	14,580	40	2,055	72,057	360,161
Saginaw-Saginaw Township North	2	789	38,953	187,256	329,449	513	903	4.8	37,217	31	3,475	126,482	709,630
South Bend-Mishawaka	1	25	1,034	3,300	14,318	9	39	3.2	1,337	0	0	7,152	76,684
Warren-Farmington Hills-Troy . . .	24	5,508	281,161	1,421,744	2,597,327	3,895	7,114	5.1	271,961	409	27,627	834,842	5,349,289

TABLE 8

U.S. CENSUS DIVISION 4, EAST NORTH CENTRAL

U.S. Community Hospitals
(Nonfederal, short-term general and other special hospitals)

2006 Utilization, Personnel and Finances

FULL-TIME EQUIVALENT PERSONNEL					FULL-TIME EQUIV. TRAINEES			EXPENSES						
								LABOR				TOTAL		
Physicians and Dentists	Registered Nurses	Licensed Practical Nurses	Other Salaried Personnel	Total Personnel	Medical and Dental Residents	Other Trainees	Total Trainees	Payroll (in thousands)	Employee Benefits (in thousands)	Total (in thousands)	Percent of Total	Amount (in thousands)	Adjusted per Admission	Adjusted per Inpatient Day
82,249	1,138,633	112,897	2,419,268	4,343,480	85,320	7,428	92,748	$225,892,043	$57,781,527	$283,673,571	51.4	$551,835,328	$8,970.31	$1,612.23
9,876	143,037	32,484	356,147	641,178	1,422	280	1,702	27,189,409	7,290,060	34,479,464	53.5	64,488,354	5,979.83	914.81
72,373	995,596	80,413	2,063,121	3,702,302	83,898	7,148	91,046	198,702,635	50,491,466	249,194,107	51.1	487,346,974	9,605.99	1,793.12
18,603	190,850	14,733	428,179	749,195	19,027	1,509	20,536	38,537,476	10,331,996	48,869,466	51.8	94,345,981	8,736.39	1,674.54
1,761	24,376	3,837	64,637	109,886	190	81	271	4,896,413	1,455,014	6,351,423	53.7	11,837,975	6,071.00	1,023.48
16,842	166,474	10,896	363,542	639,309	18,837	1,428	20,265	33,641,063	8,876,982	42,518,043	51.5	82,508,007	9,323.70	1,842.73
4,453	48,940	2,876	109,995	192,526	5,577	167	5,744	9,876,014	2,622,444	12,498,455	51.9	24,077,973	8,604.94	1,675.73
263	5,262	931	13,325	23,156	61	2	63	950,280	291,686	1,241,965	52.8	2,353,124	5,859.39	1,050.75
4,190	43,678	1,945	96,670	169,370	5,516	165	5,681	8,925,734	2,330,758	11,256,490	51.8	21,724,848	9,065.02	1,791.12
38	436	20	1,237	1,992	16	0	16	93,428	23,887	117,314	48.2	243,441	8,430.57	2,078.79
5	974	34	1,782	3,139	24	0	24	143,404	34,547	177,951	41.4	430,188	9,765.69	1,739.15
3,702	31,863	1,183	70,099	122,789	5,047	131	5,178	6,704,257	1,693,049	8,397,304	52.7	15,941,436	9,326.63	1,862.11
5	191	34	570	918	1	0	1	37,499	9,225	46,725	43.3	107,810	6,182.11	1,040.88
36	809	40	2,010	3,273	0	0	0	125,362	33,586	158,948	47.2	336,507	6,282.93	1,161.45
39	783	83	1,651	3,008	30	2	32	129,929	37,682	167,611	51.1	327,972	9,004.04	1,658.47
37	530	43	1,321	2,184	1	1	2	102,849	25,941	128,790	43.2	297,791	7,754.57	1,713.50
47	1,489	109	2,918	5,548	8	1	9	331,476	86,760	418,237	51.2	817,088	8,792.42	2,004.08
205	2,394	78	4,571	8,435	192	4	196	405,639	118,316	523,954	52.1	1,005,383	9,777.80	1,732.48
54	1,409	67	3,078	5,579	0	19	19	280,299	80,765	361,064	51.2	704,824	9,716.75	1,961.51
2	1,063	126	3,176	5,029	197	0	197	257,382	90,329	347,711	48.0	724,411	10,654.67	2,123.39
20	1,737	128	4,257	7,476	0	7	7	314,210	96,671	410,881	52.1	787,996	5,956.81	1,050.11
1,568	25,955	2,887	57,100	101,613	1,289	211	1,500	5,049,214	1,346,807	6,396,024	50.6	12,642,921	8,726.27	1,699.49
348	3,590	683	9,233	16,278	17	51	68	716,710	205,901	922,611	54.2	1,701,909	5,904.18	1,394.98
1,220	22,365	2,204	47,867	85,335	1,272	160	1,432	4,332,505	1,140,906	5,473,413	50.0	10,941,012	9,427.20	1,759.22
43	273	64	1,087	1,617	0	0	0	76,835	20,920	97,754	56.9	171,698	6,772.04	1,076.98
17	573	87	1,217	2,445	0	0	0	110,713	34,330	145,043	56.0	258,993	8,343.84	1,948.41
5	113	30	373	613	0	0	0	28,001	9,479	37,480	59.6	62,836	5,379.77	1,308.89
0	300	43	969	1,465	0	0	0	67,814	19,770	87,584	51.3	170,797	8,651.43	1,944.65
65	746	53	1,593	2,730	0	0	0	132,822	54,377	187,199	51.5	363,463	9,821.74	2,250.50
149	1,480	118	3,606	6,289	36	8	44	288,651	79,718	368,369	51.1	721,391	9,655.11	1,610.00
17	2,190	170	3,839	6,985	0	0	0	355,211	94,406	449,617	46.5	967,220	9,516.88	1,606.25
212	2,784	225	7,443	12,088	78	42	120	625,972	156,997	782,969	51.7	1,515,280	8,350.54	1,581.60
488	8,761	789	16,741	31,430	937	65	1,002	1,695,321	412,779	2,108,101	49.4	4,266,361	11,260.28	1,987.80
39	525	87	1,246	2,325	13	0	13	101,309	28,660	129,969	52.6	246,989	7,940.25	1,228.94
38	619	40	1,259	2,249	50	9	59	108,958	27,915	136,874	50.6	270,382	9,673.08	2,013.82
28	849	131	2,004	3,626	0	0	0	159,090	35,172	194,261	52.4	371,029	5,858.38	1,355.07
40	399	19	1,044	1,756	0	0	0	102,397	32,966	135,363	50.0	270,866	9,096.48	1,640.68
5	497	76	1,206	2,009	75	35	110	91,062	29,839	120,901	48.2	251,081	7,759.72	1,406.84
34	1,379	53	2,548	4,570	66	1	67	241,153	65,179	306,332	46.4	659,550	10,673.37	2,308.87
40	877	219	1,692	3,138	17	0	17	147,195	38,399	185,597	49.7	373,076	7,073.20	1,576.16
5,190	40,389	2,398	95,586	163,221	4,518	323	4,841	8,618,409	2,301,411	10,919,816	52.7	20,701,789	8,770.96	1,607.91
582	5,211	944	16,177	26,191	75	3	78	1,182,128	355,345	1,537,473	54.3	2,830,404	6,471.24	896.62
4,608	35,178	1,454	79,409	137,030	4,443	320	4,763	7,436,281	1,946,065	9,382,343	52.5	17,871,385	9,294.05	1,838.96
1,606	4,635	105	9,872	16,770	1,123	5	1,128	794,053	237,771	1,031,824	52.6	1,963,203	13,028.61	2,596.32
11	530	20	1,275	2,036	0	0	0	103,038	31,100	134,138	51.4	260,870	6,450.63	1,574.53
7	334	53	888	1,470	9	0	9	82,204	21,614	103,818	49.1	211,649	7,729.49	1,699.76
1,267	8,376	162	18,787	33,559	1,521	98	1,619	2,064,911	472,231	2,537,139	50.7	5,008,957	10,495.08	2,020.10
102	2,213	145	3,773	7,004	337	0	337	401,196	143,784	544,980	56.8	959,150	8,171.60	1,829.42
213	3,259	200	8,061	13,774	77	2	79	673,335	181,859	855,193	52.8	1,620,471	9,838.27	1,802.58
29	425	50	1,124	1,855	5	1	6	82,058	21,180	103,238	52.9	195,014	7,208.06	1,836.22
34	557	84	1,916	2,843	0	0	0	120,363	28,522	148,885	55.6	267,748	6,944.74	1,466.28
80	1,449	31	3,763	5,887	0	0	0	336,631	99,692	436,323	54.1	807,074	10,683.78	1,839.85
155	1,841	62	4,350	7,125	222	2	224	400,070	108,162	508,232	57.0	891,947	8,427.08	1,843.77
13	276	44	885	1,399	0	0	0	54,824	16,758	71,582	55.4	129,237	6,017.74	1,414.40
59	576	43	1,610	2,546	15	2	17	145,026	48,051	193,077	54.4	355,058	6,626.82	1,606.40
6	498	65	1,811	2,727	0	0	0	115,062	38,494	153,557	56.5	271,552	8,692.99	892.33
98	1,248	131	3,269	5,373	0	38	38	239,803	65,485	305,288	50.8	600,878	8,762.72	1,823.89
5	34	0	139	202	0	0	0	9,973	3,482	13,455	63.9	21,066	4,695.94	1,471.29
923	8,927	259	17,886	32,460	1,134	172	1,306	1,813,733	427,881	2,241,614	52.0	4,307,512	8,304.79	1,658.44

Table continues

MSAs

MSAs

CLASSIFICATION	Hospitals	Beds	Admissions	Inpatient Days	Adjusted Patient Days	Average Daily Census	Adjusted Average Daily Census	Average Stay (days)	Surgical Operations	NEWBORNS		OUTPATIENT VISITS	
										Bassinets	Births	Emergency	Total
Ohio	171	32,822	1,542,333	7,742,312	14,500,863	21,216	39,729	5.0	1,197,406	2,674	147,992	5,840,398	32,686,517
Nonmetropolitan	54	4,480	184,105	843,911	2,116,169	2,312	5,799	4.6	179,687	608	22,157	1,111,506	5,523,778
Metropolitan	117	28,342	1,358,228	6,898,401	12,384,694	18,904	33,930	5.1	1,017,719	2,066	125,835	4,728,892	27,162,739
Akron	9	1,874	94,662	477,270	842,426	1,307	2,308	5.0	69,178	111	8,052	319,470	1,940,344
Canton-Massillon	5	1,421	57,750	313,507	573,004	860	1,570	5.4	47,326	92	4,967	199,842	1,330,285
Cincinnati-Middletown	18	4,281	217,977	1,032,583	1,713,188	2,830	4,693	4.7	154,726	327	24,178	735,668	3,236,811
Cleveland-Elyria-Mentor	28	7,264	357,063	1,937,874	3,632,016	5,312	9,952	5.4	291,814	451	27,418	1,092,263	9,194,875
Columbus	16	4,714	234,271	1,123,934	2,003,454	3,078	5,490	4.8	153,875	370	27,463	916,183	4,279,421
Dayton	9	2,496	117,133	588,047	1,017,731	1,611	2,788	5.0	101,242	203	11,771	414,291	1,870,184
Lima	4	670	27,780	126,654	230,906	347	632	4.6	14,028	58	2,555	101,465	618,370
Mansfield	1	317	16,442	80,010	144,228	219	395	4.9	9,038	38	1,422	68,997	274,356
Parkersburg-Marietta-Vienna	2	173	8,284	34,231	89,774	94	246	4.1	13,484	16	634	42,628	209,437
Sandusky	1	240	10,124	55,155	117,565	151	322	5.4	8,899	20	768	45,182	328,766
Springfield	2	369	18,121	80,906	143,742	222	393	4.5	9,996	31	1,641	79,717	234,080
Toledo	12	2,513	109,644	569,742	1,037,668	1,562	2,843	5.2	84,291	204	9,561	426,117	2,088,362
Weirton-Steubenville	1	315	11,619	67,752	133,441	186	366	5.8	5,531	19	608	48,778	205,613
Wheeling	3	269	8,999	68,682	145,036	188	397	7.6	6,820	10	438	34,777	286,823
Youngstown-Warren-Boardman	6	1,426	68,359	342,054	560,515	937	1,535	5.0	47,471	116	4,359	203,514	1,065,012
Wisconsin	124	14,123	609,108	3,210,210	7,157,563	8,798	19,609	5.3	645,428	1,271	68,461	2,091,172	12,512,050
Nonmetropolitan	57	4,103	118,690	973,399	2,833,953	2,667	7,765	8.2	117,444	332	12,773	514,291	3,266,090
Metropolitan	67	10,020	490,418	2,236,811	4,323,610	6,131	11,844	4.6	527,984	939	55,688	1,576,881	9,245,960
Appleton	4	389	17,556	74,164	157,753	204	432	4.2	31,236	46	2,326	67,580	319,251
Duluth	1	25	673	4,891	19,956	13	55	7.3	1,704	0	0	12,503	50,935
Eau Claire	5	575	24,295	121,634	247,283	334	677	5.0	16,840	40	2,427	67,292	391,950
Fond du Lac	3	225	9,173	37,970	126,277	104	346	4.1	13,697	3	1,076	38,079	253,262
Green Bay	5	712	33,411	140,954	280,763	386	769	4.2	51,523	94	4,544	133,504	496,327
Janesville	3	404	14,694	87,182	181,922	238	499	5.9	15,685	33	2,074	186,298	908,724
La Crosse	2	449	22,032	90,745	161,638	248	443	4.1	22,452	46	2,280	43,551	244,196
Lake County-Kenosha County	3	451	23,299	97,067	208,565	266	571	4.2	19,705	61	2,681	133,196	734,794
Madison	7	1,444	69,613	365,118	701,456	1,002	1,923	5.2	114,581	96	7,574	151,766	1,268,556
Milwaukee-Waukesha-West Allis	20	3,840	202,290	910,885	1,561,005	2,497	4,275	4.5	165,015	334	21,654	536,862	3,457,070
Minneapolis-St. Paul-Bloomington	4	100	5,561	16,223	45,854	45	127	2.9	6,588	25	855	22,567	102,732
Oshkosh-Neenah	4	442	18,976	74,674	148,446	205	406	3.9	28,218	62	2,657	52,074	192,201
Racine	2	454	20,612	107,562	296,857	294	813	5.2	14,251	45	2,242	66,920	556,940
Sheboygan	2	220	10,579	38,885	83,027	106	227	3.7	14,369	28	1,605	31,495	166,899
Wausau	2	290	17,654	68,857	102,808	189	281	3.9	12,120	26	1,693	33,194	102,123

TABLE **8**

U.S. CENSUS DIVISION 4, EAST NORTH CENTRAL CONTINUED

U.S. Community Hospitals
(Nonfederal, short-term general and other special hospitals)

2006 Utilization, Personnel and Finances

	FULL-TIME EQUIVALENT PERSONNEL				FULL-TIME EQUIV. TRAINEES			EXPENSES						
								LABOR				TOTAL		
Physicians and Dentists	Registered Nurses	Licensed Practical Nurses	Other Salaried Personnel	Total Personnel	Medical and Dental Residents	Other Trainees	Total Trainees	Payroll (in thousands)	Employee Benefits (in thousands)	Total (in thousands)	Percent of Total	Amount (in thousands)	Adjusted per Admission	Adjusted per Inpatient Day
6,674	54,755	5,340	115,580	209,246	7,095	409	7,504	10,666,266	2,797,926	13,464,191	52.4	25,712,642	8,781.99	1,773.18
324	6,546	971	14,926	26,756	37	2	39	1,167,076	352,441	1,519,516	53.9	2,821,228	5,804.84	1,333.18
6,350	48,209	4,369	100,654	182,490	7,058	407	7,465	9,499,191	2,445,485	11,944,675	52.2	22,891,414	9,374.55	1,848.36
315	3,705	468	7,753	13,708	444	46	490	641,161	160,959	802,119	53.0	1,513,576	8,975.14	1,796.69
70	1,851	226	4,710	7,722	92	0	92	333,136	89,062	422,197	52.1	810,378	7,708.27	1,414.26
654	7,114	391	15,417	26,565	831	245	1,076	1,278,789	331,926	1,610,715	47.3	3,408,613	9,182.76	1,989.63
2,357	12,362	1,599	30,842	52,526	2,399	111	2,510	3,112,624	750,372	3,862,995	56.9	6,789,981	10,209.70	1,869.48
2,597	9,123	278	13,843	31,118	2,355	0	2,355	1,621,610	429,056	2,050,667	49.5	4,146,819	9,746.83	2,069.83
68	4,017	255	8,906	15,799	408	1	409	786,841	192,009	978,851	52.1	1,880,366	9,174.76	1,847.61
9	991	128	2,061	3,605	0	0	0	166,374	52,893	219,267	52.0	421,345	8,190.37	1,824.75
1	491	141	1,437	2,228	0	0	0	100,786	34,447	135,233	56.1	240,974	8,130.31	1,670.79
5	294	67	553	1,146	1	0	1	55,470	23,296	78,765	54.7	143,899	6,627.30	1,602.90
1	342	107	832	1,390	19	0	19	64,438	19,447	83,885	54.1	155,089	7,186.72	1,319.18
3	547	22	1,119	1,912	0	0	0	88,745	21,877	110,621	47.7	232,033	7,199.28	1,614.23
124	4,594	395	8,044	15,009	380	0	380	767,740	205,617	973,357	51.1	1,904,238	9,996.16	1,835.11
9	384	32	749	1,438	0	0	0	57,080	19,822	76,903	53.7	143,125	6,254.37	1,072.57
26	294	66	595	1,220	0	0	0	46,239	12,713	58,951	54.6	107,904	5,514.31	743.98
111	2,100	194	3,793	7,104	129	4	133	378,159	101,989	480,149	48.3	993,074	8,875.45	1,771.72
718	20,811	1,232	49,918	82,589	548	399	947	4,327,572	1,263,409	5,590,980	49.9	11,210,657	8,868.76	1,566.27
244	3,767	308	10,976	17,505	0	23	23	880,220	249,641	1,129,858	53.0	2,131,310	6,330.51	752.06
474	17,044	924	38,942	65,084	548	376	924	3,447,352	1,013,767	4,461,122	49.1	9,079,347	9,790.24	2,099.95
1	570	59	1,225	2,088	0	9	9	118,366	32,108	150,475	53.0	283,835	7,485.50	1,799.24
0	30	11	117	188	0	0	0	8,850	3,188	12,038	64.5	18,668	6,798.16	935.44
2	831	43	1,944	3,192	0	12	12	148,542	48,688	197,230	55.2	356,988	7,575.82	1,443.64
28	334	61	811	1,378	0	2	2	81,469	20,187	101,656	42.8	237,678	7,803.71	1,882.19
68	1,452	110	3,183	5,370	0	6	6	279,778	79,616	359,394	52.2	688,919	10,225.29	2,453.74
44	777	80	1,838	3,127	10	2	12	173,905	51,483	225,389	55.2	408,220	14,088.70	2,243.93
12	776	46	1,521	2,655	17	9	26	130,394	46,575	176,969	49.3	359,055	9,198.74	2,221.35
60	773	67	2,006	3,320	6	9	15	175,316	46,728	222,044	53.4	416,077	8,244.22	1,994.95
26	2,355	75	6,033	9,625	347	139	486	537,469	170,366	707,835	53.4	1,326,108	11,454.18	1,890.51
206	6,728	245	14,575	24,770	168	152	320	1,289,622	382,027	1,671,648	44.7	3,743,674	10,752.31	2,398.25
0	151	8	428	681	0	0	0	36,875	8,319	45,195	47.8	94,601	6,027.87	2,063.10
15	652	33	1,149	2,087	0	16	16	116,755	32,172	148,926	50.9	292,656	7,604.62	1,971.47
0	700	64	2,097	3,225	0	9	9	181,821	49,619	231,441	57.5	402,780	7,154.94	1,356.82
0	258	9	673	1,089	0	11	11	53,969	14,870	68,839	51.2	134,544	5,964.11	1,620.49
12	657	13	1,342	2,289	0	0	0	114,221	27,821	142,043	45.0	315,543	11,991.46	3,069.25

MSAs

TABLE 8

U.S. CENSUS DIVISION 5, EAST SOUTH CENTRAL

U.S. Community Hospitals
(Nonfederal, short-term general and other special hospitals)

2006 Utilization, Personnel and Finances

CLASSIFICATION	Hospitals	Beds	Admissions	Inpatient Days	Adjusted Patient Days	Average Daily Census	Adjusted Average Daily Census	Average Stay (days)	Surgical Operations	NEWBORNS Bassinets	Births	OUTPATIENT VISITS Emergency	Total
UNITED STATES	4,927	802,658	35,377,659	196,366,512	342,281,133	538,496	938,580	5.6	27,330,824	57,832	4,075,193	118,374,029	599,553,025
Nonmetropolitan	2,001	145,328	4,662,402	30,375,652	70,493,783	83,319	193,322	6.5	4,130,326	11,655	481,086	22,555,781	112,987,297
Metropolitan	2,926	657,330	30,715,257	165,990,860	271,787,350	455,177	745,258	5.4	23,200,498	46,177	3,594,107	95,818,248	486,565,728
CENSUS DIVISION 5, EAST SOUTH CENTRAL	437	63,514	2,565,449	14,300,824	25,241,478	39,259	69,300	5.6	2,045,567	4,385	237,866	8,840,824	31,918,915
Nonmetropolitan	236	22,155	740,199	4,552,163	9,367,674	12,528	25,771	6.1	575,905	1,544	64,534	3,356,595	10,939,993
Metropolitan	201	41,359	1,825,250	9,748,661	15,873,804	26,731	43,529	5.3	1,469,662	2,841	173,332	5,484,229	20,978,922
Alabama	109	15,639	683,726	3,556,939	5,926,986	9,791	16,318	5.2	597,564	1,396	59,456	2,192,221	8,023,354
Nonmetropolitan	49	3,766	138,959	691,627	1,423,696	1,942	3,980	5.0	128,463	330	12,033	593,367	2,136,216
Metropolitan	60	11,873	544,767	2,865,312	4,503,290	7,849	12,338	5.3	469,101	1,066	47,423	1,598,854	5,887,138
Anniston-Oxford	3	431	23,281	102,477	155,579	280	427	4.4	14,956	39	1,858	85,687	201,303
Auburn-Opelika	1	389	16,206	106,780	196,723	293	539	6.6	11,414	35	1,605	39,246	103,480
Birmingham-Hoover	19	4,447	197,360	1,083,256	1,625,851	2,967	4,456	5.5	187,797	377	15,441	507,267	2,371,982
Columbus	1	38	696	10,370	10,739	28	29	14.9	0	0	0	0	2,333
Decatur	4	514	18,484	85,112	137,500	233	376	4.6	12,694	42	1,973	82,947	279,725
Dothan	4	802	35,864	192,764	341,325	529	935	5.4	30,867	45	2,672	98,356	259,075
Florence-Muscle Shoals	3	543	22,601	108,714	187,455	297	514	4.8	20,468	48	1,743	89,855	228,085
Gadsden	3	490	20,348	121,918	189,680	334	520	6.0	25,222	32	1,212	53,999	140,749
Huntsville	4	982	56,771	269,778	444,487	739	1,218	4.8	48,686	78	5,316	177,335	769,796
Mobile	6	1,510	70,115	390,091	597,978	1,069	1,638	5.6	52,106	197	6,907	189,976	658,445
Montgomery	8	1,043	48,515	216,412	338,079	594	926	4.5	40,063	121	5,457	157,634	350,601
Tuscaloosa	4	684	34,526	177,640	277,894	486	760	5.1	24,828	52	3,239	116,552	521,564
Kentucky	104	14,574	612,842	3,239,168	6,028,157	8,877	16,518	5.3	551,438	985	54,614	2,191,969	8,815,306
Nonmetropolitan	64	5,933	231,966	1,203,394	2,542,486	3,298	6,969	5.2	174,651	448	17,511	1,028,618	3,770,410
Metropolitan	40	8,641	380,876	2,035,774	3,485,671	5,579	9,549	5.3	376,787	537	37,103	1,163,351	5,044,896
Bowling Green	3	601	20,910	106,694	162,753	292	445	5.1	16,518	19	2,076	58,568	143,665
Cincinnati-Middletown	5	957	46,098	214,826	381,313	589	1,044	4.7	32,390	80	5,031	192,748	770,615
Clarksville	2	164	7,722	34,102	75,798	94	208	4.4	6,115	10	836	38,508	133,658
Elizabethtown	2	308	12,897	67,597	144,951	185	397	5.2	8,631	26	1,621	51,429	256,965
Evansville	1	216	6,775	29,598	64,077	81	176	4.4	10,412	12	693	26,896	203,916
Huntington-Ashland	2	756	32,633	196,253	352,040	538	964	6.0	52,918	25	1,694	93,587	523,664
Lexington-Fayette	13	2,059	87,342	436,128	716,455	1,196	1,963	5.0	82,366	117	8,755	254,983	1,132,975
Louisville	11	3,242	147,970	864,827	1,429,582	2,369	3,917	5.8	148,934	214	14,648	381,564	1,593,805
Owensboro	1	338	18,529	85,749	158,702	235	435	4.6	18,503	34	1,749	65,068	285,633
Mississippi	94	12,973	415,577	2,697,952	4,762,120	7,405	13,077	6.5	284,636	792	42,729	1,650,523	4,218,371
Nonmetropolitan	67	7,602	215,044	1,621,242	3,052,401	4,450	8,387	7.5	147,956	456	20,774	936,676	2,390,790
Metropolitan	27	5,371	200,533	1,076,710	1,709,719	2,955	4,690	5.4	136,680	336	21,955	713,847	1,827,581
Gulfport-Biloxi	6	967	29,940	159,279	258,102	437	708	5.3	29,822	75	2,956	132,310	334,578
Hattiesburg	2	723	34,255	183,944	281,412	504	771	5.4	16,554	45	4,365	118,216	214,656
Jackson	14	2,954	102,184	572,446	924,477	1,573	2,539	5.6	73,179	148	11,015	294,250	783,899
Memphis	3	293	14,746	71,748	103,176	197	282	4.9	4,642	30	1,813	55,378	114,499
Pascagoula	2	434	19,408	89,293	142,552	244	390	4.6	12,483	38	1,806	113,693	379,949
Tennessee	130	20,328	853,304	4,806,765	8,524,215	13,186	23,387	5.6	611,929	1,212	81,067	2,806,111	10,861,884
Nonmetropolitan	56	4,854	154,230	1,035,900	2,349,091	2,838	6,435	6.7	124,835	310	14,216	797,934	2,642,577
Metropolitan	74	15,474	699,074	3,770,865	6,175,124	10,348	16,952	5.4	487,094	902	66,851	2,008,177	8,219,307
Chattanooga	6	1,353	64,423	338,528	529,509	928	1,450	5.3	53,446	30	4,744	204,196	786,407
Clarksville	1	198	9,605	37,353	70,779	102	194	3.9	5,902	16	1,741	47,867	129,699
Cleveland	2	192	6,503	44,631	90,227	122	247	6.9	5,727	0	0	29,957	121,489
Jackson	2	748	34,095	187,400	322,239	514	883	5.5	26,497	45	3,559	94,141	212,739
Johnson City	6	896	34,480	190,804	319,281	522	874	5.5	20,867	51	2,783	111,596	411,274
Kingsport-Bristol-Bristol	5	1,111	44,065	219,656	387,758	603	1,063	5.0	24,704	71	2,827	172,471	595,680
Knoxville	9	2,354	113,472	596,900	985,172	1,636	2,699	5.3	85,019	160	10,228	367,614	1,389,227
Memphis	14	3,652	166,840	1,031,882	1,561,277	2,827	4,279	6.2	84,440	221	17,644	276,994	1,375,201
Morristown	3	305	12,787	54,222	104,954	149	287	4.2	11,731	36	1,310	66,334	207,267
Nashville-Davidson—Murfreesboro	26	4,665	212,804	1,069,489	1,803,928	2,945	4,976	5.0	168,761	272	22,015	637,007	2,990,324

MSAs

TABLE 8

U.S. CENSUS DIVISION 5, EAST SOUTH CENTRAL

U.S. Community Hospitals
(Nonfederal, short-term general and other special hospitals)

2006 Utilization, Personnel and Finances

FULL-TIME EQUIVALENT PERSONNEL					FULL-TIME EQUIV. TRAINEES			EXPENSES						
								LABOR				TOTAL		
Physicians and Dentists	Registered Nurses	Licensed Practical Nurses	Other Salaried Personnel	Total Personnel	Medical and Dental Residents	Other Trainees	Total Trainees	Payroll (in thousands)	Employee Benefits (in thousands)	Total (in thousands)	Percent of Total	Amount (in thousands)	Adjusted per Admission	Adjusted per Inpatient Day
82,249	1,138,633	112,897	2,419,268	4,343,480	85,320	7,428	92,748	$225,892,043	$57,781,527	$283,673,571	51.4	$551,835,328	$8,970.31	$1,612.23
9,876	143,037	32,484	356,147	641,178	1,422	280	1,702	27,189,409	7,290,060	34,479,464	53.5	64,488,354	5,979.83	914.81
72,373	995,596	80,413	2,063,121	3,702,302	83,898	7,148	91,046	198,702,635	50,491,466	249,194,107	51.1	487,346,974	9,605.99	1,793.12
3,663	78,084	11,269	154,591	293,159	3,269	358	3,627	12,622,929	3,182,394	15,805,324	49.0	32,228,481	7,105.05	1,276.81
914	19,525	5,005	43,504	83,155	128	41	169	3,192,638	825,455	4,018,093	51.9	7,736,492	5,047.85	825.87
2,749	58,559	6,264	111,087	210,004	3,141	317	3,458	9,430,290	2,356,940	11,787,231	48.1	24,491,989	8,154.85	1,542.92
1,585	20,643	2,670	37,241	73,141	1,275	62	1,337	2,992,694	723,246	3,715,942	49.2	7,550,751	6,563.23	1,273.96
113	3,344	779	7,188	13,852	18	5	23	487,015	116,478	603,495	50.5	1,195,063	4,123.64	839.41
1,472	17,299	1,891	30,053	59,289	1,257	57	1,314	2,505,679	606,768	3,112,447	49.0	6,355,689	7,384.72	1,411.34
4	575	103	932	1,848	16	0	16	75,794	17,328	93,122	54.1	172,079	4,864.30	1,106.06
7	530	54	1,404	2,290	0	0	0	90,237	18,906	109,142	52.6	207,636	6,954.35	1,055.47
1,190	6,659	497	11,538	23,548	879	16	895	1,047,886	237,802	1,285,690	46.7	2,753,750	9,218.90	1,693.73
0	7	6	78	105	0	0	0	4,419	758	5,176	62.6	8,265	11,463.93	769.67
18	447	86	924	1,668	1	0	1	65,205	18,401	83,606	50.5	165,461	5,534.19	1,203.36
26	1,069	253	1,773	3,768	0	0	0	143,525	32,709	176,235	45.7	386,000	6,108.26	1,130.89
18	646	88	844	1,995	8	0	8	76,971	23,150	100,120	45.1	222,001	5,692.47	1,184.29
8	538	103	696	1,716	0	0	0	79,545	19,185	98,730	48.7	202,589	6,400.30	1,068.05
66	2,232	196	3,577	6,669	6	0	6	246,514	85,370	331,884	49.5	670,696	7,123.62	1,508.92
97	2,240	154	4,406	7,767	327	7	334	319,443	85,464	404,906	53.8	751,931	6,971.10	1,257.46
29	1,352	144	1,920	4,202	20	0	20	187,929	36,941	224,870	47.1	477,599	6,331.10	1,412.69
9	1,004	207	1,961	3,713	0	34	34	168,212	30,754	198,966	58.9	337,682	6,162.30	1,215.15
530	18,303	2,422	37,400	69,033	111	62	173	3,036,140	798,182	3,834,323	48.3	7,943,140	6,796.39	1,317.67
291	6,107	1,475	13,749	25,764	34	23	57	981,254	271,553	1,252,807	52.0	2,410,039	4,802.49	947.91
239	12,196	947	23,651	43,269	77	39	116	2,054,886	526,629	2,581,516	46.7	5,533,100	8,296.77	1,587.38
0	630	41	1,442	2,420	0	0	0	113,165	27,638	140,803	49.6	283,848	8,908.40	1,744.04
66	1,330	126	2,572	4,718	25	1	26	258,251	71,166	329,416	54.1	609,210	7,369.36	1,597.66
1	237	45	485	850	0	0	0	32,426	9,007	41,433	45.6	90,819	5,335.10	1,198.18
7	385	21	869	1,433	0	0	0	63,638	17,859	81,497	53.2	153,301	5,409.56	1,057.61
9	239	27	646	1,057	4	0	4	39,971	15,649	55,620	59.4	93,678	6,386.97	1,461.96
46	851	183	1,889	3,487	4	0	4	165,081	54,365	219,446	47.9	458,343	7,523.19	1,301.96
30	3,008	174	5,554	10,398	0	0	0	485,649	117,066	602,715	44.8	1,345,294	9,042.90	1,877.71
72	4,999	280	9,126	16,936	44	38	82	813,562	186,913	1,000,476	44.0	2,275,587	9,162.71	1,591.78
8	517	50	1,068	1,970	0	0	0	83,143	26,966	110,110	49.4	223,020	6,503.36	1,405.27
600	11,887	2,039	24,506	48,720	445	1	446	2,106,870	522,766	2,629,635	50.2	5,237,172	7,294.54	1,099.76
383	5,834	1,459	12,909	25,234	52	1	53	1,051,936	262,444	1,314,379	51.5	2,551,033	6,373.73	835.75
217	6,053	580	11,597	23,486	393	0	393	1,054,934	260,322	1,315,256	49.0	2,686,139	8,454.53	1,571.10
65	1,178	75	1,473	3,612	2	0	2	195,019	50,715	245,733	53.4	460,206	9,413.48	1,783.04
22	1,005	95	1,800	3,851	0	0	0	161,371	42,009	203,380	48.4	419,897	8,020.18	1,492.11
85	2,750	307	6,519	12,256	390	0	390	516,603	119,714	636,318	46.5	1,368,639	8,353.92	1,480.45
0	432	60	634	1,380	0	0	0	58,815	15,850	74,666	47.9	155,865	7,342.42	1,510.67
45	688	43	1,171	2,387	1	0	1	123,126	32,034	155,159	55.1	281,532	8,962.28	1,974.94
948	27,251	4,138	55,444	102,265	1,438	233	1,671	4,487,225	1,138,201	5,625,424	48.9	11,497,418	7,670.84	1,348.79
127	4,240	1,292	9,658	18,305	24	12	36	672,433	174,980	847,412	53.6	1,580,357	4,637.88	672.75
821	23,011	2,846	45,786	83,960	1,414	221	1,635	3,814,791	963,221	4,778,012	48.2	9,917,061	8,563.23	1,605.97
42	2,219	208	4,764	8,151	144	0	144	364,246	100,355	464,601	49.9	931,136	9,136.22	1,758.49
2	291	53	546	1,028	0	0	0	42,882	9,810	52,692	57.0	92,501	5,082.49	1,306.90
23	209	41	503	910	9	0	9	38,612	10,715	49,327	53.5	92,220	6,844.81	1,022.09
9	1,143	221	2,606	4,483	3	0	3	180,108	51,990	232,097	55.1	421,572	7,230.46	1,308.26
60	960	223	1,580	3,266	0	72	72	143,453	30,485	173,937	43.3	401,598	7,340.75	1,257.82
5	1,185	209	2,591	4,629	0	7	7	184,432	47,335	231,767	46.9	493,892	6,214.83	1,273.71
131	4,133	484	8,086	15,158	128	90	218	604,478	147,931	752,409	47.4	1,587,064	8,423.55	1,610.95
421	5,265	422	11,065	19,921	570	42	612	996,268	249,305	1,245,573	50.3	2,476,340	9,732.97	1,586.10
14	370	54	682	1,321	5	0	5	52,489	12,382	64,871	50.9	127,470	5,111.28	1,214.54
114	7,236	931	13,363	25,093	555	10	565	1,207,824	302,914	1,510,738	45.9	3,293,267	9,041.23	1,825.61

MSAs

TABLE 8

U.S. CENSUS DIVISION 6, WEST NORTH CENTRAL

U.S. Community Hospitals
(Nonfederal, short-term general and other special hospitals)

2006 Utilization, Personnel and Finances

CLASSIFICATION	Hospitals	Beds	Admissions	Inpatient Days	Adjusted Patient Days	Average Daily Census	Adjusted Average Daily Census	Average Stay (days)	Surgical Operations	NEWBORNS Bassinets	Births	OUTPATIENT VISITS Emergency	Total
UNITED STATES	4,927	802,658	35,377,659	196,366,512	342,281,133	538,496	938,580	5.6	27,330,824	57,832	4,075,193	118,374,029	599,553,025
Nonmetropolitan	2,001	145,328	4,662,402	30,375,652	70,493,783	83,319	193,322	6.5	4,130,326	11,655	481,086	22,555,781	112,987,297
Metropolitan	2,926	657,330	30,715,257	165,990,860	271,787,350	455,177	745,258	5.4	23,200,498	46,177	3,594,107	95,818,248	486,565,728
CENSUS DIVISION 6, WEST NORTH CENTRAL	674	70,501	2,560,628	16,030,245	32,319,232	43,941	88,592	6.3	2,135,784	4,874	278,721	7,485,813	50,419,890
Nonmetropolitan	465	28,339	659,704	5,956,633	14,480,281	16,336	39,710	9.0	612,512	2,127	72,748	2,482,365	19,360,032
Metropolitan	209	42,162	1,900,924	10,073,612	17,838,951	27,605	48,882	5.3	1,523,272	2,747	205,973	5,003,448	31,059,858
Iowa	117	10,500	363,077	2,267,449	5,333,844	6,207	14,614	6.2	434,702	731	39,560	1,122,636	10,295,093
Nonmetropolitan	84	4,605	119,289	976,384	2,825,718	2,671	7,740	8.2	136,798	340	11,695	476,507	4,440,775
Metropolitan	33	5,895	243,788	1,291,065	2,508,126	3,536	6,874	5.3	297,904	391	27,865	646,129	5,854,318
Ames	2	276	10,322	62,559	134,380	172	368	6.1	9,657	17	1,318	22,288	154,214
Cedar Rapids	4	803	29,472	182,539	436,122	501	1,196	6.2	36,219	54	3,623	98,682	809,909
Davenport-Moline-Rock Island . . .	2	518	23,062	108,962	181,753	298	498	4.7	11,938	33	2,676	72,575	216,188
Des Moines	8	1,468	70,218	346,872	569,612	949	1,561	4.9	49,111	121	9,197	176,231	1,567,890
Dubuque	3	465	13,999	72,622	129,186	199	354	5.2	14,178	36	1,609	47,576	140,845
Iowa City	3	954	35,972	230,862	437,963	632	1,200	6.4	104,754	39	2,896	63,408	1,265,428
Omaha-Council Bluffs	3	304	14,491	60,272	107,160	165	294	4.2	13,172	21	1,166	47,366	185,336
Sioux City	2	405	20,270	94,178	150,370	258	412	4.6	16,534	31	2,647	49,547	411,531
Waterloo-Cedar Falls	6	702	25,982	132,199	361,580	362	991	5.1	42,341	39	2,733	68,456	1,102,977
Kansas	129	10,019	332,524	2,024,257	3,993,672	5,547	10,942	6.1	243,737	722	40,729	972,761	6,146,257
Nonmetropolitan	100	5,263	118,752	1,028,878	2,309,753	2,821	6,328	8.7	100,062	357	12,084	380,268	3,096,834
Metropolitan	29	4,756	213,772	995,379	1,683,919	2,726	4,614	4.7	143,675	365	28,645	592,493	3,049,423
Kansas City	13	2,032	93,272	438,238	769,068	1,201	2,108	4.7	73,221	193	14,185	259,723	1,477,616
Lawrence	1	149	6,446	23,882	73,253	65	201	3.7	4,238	13	1,105	31,606	202,008
Topeka	5	786	26,578	140,227	272,213	384	746	5.3	19,337	40	3,158	94,938	495,425
Wichita	10	1,789	87,476	393,032	569,385	1,076	1,559	4.5	46,879	119	10,197	206,226	874,374
Minnesota	131	15,843	633,225	3,955,503	7,896,338	10,834	21,637	6.2	483,517	1,228	71,999	1,711,528	10,109,186
Nonmetropolitan	82	5,856	125,694	1,368,527	3,303,769	3,748	9,054	10.9	129,352	446	16,912	536,373	3,447,959
Metropolitan	49	9,987	507,531	2,586,976	4,592,569	7,086	12,583	5.1	354,165	782	55,087	1,175,155	6,661,227
Duluth	10	1,475	48,847	365,060	714,337	999	1,956	7.5	45,249	95	3,960	116,965	633,030
Grand Forks	2	259	1,931	71,370	288,722	195	791	37.0	3,074	8	206	9,023	101,111
Minneapolis-St. Paul-Bloomington .	29	6,229	354,061	1,574,289	2,587,834	4,313	7,092	4.4	256,496	579	45,505	902,795	4,724,660
Rochester	4	1,343	75,388	403,045	644,416	1,104	1,766	5.3	34,343	49	2,435	92,134	778,481
St. Cloud	4	681	27,304	173,212	357,260	475	978	6.3	15,003	51	2,981	54,238	423,945
Missouri	119	18,888	830,882	4,331,742	8,005,326	11,888	21,974	5.2	603,216	1,193	79,240	2,641,586	16,338,186
Nonmetropolitan	53	3,915	148,641	698,642	1,655,307	1,928	4,573	4.7	108,579	359	14,942	641,282	4,492,111
Metropolitan	66	14,973	682,241	3,633,100	6,350,019	9,960	17,401	5.3	494,637	834	64,298	2,000,304	11,846,075
Columbia	4	876	38,539	208,338	297,799	570	816	5.4	29,481	41	3,598	70,445	863,729
Jefferson City	3	336	19,657	81,778	151,511	224	416	4.2	13,479	38	1,902	69,519	531,361
Joplin	4	753	37,286	176,556	340,633	484	933	4.7	22,679	52	3,445	159,105	1,015,758
Kansas City	21	3,669	150,581	835,967	1,575,878	2,292	4,316	5.6	125,284	219	16,303	543,775	2,733,779
Springfield	4	1,335	67,638	338,735	690,082	929	1,891	5.0	59,162	84	6,849	255,542	1,491,149
St. Joseph	1	350	18,878	85,448	145,918	234	400	4.5	8,928	20	1,706	46,382	604,465
St. Louis	29	7,654	349,662	1,906,278	3,148,198	5,227	8,629	5.5	235,624	380	30,495	855,536	4,605,834
Nebraska	85	7,375	215,219	1,666,078	3,273,738	4,570	8,969	7.7	198,953	590	26,226	551,914	4,049,105
Nonmetropolitan	69	3,858	81,025	776,257	1,869,505	2,131	5,122	9.6	78,691	371	9,510	228,315	2,056,781
Metropolitan	16	3,517	134,194	889,821	1,404,233	2,439	3,847	6.6	120,262	219	16,716	323,599	1,992,324
Lincoln	4	1,080	39,761	289,887	440,316	794	1,207	7.3	26,246	57	4,992	91,114	443,717
Omaha-Council Bluffs	12	2,437	94,433	599,934	963,917	1,645	2,640	6.4	94,016	162	11,724	232,485	1,548,607
North Dakota	41	3,550	88,737	762,500	1,687,312	2,093	4,623	8.6	72,834	189	9,587	263,144	1,709,284
Nonmetropolitan	35	2,162	30,067	456,998	1,100,591	1,255	3,015	15.2	26,088	95	3,002	109,255	798,803
Metropolitan	6	1,388	58,670	305,502	586,721	838	1,608	5.2	46,746	94	6,585	153,889	910,481
Bismarck	2	503	19,252	89,999	187,724	247	515	4.7	15,369	27	1,915	37,885	527,649
Fargo	2	533	26,587	130,707	207,298	358	568	4.9	21,595	43	3,195	59,961	267,316
Grand Forks	2	352	12,831	84,796	191,699	233	525	6.6	9,782	24	1,475	56,043	115,516
South Dakota	52	4,326	96,964	1,022,716	2,129,002	2,802	5,833	10.5	98,825	221	11,380	222,244	1,772,779
Nonmetropolitan	42	2,680	36,236	650,947	1,415,638	1,782	3,878	18.0	32,942	159	4,603	110,365	1,026,769
Metropolitan	10	1,646	60,728	371,769	713,364	1,020	1,955	6.1	65,883	62	6,777	111,879	746,010
Rapid City	3	507	16,017	114,642	193,537	315	530	7.2	9,768	18	2,233	53,694	192,757
Sioux Falls	7	1,139	44,711	257,127	519,827	705	1,425	5.8	56,115	44	4,544	58,185	553,253

TABLE 8

U.S. CENSUS DIVISION 6, WEST NORTH CENTRAL

U.S. Community Hospitals
(Nonfederal, short-term general and other special hospitals)

2006 Utilization, Personnel and Finances

	FULL-TIME EQUIVALENT PERSONNEL				FULL-TIME EQUIV. TRAINEES			EXPENSES						
								LABOR				TOTAL		
Physicians and Dentists	Registered Nurses	Licensed Practical Nurses	Other Salaried Personnel	Total Personnel	Medical and Dental Residents	Other Trainees	Total Trainees	Payroll (in thousands)	Employee Benefits (in thousands)	Total (in thousands)	Percent of Total	Amount (in thousands)	Adjusted per Admission	Adjusted per Inpatient Day
82,249	1,138,633	112,897	2,419,268	4,343,480	85,320	7,428	92,748	$225,892,043	$57,781,527	$283,673,571	51.4	$551,835,328	$8,970.31	$1,612.23
9,876	143,037	32,484	356,147	641,178	1,422	280	1,702	27,189,409	7,290,060	34,479,464	53.5	64,488,354	5,979.83	914.81
72,373	995,596	80,413	2,063,121	3,702,302	83,898	7,148	91,046	198,702,635	50,491,466	249,194,107	51.1	487,346,974	9,605.99	1,793.12
6,641	87,414	10,983	196,998	349,689	3,099	295	3,394	17,373,850	4,018,999	21,392,841	51.0	41,972,966	8,434.42	1,298.70
1,849	23,152	5,579	60,856	108,639	68	23	91	4,497,271	1,083,442	5,580,714	54.2	10,305,381	6,302.82	711.68
4,792	64,262	5,404	136,142	241,050	3,031	272	3,303	12,876,580	2,935,557	15,812,127	49.9	31,667,584	9,477.49	1,775.19
951	13,825	1,294	32,171	55,566	596	12	608	2,412,051	644,904	3,056,956	52.4	5,830,165	7,241.06	1,093.05
301	4,845	755	12,182	21,287	22	0	22	839,547	213,980	1,053,528	54.4	1,934,862	5,636.48	684.73
650	8,980	539	19,989	34,279	574	12	586	1,572,504	430,924	2,003,428	51.4	3,895,303	8,433.60	1,553.07
4	305	15	629	1,145	0	0	0	52,942	14,473	67,414	50.2	134,323	6,583.18	999.58
26	1,041	96	2,307	4,007	0	0	0	171,355	48,976	220,330	52.4	420,466	6,511.68	964.10
5	718	13	994	1,993	5	0	5	100,622	28,416	129,039	39.4	327,237	8,463.39	1,800.45
289	2,795	90	6,106	10,396	154	4	158	451,195	111,802	562,997	53.2	1,058,673	9,126.49	1,858.59
9	523	14	1,103	1,767	0	0	0	72,494	17,760	90,254	47.2	191,106	7,583.26	1,479.31
106	1,700	26	3,964	6,827	412	8	420	334,332	116,814	451,145	52.9	852,780	12,672.64	1,947.15
11	401	23	937	1,520	0	0	0	69,593	18,311	87,904	50.4	174,480	6,693.53	1,628.22
79	640	47	1,609	2,598	0	0	0	123,024	28,162	151,186	53.6	282,292	8,665.90	1,877.31
121	857	215	2,340	4,026	3	0	3	196,947	46,211	243,159	53.6	453,946	6,384.35	1,255.45
624	10,932	1,294	22,397	42,040	116	39	155	1,947,757	460,295	2,408,048	52.2	4,612,907	7,183.65	1,155.05
206	3,982	743	9,741	18,127	5	6	11	711,645	167,395	879,038	54.7	1,606,647	6,029.42	695.59
418	6,950	551	12,656	23,913	111	33	144	1,236,112	292,900	1,529,010	50.9	3,006,259	8,002.35	1,785.28
166	3,540	104	5,686	10,993	1	17	18	578,789	140,892	719,682	49.6	1,450,062	8,358.86	1,885.48
16	211	27	471	864	0	0	0	46,374	10,318	56,692	51.8	109,444	5,535.29	1,494.05
174	914	310	2,642	4,622	0	9	9	233,681	52,700	286,381	56.3	509,117	9,265.60	1,870.29
62	2,285	110	3,857	7,434	110	7	117	377,268	88,989	466,255	49.7	937,637	7,355.34	1,646.75
1,643	19,083	2,633	42,786	77,441	621	111	732	4,762,339	1,219,764	5,982,101	55.0	10,886,427	9,361.42	1,378.67
447	4,227	1,333	11,572	21,186	11	5	16	992,503	256,191	1,248,693	56.1	2,226,361	7,126.59	673.89
1,196	14,856	1,300	31,214	56,255	610	106	716	3,769,836	963,574	4,733,408	54.7	8,660,066	10,182.31	1,885.67
152	1,299	257	3,379	5,829	1	1	2	357,069	109,625	466,693	57.6	809,941	9,190.40	1,133.84
8	89	76	264	607	0	0	0	24,529	5,320	29,849	59.5	50,161	6,964.89	173.73
804	10,806	564	22,292	39,914	495	86	581	2,757,327	683,901	3,441,227	54.5	6,309,155	10,755.78	2,438.01
210	1,774	182	3,247	6,289	102	19	121	448,590	118,487	567,078	52.8	1,074,803	8,973.96	1,667.87
22	888	221	2,032	3,616	12	0	12	182,321	46,240	228,561	54.9	416,006	8,521.56	1,164.43
2,107	27,816	3,313	61,510	108,082	1,702	121	1,823	5,188,144	981,903	6,170,039	45.7	13,503,914	8,822.20	1,686.87
493	4,567	1,232	12,394	20,889	30	10	40	855,990	179,932	1,035,918	49.6	2,088,640	5,979.49	1,261.78
1,614	23,249	2,081	49,116	87,193	1,672	111	1,783	4,332,154	801,971	5,134,121	45.0	11,415,274	9,662.71	1,797.68
17	1,249	221	3,008	5,037	325	0	325	252,723	50,236	302,959	41.8	724,128	12,979.76	2,431.60
64	572	126	1,291	2,325	10	0	10	105,404	19,137	124,541	44.5	279,694	7,671.89	1,846.03
231	1,298	239	2,957	5,481	16	0	16	249,947	30,335	280,282	49.4	567,829	7,882.03	1,666.98
306	5,617	385	11,334	19,583	182	109	291	1,024,383	193,291	1,217,672	47.5	2,563,716	9,776.00	1,626.85
230	2,724	288	7,668	12,487	24	0	24	516,679	95,024	611,703	42.6	1,436,247	10,450.52	2,081.27
95	622	155	1,407	2,551	0	0	0	150,996	31,180	182,176	53.1	343,274	10,648.13	2,352.52
671	11,167	667	21,451	39,729	1,115	2	1,117	2,032,023	382,767	2,414,788	43.9	5,500,386	9,399.64	1,747.15
477	8,623	1,334	19,127	34,420	27	2	29	1,585,483	389,561	1,975,045	51.1	3,862,461	9,496.05	1,179.83
173	3,079	900	7,921	14,442	0	1	1	590,040	149,580	739,623	55.0	1,344,627	6,932.64	719.24
304	5,544	434	11,206	19,978	27	1	28	995,444	239,981	1,235,422	49.1	2,517,834	11,832.59	1,793.03
103	1,501	215	3,679	6,251	0	0	0	273,902	87,070	360,971	54.5	662,297	11,315.51	1,504.14
201	4,043	219	7,527	13,727	27	1	28	721,541	152,912	874,451	47.1	1,855,537	12,028.79	1,925.00
521	3,230	842	9,033	15,632	17	0	17	747,155	143,703	890,858	54.6	1,630,169	8,065.95	966.13
176	1,087	417	3,531	6,363	0	0	0	252,808	49,981	302,787	57.2	529,519	6,163.79	481.12
345	2,143	425	5,502	9,269	17	0	17	494,347	93,723	588,071	53.4	1,100,650	9,472.28	1,875.93
172	748	172	2,011	3,513	0	0	0	179,076	27,523	206,599	55.7	370,973	9,163.90	1,976.16
0	987	175	1,420	2,807	0	0	0	146,489	28,408	174,897	43.8	399,270	9,585.16	1,926.07
173	408	78	2,071	2,949	17	0	17	168,783	37,792	206,575	62.5	330,408	9,700.76	1,723.58
318	3,905	273	9,974	16,508	20	10	30	730,922	178,868	909,794	55.2	1,646,923	7,265.83	773.57
53	1,365	199	3,515	6,345	0	1	1	254,739	66,383	321,127	55.9	574,725	6,863.86	405.98
265	2,540	74	6,459	10,163	20	9	29	476,182	112,485	588,667	54.9	1,072,198	7,501.30	1,503.02
16	673	50	1,429	2,469	20	9	29	124,845	20,472	145,316	52.4	277,393	10,159.05	1,433.28
249	1,867	24	5,030	7,694	0	0	0	351,338	92,013	443,351	55.8	794,805	6,873.69	1,528.98

MSAs

TABLE 8

U.S. CENSUS DIVISION 7, WEST SOUTH CENTRAL

U.S. Community Hospitals
(Nonfederal, short-term general and other special hospitals)

2006 Utilization, Personnel and Finances

CLASSIFICATION	Hospitals	Beds	Admissions	Inpatient Days	Adjusted Patient Days	Average Daily Census	Adjusted Average Daily Census	Average Stay (days)	Surgical Operations	NEWBORNS Bassinets	NEWBORNS Births	OUTPATIENT VISITS Emergency	OUTPATIENT VISITS Total
UNITED STATES	4,927	802,658	35,377,659	196,366,512	342,281,133	538,496	938,580	5.6	27,330,824	57,832	4,075,193	118,374,029	599,553,025
Nonmetropolitan	2,001	145,328	4,662,402	30,375,652	70,493,783	83,319	193,322	6.5	4,130,326	11,655	481,086	22,555,781	112,987,297
Metropolitan	2,926	657,330	30,715,257	165,990,860	271,787,350	455,177	745,258	5.4	23,200,498	46,177	3,594,107	95,818,248	486,565,728
CENSUS DIVISION 7, WEST SOUTH CENTRAL	745	94,910	3,979,239	20,852,125	33,970,679	57,325	93,389	5.2	2,798,937	7,148	540,951	13,210,287	52,220,979
Nonmetropolitan	315	16,935	622,796	2,835,553	5,998,104	7,790	16,480	4.6	421,265	1,463	64,432	2,869,994	11,365,744
Metropolitan	430	77,975	3,356,443	18,016,572	27,972,575	49,535	76,909	5.4	2,377,672	5,685	476,519	10,340,293	40,855,235
Arkansas	84	9,309	373,067	1,943,363	3,402,957	5,330	9,325	5.2	253,270	610	39,232	1,267,198	5,085,474
Nonmetropolitan	49	3,344	116,117	611,723	1,342,446	1,681	3,683	5.3	77,689	268	11,029	493,030	1,717,984
Metropolitan	35	5,965	256,950	1,331,640	2,060,511	3,649	5,642	5.2	175,581	342	28,203	774,168	3,367,490
Fayetteville-Springdale-Rogers	9	841	43,117	189,945	287,220	521	787	4.4	27,683	77	7,014	154,399	417,564
Fort Smith	5	872	33,312	182,453	274,933	500	753	5.5	30,213	43	3,537	116,373	251,398
Hot Springs	3	483	19,551	108,252	159,169	297	436	5.5	12,020	24	1,978	61,296	445,971
Jonesboro	3	476	24,797	115,548	181,252	316	496	4.7	13,829	32	2,031	67,086	253,117
Little Rock-North Little Rock	13	2,834	119,449	651,494	1,005,758	1,785	2,754	5.5	82,638	118	11,544	317,107	1,787,181
Memphis	1	130	4,038	19,699	36,303	54	99	4.9	3,694	12	773	20,328	57,045
Pine Bluff	1	329	12,686	64,249	115,876	176	317	5.1	5,504	36	1,326	37,579	155,214
Louisiana	132	15,864	623,144	3,556,169	5,865,732	9,872	16,281	5.7	458,600	1,059	69,455	2,096,962	9,861,651
Nonmetropolitan	51	3,164	117,411	550,400	1,077,537	1,506	2,952	4.7	93,999	241	10,907	541,051	1,746,962
Metropolitan	81	12,700	505,733	3,005,769	4,788,195	8,366	13,329	5.9	364,601	818	58,548	1,555,911	8,114,689
Alexandria	6	717	34,497	186,831	295,768	513	810	5.4	23,074	61	3,213	122,645	418,745
Baton Rouge	16	2,682	94,925	686,994	1,083,134	1,883	2,968	7.2	57,540	145	11,455	285,919	996,698
Houma-Bayou Cane-Thibodaux	5	593	27,490	124,995	235,023	341	645	4.5	24,708	61	3,411	128,581	513,053
Lafayette	7	1,066	43,987	229,797	328,832	631	901	5.2	23,701	88	5,029	151,029	505,029
Lake Charles	8	855	32,611	157,167	275,787	433	761	4.8	25,013	49	2,593	101,880	387,212
Monroe	11	1,239	46,159	274,336	495,258	753	1,358	5.9	34,393	85	6,271	132,272	528,820
New Orleans-Metairie-Kenner	18	3,422	143,181	842,705	1,320,119	2,433	3,819	5.9	109,496	209	18,310	446,485	3,608,550
Shreveport-Bossier City	10	2,126	82,883	502,944	754,274	1,379	2,067	6.1	66,676	120	8,266	187,100	1,156,582
Oklahoma	112	10,773	454,085	2,307,539	3,904,745	6,343	10,739	5.1	301,618	830	47,489	1,554,914	5,334,806
Nonmetropolitan	66	3,758	145,641	664,411	1,352,438	1,839	3,747	4.6	94,212	347	14,163	610,004	2,236,005
Metropolitan	46	7,015	308,444	1,643,128	2,552,307	4,504	6,992	5.3	207,406	483	33,326	944,910	3,098,801
Fort Smith	2	79	3,412	12,379	26,783	34	73	3.6	2,191	9	443	17,802	43,139
Lawton	2	449	14,415	84,937	145,603	233	399	5.9	9,896	37	1,436	56,623	188,235
Oklahoma City	20	3,728	159,704	887,359	1,352,567	2,430	3,705	5.6	101,778	272	17,305	511,851	1,773,186
Tulsa	22	2,759	130,913	658,453	1,027,354	1,807	2,815	5.0	93,541	165	14,142	358,634	1,094,241
Texas	417	58,964	2,528,943	13,045,054	20,797,245	35,780	57,044	5.2	1,785,449	4,649	384,775	8,291,213	31,939,048
Nonmetropolitan	149	6,669	243,627	1,009,019	2,225,683	2,764	6,098	4.1	155,365	607	28,333	1,225,909	5,664,793
Metropolitan	268	52,295	2,285,316	12,036,035	18,571,562	33,016	50,946	5.3	1,630,084	4,042	356,442	7,065,304	26,274,255
Abilene	5	631	25,556	136,351	214,159	374	587	5.3	13,567	46	2,870	81,355	367,669
Amarillo	5	987	39,512	209,208	297,674	580	822	5.3	26,133	54	4,705	94,667	316,145
Austin-Round Rock	18	2,281	115,773	577,938	873,509	1,597	2,424	5.0	91,890	191	20,691	453,118	1,264,525
Beaumont-Port Arthur	9	1,784	60,710	319,679	494,604	877	1,359	5.3	39,233	91	5,228	195,849	610,331
Brownsville-Harlingen	4	948	48,954	213,129	306,178	584	839	4.4	23,403	92	8,111	99,243	194,248
College Station-Bryan	3	434	21,558	95,031	164,815	261	451	4.4	17,032	60	3,561	81,303	309,786
Corpus Christi	5	1,457	59,541	321,260	499,211	880	1,368	5.4	43,564	98	7,384	182,622	608,766
Dallas-Plano-Irving	47	9,068	391,348	2,038,036	3,012,087	5,590	8,257	5.2	252,633	775	69,351	1,311,522	4,421,711
El Paso	8	1,666	76,524	376,200	560,276	1,031	1,536	4.9	42,264	164	15,833	217,803	1,079,299
Fort Worth-Arlington	23	4,073	202,828	1,045,674	1,618,709	2,867	4,434	5.2	167,683	394	35,381	730,068	2,413,492
Houston-Sugar Land-Baytown	57	13,053	554,777	3,133,577	4,914,615	8,582	13,468	5.6	407,434	959	87,454	1,549,250	7,537,042
Killeen-Temple-Fort Hood	5	992	36,571	208,785	479,682	572	1,315	5.7	35,142	44	4,335	130,085	1,181,751
Laredo	2	483	24,580	122,195	182,009	335	499	5.0	14,533	65	6,379	58,003	226,154
Longview	5	639	29,401	128,867	215,352	353	590	4.4	19,842	67	3,862	133,339	266,486
Lubbock	6	1,504	56,253	306,764	464,228	840	1,272	5.5	40,846	45	5,330	153,324	591,638
McAllen-Edinburg-Mission	8	1,959	88,791	415,283	557,124	1,138	1,525	4.7	64,847	151	17,099	136,857	394,122
Midland	5	425	14,270	80,212	137,581	230	393	5.6	13,537	34	2,553	61,268	163,468
Odessa	4	489	18,769	101,606	153,187	279	419	5.4	12,279	39	3,481	66,666	212,850
San Angelo	2	443	18,213	86,300	147,724	236	405	4.7	14,601	35	2,080	67,968	208,924
San Antonio	24	5,042	235,283	1,189,375	1,793,965	3,259	4,916	5.1	165,042	418	34,446	734,410	2,024,089
Sherman-Denison	2	395	20,462	99,619	153,660	273	421	4.9	18,188	37	1,581	66,895	140,678
Texarkana TX-Texarkana AR	5	612	29,613	152,480	219,097	417	600	5.1	14,346	46	2,627	96,237	333,357
Tyler	6	1,041	46,702	254,012	395,639	696	1,084	5.4	30,525	36	3,366	93,349	618,154
Victoria	3	549	21,976	99,721	170,027	274	465	4.5	19,402	34	2,461	72,188	210,511
Waco	2	833	28,120	231,905	393,070	636	1,077	8.2	26,876	51	3,947	118,108	401,284
Wichita Falls	5	507	19,231	92,828	153,380	255	420	4.8	15,242	16	2,326	79,807	177,775

MSAs

TABLE 8

U.S. CENSUS DIVISION 7, WEST SOUTH CENTRAL

U.S. Community Hospitals
(Nonfederal, short-term general and other special hospitals)

2006 Utilization, Personnel and Finances

FULL-TIME EQUIVALENT PERSONNEL					FULL-TIME EQUIV. TRAINEES			EXPENSES						
								LABOR				TOTAL		
Physicians and Dentists	Registered Nurses	Licensed Practical Nurses	Other Salaried Personnel	Total Personnel	Medical and Dental Residents	Other Trainees	Total Trainees	Payroll (in thousands)	Employee Benefits (in thousands)	Total (in thousands)	Percent of Total	Amount (in thousands)	Adjusted per Admission	Adjusted per Inpatient Day
82,249	1,138,633	112,897	2,419,268	4,343,480	85,320	7,428	92,748	$225,892,043	$57,781,527	$283,673,571	51.4	$551,835,328	$8,970.31	$1,612.23
9,876	143,037	32,484	356,147	641,178	1,422	280	1,702	27,189,409	7,290,060	34,479,464	53.5	64,488,354	5,979.83	914.81
72,373	995,596	80,413	2,063,121	3,702,302	83,898	7,148	91,046	198,702,635	50,491,466	249,194,107	51.1	487,346,974	9,605.99	1,793.12
3,544	118,345	20,867	239,217	446,986	4,489	1,295	5,784	21,112,176	4,840,693	25,952,866	48.2	53,806,426	8,044.91	1,583.91
513	14,547	6,557	37,051	70,098	39	77	116	2,654,999	637,921	3,292,919	52.1	6,325,794	4,686.63	1,054.63
3,031	103,798	14,310	202,166	376,888	4,450	1,218	5,668	18,457,177	4,202,772	22,659,947	47.7	47,480,632	8,893.99	1,697.40
293	11,355	3,003	22,521	42,985	29	59	88	1,773,057	410,137	2,183,194	49.2	4,437,597	6,686.61	1,304.04
118	3,096	1,405	6,722	13,659	1	58	59	493,285	115,386	608,671	53.1	1,146,601	4,404.26	854.11
175	8,259	1,598	15,799	29,326	28	1	29	1,279,772	294,751	1,574,523	47.8	3,290,996	8,159.86	1,597.17
37	1,101	220	2,184	4,060	0	0	0	198,130	39,414	237,545	47.8	497,217	7,348.65	1,731.14
34	935	199	2,028	3,721	28	1	29	134,716	34,281	168,996	48.1	351,417	6,894.72	1,278.19
24	552	172	1,038	2,056	0	0	0	90,874	25,451	116,325	52.5	221,743	7,585.64	1,393.13
3	734	208	1,075	2,413	0	0	0	82,659	19,007	101,666	41.3	246,098	6,179.33	1,357.77
61	4,450	627	8,504	15,222	0	0	0	695,387	159,522	854,910	48.0	1,779,894	9,605.21	1,769.70
7	125	53	271	487	0	0	0	20,050	2,741	22,790	46.9	48,576	6,527.22	1,338.06
9	362	119	699	1,367	0	0	0	57,957	14,334	72,291	49.5	146,051	6,383.35	1,260.41
1,327	18,279	3,154	39,461	72,913	1,101	61	1,162	3,101,023	710,907	3,811,931	50.5	7,552,791	6,973.00	1,287.61
173	2,863	924	7,445	13,368	20	1	21	497,721	115,802	613,521	55.6	1,102,847	4,631.14	1,023.49
1,154	15,416	2,230	32,016	59,545	1,081	60	1,141	2,603,302	595,105	3,198,410	49.6	6,449,944	7,632.97	1,347.05
66	1,035	174	2,017	3,884	26	8	34	153,561	38,054	191,616	45.2	423,671	7,736.17	1,432.44
144	2,695	451	6,754	11,617	35	36	71	499,888	106,735	606,623	50.4	1,203,286	7,651.96	1,110.93
23	740	123	1,880	3,194	0	0	0	133,027	35,158	168,185	48.0	350,654	6,729.88	1,492.00
20	1,142	246	2,293	4,350	9	0	9	184,663	49,526	234,190	45.3	516,765	8,132.90	1,571.52
27	893	168	1,709	3,388	17	0	17	149,424	39,089	188,514	48.4	389,149	6,659.98	1,411.05
72	1,370	263	2,451	5,043	51	5	56	203,375	56,092	259,467	47.2	549,350	5,124.77	1,109.22
187	5,050	561	9,749	18,195	340	3	343	908,387	183,652	1,092,039	50.0	2,184,052	9,678.21	1,654.44
615	2,491	244	5,163	9,874	603	8	611	370,977	86,799	457,776	55.0	833,018	6,608.26	1,104.40
545	11,396	2,551	26,605	48,573	224	147	371	2,136,982	509,599	2,646,581	49.1	5,384,899	6,789.88	1,379.07
203	3,165	1,273	8,220	15,388	18	18	36	600,082	150,590	750,672	51.2	1,465,922	4,813.86	1,083.91
342	8,231	1,278	18,385	33,185	206	129	335	1,536,900	359,008	1,895,909	48.4	3,918,977	8,021.55	1,535.46
10	77	30	208	388	0	0	0	10,983	2,798	13,780	55.7	24,746	3,453.22	923.94
77	282	218	1,213	1,952	0	0	0	88,684	17,921	106,604	51.9	205,506	8,212.04	1,411.42
178	4,610	514	9,585	17,131	82	68	150	808,514	192,433	1,000,948	47.6	2,104,859	8,448.06	1,556.20
77	3,262	516	7,379	13,714	124	61	185	628,720	145,856	774,577	48.9	1,583,865	7,643.69	1,541.69
1,379	77,315	12,159	150,630	282,515	3,135	1,028	4,163	14,101,114	3,210,050	17,311,160	47.5	36,431,139	8,782.02	1,751.73
19	5,423	2,955	14,664	27,683	0	0	0	1,063,911	256,142	1,320,055	50.6	2,610,424	4,774.39	1,172.86
1,360	71,892	9,204	135,966	254,832	3,135	1,028	4,163	13,037,204	2,953,908	15,991,105	47.3	33,820,716	9,390.41	1,821.10
5	791	252	1,514	3,171	0	22	22	114,479	24,051	138,530	49.4	280,487	6,914.00	1,309.71
18	1,369	173	2,055	4,149	0	0	0	179,329	36,342	215,670	41.0	525,546	9,077.26	1,765.51
48	3,325	346	4,746	10,444	54	25	79	612,008	112,164	724,172	44.4	1,631,823	8,751.18	1,868.12
16	1,725	304	2,766	5,791	9	2	11	278,831	64,701	343,533	47.7	719,968	7,486.26	1,455.65
24	839	246	1,833	3,290	30	27	57	185,734	36,079	221,814	46.3	479,125	6,736.00	1,564.86
0	650	151	1,280	2,345	0	0	0	96,951	27,812	124,763	47.5	262,752	7,044.28	1,594.22
1	1,696	289	3,245	5,926	88	6	94	297,457	66,585	364,041	48.2	755,234	8,118.17	1,532.85
188	13,899	884	21,444	43,497	1,357	71	1,428	2,459,643	517,312	2,976,954	48.5	6,135,719	10,242.02	2,037.03
10	1,857	151	3,422	6,516	0	0	0	312,949	68,231	381,179	39.7	959,774	8,353.78	1,713.04
46	6,699	782	10,865	21,828	182	64	246	1,140,879	271,746	1,412,623	48.3	2,923,648	9,074.97	1,806.16
831	20,104	1,842	43,911	77,230	707	743	1,450	4,193,742	1,040,541	5,234,283	49.4	10,594,238	11,878.27	2,155.66
0	1,212	283	3,141	5,510	343	51	394	244,888	61,260	306,147	54.6	560,630	7,225.55	1,168.75
0	419	65	1,075	1,854	0	0	0	77,725	14,957	92,683	39.9	232,400	6,333.10	1,276.86
2	882	97	1,203	2,691	0	0	0	116,525	25,041	141,566	42.7	331,167	6,670.17	1,537.80
0	1,925	344	3,667	6,564	0	0	0	296,867	60,719	357,587	42.4	843,301	9,718.03	1,816.57
0	1,881	242	3,303	6,275	0	0	0	303,919	63,504	367,423	43.1	852,117	6,993.16	1,529.49
2	483	109	978	1,912	0	0	0	84,149	19,527	103,675	45.1	229,823	8,879.31	1,670.46
0	510	116	1,030	1,929	0	0	0	88,217	37,338	125,555	54.5	230,240	7,784.44	1,503.00
0	410	104	1,087	1,900	0	0	0	74,124	19,474	93,598	47.3	197,965	6,360.33	1,340.10
45	6,734	1,197	12,465	23,030	343	5	348	1,083,496	205,707	1,289,202	42.9	3,005,113	8,319.37	1,675.12
1	415	123	1,457	2,168	0	0	0	93,247	18,915	112,162	50.6	221,817	7,023.52	1,443.56
0	762	217	1,212	2,614	0	3	3	113,494	24,679	138,173	47.2	292,858	6,630.55	1,336.66
100	1,482	352	4,589	7,124	22	0	22	280,910	66,644	347,555	46.0	756,171	10,063.36	1,911.27
0	584	152	1,106	2,082	0	9	9	87,554	21,001	108,554	48.4	224,204	5,878.77	1,318.64
23	698	143	1,500	2,790	0	0	0	127,116	29,521	156,637	47.3	330,816	6,811.39	841.62
0	541	240	1,072	2,202	0	0	0	92,973	20,054	113,026	46.4	243,778	7,372.90	1,589.37

MSAs

TABLE 8

U.S. CENSUS DIVISION 8, MOUNTAIN

U.S. Community Hospitals
(Nonfederal, short-term general and other special hospitals)

2006 Utilization, Personnel and Finances

MSAs

CLASSIFICATION	Hospitals	Beds	Admissions	Inpatient Days	Adjusted Patient Days	Average Daily Census	Adjusted Average Daily Census	Average Stay (days)	Surgical Operations	NEWBORNS Bassinets	Births	OUTPATIENT VISITS Emergency	Total
UNITED STATES	4,927	802,658	35,377,659	196,366,512	342,281,133	538,496	938,580	5.6	27,330,824	57,832	4,075,193	118,374,029	599,553,025
Nonmetropolitan	2,001	145,328	4,662,402	30,375,652	70,493,783	83,319	193,322	6.5	4,130,326	11,655	481,086	22,555,781	112,987,297
Metropolitan	2,926	657,330	30,715,257	165,990,860	271,787,350	455,177	745,258	5.4	23,200,498	46,177	3,594,107	95,818,248	486,565,728
CENSUS DIVISION 8, MOUNTAIN	365	43,792	2,013,762	10,300,681	17,918,026	28,265	49,146	5.1	1,483,417	3,992	312,461	6,901,098	32,102,950
Nonmetropolitan	196	10,275	286,405	2,066,762	4,992,493	5,668	13,678	7.2	262,969	905	43,577	1,569,832	8,083,133
Metropolitan	169	33,517	1,727,357	8,233,919	12,925,533	22,597	35,468	4.8	1,220,448	3,087	268,884	5,331,266	24,019,817
Arizona	66	11,947	664,773	3,023,329	4,642,693	8,319	12,771	4.5	443,028	989	96,797	2,073,320	6,555,635
Nonmetropolitan	16	997	47,544	215,859	482,367	592	1,320	4.5	35,784	79	6,366	248,570	978,126
Metropolitan	50	10,950	617,229	2,807,470	4,160,326	7,727	11,451	4.5	407,244	910	90,431	1,824,750	5,577,509
Flagstaff	3	357	16,514	74,900	139,454	206	382	4.5	11,874	49	2,354	98,563	360,138
Phoenix-Mesa-Scottsdale	32	7,704	436,285	1,994,624	2,892,153	5,499	7,976	4.6	285,498	657	67,295	1,168,349	3,443,158
Prescott	2	262	16,440	58,818	103,483	161	284	3.6	10,867	23	2,021	76,962	186,190
Tucson	11	2,253	127,777	596,702	898,188	1,635	2,461	4.7	86,759	162	15,155	421,752	1,441,820
Yuma	2	374	20,213	82,426	127,048	226	348	4.1	12,246	19	3,606	59,124	146,203
Colorado	73	9,518	420,547	2,164,588	3,899,714	5,940	10,690	5.1	309,087	1,001	66,612	1,496,363	7,264,370
Nonmetropolitan	37	1,538	44,033	297,985	873,026	823	2,396	6.8	41,763	144	7,251	237,998	1,455,682
Metropolitan	36	7,980	376,514	1,866,603	3,026,688	5,117	8,294	5.0	267,324	857	59,361	1,258,365	5,808,688
Boulder	4	627	35,180	139,330	243,849	383	668	4.0	23,101	98	7,662	125,733	770,619
Colorado Springs	3	857	52,402	241,882	374,338	663	1,025	4.6	31,136	129	7,047	177,214	625,909
Denver-Aurora	20	4,729	209,930	1,083,405	1,739,720	2,970	4,767	5.2	157,103	480	33,977	688,874	2,603,964
Fort Collins-Loveland	3	473	24,405	111,110	191,918	304	526	4.6	19,560	49	3,872	75,200	653,724
Grand Junction	3	450	15,820	107,864	189,605	296	520	6.8	11,180	18	2,153	52,753	510,387
Greeley	1	301	16,166	68,762	107,652	188	295	4.3	7,340	38	2,232	43,282	316,162
Pueblo	2	543	22,611	114,250	179,606	313	493	5.1	17,904	45	2,418	95,309	327,923
Idaho	38	3,303	141,839	678,059	1,378,654	1,856	3,779	4.8	106,361	269	21,341	511,381	2,703,605
Nonmetropolitan	24	1,071	35,903	209,371	543,729	572	1,491	5.8	31,023	100	5,970	157,872	833,825
Metropolitan	14	2,232	105,936	468,688	834,925	1,284	2,288	4.4	75,338	169	15,371	353,509	1,869,780
Boise City-Nampa	7	1,174	59,457	243,164	466,799	666	1,279	4.1	47,912	98	9,835	215,330	1,162,870
Coeur d'Alene	1	246	12,677	52,689	93,632	144	257	4.2	6,186	18	1,640	47,209	158,689
Idaho Falls	2	299	12,115	66,251	95,430	182	262	5.5	11,813	10	1,357	37,698	170,514
Lewiston	1	156	12,160	27,775	44,633	76	122	2.3	4,583	15	705	12,129	79,413
Logan	1	65	703	14,563	22,972	40	63	20.7	385	5	121	3,141	4,093
Pocatello	2	292	8,824	64,246	111,459	176	305	7.3	4,459	23	1,713	38,002	294,201
Montana	52	4,089	106,826	975,390	1,948,852	2,674	5,338	9.1	76,228	234	10,681	333,504	2,901,878
Nonmetropolitan	46	2,599	49,404	612,593	1,306,835	1,679	3,579	12.4	37,700	151	5,177	191,787	1,213,377
Metropolitan	6	1,490	57,422	362,797	642,017	995	1,759	6.3	38,528	83	5,504	141,717	1,688,501
Billings	3	674	28,342	180,142	378,371	494	1,037	6.4	18,985	38	2,461	53,271	1,279,860
Great Falls	1	480	14,087	116,704	160,244	320	439	8.3	8,586	24	1,398	35,584	114,858
Missoula	2	336	14,993	65,951	103,402	181	283	4.4	10,957	21	1,645	52,862	293,783
Nevada	33	4,826	245,649	1,307,303	1,898,441	3,578	5,200	5.3	155,099	290	32,737	697,906	2,387,808
Nonmetropolitan	11	337	8,559	68,343	172,222	186	471	8.0	8,982	34	1,378	65,777	375,058
Metropolitan	22	4,489	237,090	1,238,960	1,726,219	3,392	4,729	5.2	146,117	256	31,359	632,129	2,012,750
Carson City	1	172	10,328	41,392	61,662	113	169	4.0	3,018	12	1,035	33,380	138,051
Las Vegas-Paradise	15	3,307	181,903	977,317	1,338,068	2,677	3,666	5.4	110,998	194	23,533	452,453	1,281,186
Reno-Sparks	6	1,010	44,859	220,251	326,489	602	894	4.9	32,101	50	6,791	146,296	593,513
New Mexico	36	3,525	160,792	762,267	1,456,684	2,092	3,990	4.7	136,590	390	24,275	777,671	4,344,119
Nonmetropolitan	22	1,439	51,726	221,106	488,741	608	1,338	4.3	55,247	163	8,223	382,160	1,804,759
Metropolitan	14	2,086	109,066	541,161	967,943	1,484	2,652	5.0	81,343	227	16,052	395,511	2,539,360
Albuquerque	10	1,425	69,951	377,156	695,236	1,035	1,905	5.4	53,644	135	10,121	251,754	2,035,080
Farmington	1	186	10,281	42,171	74,035	116	203	4.1	5,069	22	1,388	40,054	178,709
Las Cruces	2	295	17,123	75,129	112,968	205	309	4.4	17,589	46	2,916	52,702	203,286
Santa Fe	1	180	11,711	46,705	85,704	128	235	4.0	5,041	24	1,627	51,001	122,285

TABLE 8

U.S. CENSUS DIVISION 8, MOUNTAIN

U.S. Community Hospitals
(Nonfederal, short-term general and other special hospitals)

2006 Utilization, Personnel and Finances

FULL-TIME EQUIVALENT PERSONNEL					FULL-TIME EQUIV. TRAINEES			EXPENSES						
								LABOR				TOTAL		
Physicians and Dentists	Registered Nurses	Licensed Practical Nurses	Other Salaried Personnel	Total Personnel	Medical and Dental Residents	Other Trainees	Total Trainees	Payroll (in thousands)	Employee Benefits (in thousands)	Total (in thousands)	Percent of Total	Amount (in thousands)	Adjusted per Admission	Adjusted per Inpatient Day
82,249	1,138,633	112,897	2,419,268	4,343,480	85,320	7,428	92,748	$225,892,043	$57,781,527	$283,673,571	51.4	$551,835,328	$8,970.31	$1,612.23
9,876	143,037	32,484	356,147	641,178	1,422	280	1,702	27,189,409	7,290,060	34,479,464	53.5	64,488,354	5,979.83	914.81
72,373	995,596	80,413	2,063,121	3,702,302	83,898	7,148	91,046	198,702,635	50,491,466	249,194,107	51.1	487,346,974	9,605.99	1,793.12
3,507	64,134	5,295	133,724	238,466	2,226	366	2,592	12,305,727	2,924,385	15,230,104	51.1	29,827,199	8,706.94	1,664.65
741	9,754	1,618	25,224	44,626	24	8	32	1,892,736	469,861	2,362,587	52.8	4,475,001	6,427.59	896.35
2,766	54,380	3,677	108,500	193,840	2,202	358	2,560	10,412,991	2,454,524	12,867,517	50.8	25,352,198	9,288.35	1,961.40
844	19,626	1,191	38,215	68,550	803	114	917	3,607,560	782,351	4,389,911	49.0	8,959,777	8,804.99	1,929.87
58	1,431	218	3,209	5,932	6	0	6	253,221	61,377	314,598	50.2	626,626	6,355.87	1,299.06
786	18,195	973	35,006	62,618	797	114	911	3,354,339	720,974	4,075,313	48.9	8,333,151	9,067.74	2,003.00
26	1,050	44	1,797	3,420	1	37	38	142,559	37,248	179,807	49.6	362,664	11,341.05	2,600.60
685	12,013	624	24,203	42,054	726	75	801	2,320,270	496,258	2,816,529	48.3	5,837,214	9,206.41	2,018.29
4	620	3	1,086	2,016	0	0	0	108,774	28,017	136,791	53.7	254,714	8,823.71	2,461.41
70	3,984	270	6,867	13,206	70	2	72	688,185	136,294	824,479	50.1	1,644,746	8,522.49	1,831.18
1	528	32	1,053	1,922	0	0	0	94,551	23,157	117,707	50.3	233,813	7,513.98	1,840.35
893	14,414	1,017	31,857	54,338	637	37	674	3,007,684	694,247	3,701,926	50.9	7,269,883	9,895.74	1,864.21
145	1,739	255	4,951	8,182	5	2	7	368,950	94,756	463,702	53.0	874,764	7,261.14	1,001.99
748	12,675	762	26,906	46,156	632	35	667	2,638,734	599,491	3,238,224	50.6	6,395,119	10,412.52	2,112.91
43	1,142	25	2,852	4,392	0	0	0	237,976	54,904	292,879	50.8	576,055	9,404.52	2,362.34
76	1,389	96	3,025	5,244	102	5	107	282,771	75,990	358,761	51.7	694,098	8,542.11	1,854.20
505	7,663	453	15,080	26,437	440	26	466	1,606,927	341,379	1,948,305	49.9	3,903,712	11,364.48	2,243.87
39	792	71	1,875	3,201	24	2	26	179,858	51,689	231,547	54.9	421,501	10,512.82	2,196.26
38	530	33	1,227	2,128	22	0	22	113,232	26,496	139,729	52.2	267,767	9,827.77	1,412.24
22	396	15	1,194	1,929	30	0	30	104,068	22,756	126,824	46.3	274,020	10,826.96	2,545.42
25	763	69	1,653	2,825	14	2	16	113,902	26,278	140,179	54.3	257,967	7,263.19	1,436.29
256	4,503	500	10,207	17,994	5	37	42	841,369	214,618	1,055,986	50.7	2,083,181	7,356.78	1,511.03
70	1,077	192	2,911	5,136	0	0	0	210,320	51,182	261,500	51.2	511,133	5,569.60	940.05
186	3,426	308	7,296	12,858	5	37	42	631,049	163,436	794,486	50.5	1,572,048	8,213.72	1,882.86
167	2,322	112	4,755	8,349	5	37	42	416,500	101,180	517,681	50.1	1,032,645	9,002.85	2,212.18
0	349	13	818	1,368	0	0	0	65,221	17,534	82,755	51.1	162,062	7,193.79	1,730.84
2	291	73	628	1,150	0	0	0	54,738	16,074	70,811	50.7	139,608	7,513.06	1,462.93
8	159	8	336	588	0	0	0	33,433	10,754	44,187	53.6	82,490	4,221.38	1,848.18
0	18	20	75	161	0	0	0	4,905	1,459	6,365	69.3	9,184	8,281.32	399.79
9	287	82	684	1,242	0	0	0	56,251	16,435	72,687	49.8	146,060	9,782.30	1,310.43
475	3,446	645	9,534	16,609	0	3	3	789,322	180,077	969,398	53.8	1,800,737	8,340.76	924.00
148	1,683	314	4,874	8,513	0	0	0	341,297	81,457	422,753	54.8	771,231	6,627.52	590.15
327	1,763	331	4,660	8,096	0	3	3	448,025	98,620	546,645	53.1	1,029,505	10,343.88	1,603.55
278	851	237	2,515	4,441	0	0	0	258,722	54,651	313,374	55.3	566,427	9,981.62	1,497.02
7	477	31	1,031	1,822	0	0	0	76,951	19,254	96,205	51.9	185,290	9,579.19	1,156.30
42	435	63	1,114	1,833	0	3	3	112,352	24,714	137,066	49.3	277,788	11,852.03	2,686.49
104	6,133	505	10,349	19,656	30	11	41	1,217,475	322,890	1,540,365	52.6	2,930,774	8,277.85	1,543.78
19	253	59	713	1,277	1	1	2	74,458	15,665	90,122	52.2	172,499	7,684.39	1,001.61
85	5,880	446	9,636	18,379	29	10	39	1,143,017	307,225	1,450,243	52.6	2,758,275	8,318.03	1,597.87
0	245	6	534	969	0	9	9	57,563	14,128	71,692	46.3	154,925	10,069.20	2,512.48
84	4,625	401	6,953	13,642	29	1	30	835,648	235,288	1,070,935	55.9	1,915,764	7,679.68	1,431.74
1	1,010	39	2,149	3,768	0	0	0	249,806	57,809	307,616	44.7	687,585	10,299.82	2,106.00
585	5,917	652	12,006	22,690	35	86	121	1,146,754	260,726	1,407,483	55.6	2,532,321	7,979.33	1,738.41
185	1,750	276	4,046	7,417	11	1	12	314,031	76,515	390,548	52.4	745,910	6,031.41	1,526.19
400	4,167	376	7,960	15,273	24	85	109	832,722	184,211	1,016,935	56.9	1,786,410	9,223.09	1,845.57
332	2,890	321	5,720	10,980	3	83	86	612,740	129,402	742,145	58.2	1,275,365	9,935.69	1,834.43
32	362	5	734	1,290	0	0	0	67,815	18,840	86,655	57.4	150,847	8,357.66	2,037.51
9	535	6	634	1,472	14	0	14	79,522	17,178	96,699	51.6	187,512	7,271.30	1,659.87
27	380	44	872	1,531	7	2	9	72,645	18,791	91,436	52.9	172,686	8,035.63	2,014.91

Table continues

MSAs

TABLE **8**

U.S. CENSUS DIVISION 8, MOUNTAIN CONTINUED

U.S. Community Hospitals
(Nonfederal, short-term general and other special hospitals)

2006 Utilization, Personnel and Finances

CLASSIFICATION	Hospitals	Beds	Admissions	Inpatient Days	Adjusted Patient Days	Average Daily Census	Adjusted Average Daily Census	Average Stay (days)	Surgical Operations	NEWBORNS		OUTPATIENT VISITS	
										Bassinets	Births	Emergency	Total
Utah	43	4,528	220,750	968,656	1,795,390	2,654	4,919	4.4	217,594	644	53,194	789,653	4,981,695
Nonmetropolitan	18	658	17,412	107,841	350,661	295	960	6.2	24,323	99	4,665	127,739	616,664
Metropolitan	25	3,870	203,338	860,815	1,444,729	2,359	3,959	4.2	193,271	545	48,529	661,914	4,365,031
Logan	2	142	7,864	24,856	55,162	68	151	3.2	7,611	21	2,626	24,308	274,234
Ogden-Clearfield	4	704	37,652	143,006	235,382	392	645	3.8	27,236	109	9,129	138,005	541,095
Provo-Orem	6	666	35,962	140,280	233,443	384	640	3.9	32,358	136	11,631	113,039	746,987
Salt Lake City	12	2,113	107,906	500,600	837,995	1,372	2,296	4.6	118,998	263	22,386	346,800	2,451,581
St. George	1	245	13,954	52,073	82,747	143	227	3.7	7,068	16	2,757	39,762	351,134
Wyoming	24	2,056	52,586	421,089	897,598	1,152	2,459	8.0	39,430	175	6,824	221,300	963,840
Nonmetropolitan	22	1,636	31,824	333,664	774,912	913	2,123	10.5	28,147	135	4,547	157,929	805,642
Metropolitan	2	420	20,762	87,425	122,686	239	336	4.2	11,283	40	2,277	63,371	158,198
Casper	1	205	9,515	40,253	56,501	110	155	4.2	5,296	24	1,022	34,045	71,029
Cheyenne	1	215	11,247	47,172	66,185	129	181	4.2	5,987	16	1,255	29,326	87,169

MSAs

TABLE **8**

U.S. CENSUS DIVISION 8, MOUNTAIN CONTINUED

U.S. Community Hospitals
(Nonfederal, short-term general and other special hospitals)

2006 Utilization, Personnel and Finances

FULL-TIME EQUIVALENT PERSONNEL					FULL-TIME EQUIV. TRAINEES			EXPENSES						
								LABOR				TOTAL		
Physicians and Dentists	Registered Nurses	Licensed Practical Nurses	Other Salaried Personnel	Total Personnel	Medical and Dental Residents	Other Trainees	Total Trainees	Payroll (in thousands)	Employee Benefits (in thousands)	Total (in thousands)	Percent of Total	Amount (in thousands)	Adjusted per Admission	Adjusted per Inpatient Day
254	8,281	594	17,033	30,790	715	76	791	1,346,084	374,153	1,720,235	50.0	3,437,079	8,546.67	1,914.39
24	669	165	1,557	2,904	0	2	2	100,509	27,159	127,666	48.5	263,394	5,144.00	751.13
230	7,612	429	15,476	27,886	715	74	789	1,245,576	346,994	1,592,569	50.2	3,173,686	9,043.13	2,196.73
0	237	10	504	822	0	0	0	33,850	10,439	44,289	53.4	82,995	4,701.98	1,504.56
42	1,136	141	1,797	3,721	22	1	23	177,397	48,431	225,828	47.9	471,049	7,629.32	2,001.21
34	1,351	58	2,065	4,099	25	22	47	186,443	53,858	240,301	50.7	473,561	7,516.00	2,028.59
144	4,606	210	9,993	17,670	668	51	719	774,097	211,848	985,944	50.4	1,954,336	10,485.99	2,332.16
10	282	10	1,117	1,574	0	0	0	73,789	22,418	96,207	50.2	191,745	8,647.29	2,317.24
96	1,814	191	4,523	7,839	1	2	3	349,479	95,323	444,800	54.7	813,448	8,067.60	906.25
92	1,152	139	2,963	5,265	1	2	3	229,950	61,750	291,698	57.3	509,444	7,105.91	657.42
4	662	52	1,560	2,574	0	0	0	119,528	33,573	153,102	50.4	304,003	10,433.95	2,477.90
1	307	1	578	1,051	0	0	0	51,750	16,405	68,156	49.0	139,062	10,411.95	2,461.23
3	355	51	982	1,523	0	0	0	67,778	17,168	84,946	51.5	164,941	10,452.56	2,492.13

MSAs

TABLE 8

U.S. CENSUS DIVISION 9, PACIFIC

U.S. Community Hospitals
(Nonfederal, short-term general and other special hospitals)

2006 Utilization, Personnel and Finances

CLASSIFICATION	Hospitals	Beds	Admissions	Inpatient Days	Adjusted Patient Days	Average Daily Census	Adjusted Average Daily Census	Average Stay (days)	Surgical Operations	NEWBORNS Bassinets	NEWBORNS Births	OUTPATIENT VISITS Emergency	OUTPATIENT VISITS Total
UNITED STATES	4,927	802,658	35,377,659	196,366,512	342,281,133	538,496	938,580	5.6	27,330,824	57,832	4,075,193	118,374,029	599,553,025
Nonmetropolitan	2,001	145,328	4,662,402	30,375,652	70,493,783	83,319	193,322	6.5	4,130,326	11,655	481,086	22,555,781	112,987,297
Metropolitan.	2,926	657,330	30,715,257	165,990,860	271,787,350	455,177	745,258	5.4	23,200,498	46,177	3,594,107	95,818,248	486,565,728
CENSUS DIVISION 9, PACIFIC	549	92,077	4,491,195	23,419,759	36,783,532	64,196	100,801	5.2	3,035,077	7,164	670,591	14,623,874	76,239,809
Nonmetropolitan	125	5,922	216,941	1,287,001	3,014,891	3,529	8,260	5.9	221,653	593	30,558	1,238,311	6,593,180
Metropolitan.	424	86,155	4,274,254	22,132,758	33,768,641	60,667	92,541	5.2	2,813,424	6,571	640,033	13,385,563	69,646,629
Alaska	22	1,551	52,357	304,978	580,180	836	1,588	5.8	61,309	145	9,128	610,324	1,775,920
Nonmetropolitan	17	543	14,673	95,038	232,517	261	636	6.5	18,858	61	2,555	106,084	585,270
Metropolitan.	5	1,008	37,684	209,940	347,663	575	952	5.6	42,451	84	6,573	504,240	1,190,650
Anchorage	4	766	31,990	160,232	257,057	439	704	5.0	36,549	68	5,417	477,889	932,498
Fairbanks	1	242	5,694	49,708	90,606	136	248	8.7	5,902	16	1,156	26,351	258,152
California	357	70,021	3,428,885	18,278,223	27,297,601	50,086	74,783	5.3	2,151,923	5,081	524,279	10,276,370	53,938,435
Nonmetropolitan	33	1,637	59,789	388,593	867,535	1,065	2,378	6.5	68,730	130	7,581	404,962	2,209,744
Metropolitan.	324	68,384	3,369,096	17,889,630	26,430,066	49,021	72,405	5.3	2,083,193	4,951	516,698	9,871,408	51,728,691
Bakersfield	10	1,378	66,569	371,207	608,491	1,018	1,666	5.6	38,504	87	12,929	172,368	618,736
Chico	4	602	28,337	139,902	230,488	383	632	4.9	20,630	36	3,051	102,627	675,201
El Centro	2	272	11,354	45,352	79,461	124	217	4.0	7,960	39	2,952	76,556	239,782
Fresno	11	1,777	103,626	504,405	813,574	1,384	2,231	4.9	62,468	200	20,128	328,850	2,389,199
Hanford-Corcoran	3	181	9,078	36,687	85,556	100	234	4.0	10,354	35	1,288	71,640	331,911
Los Angeles-Long Beach-Glendale	92	21,907	1,037,527	5,601,657	7,928,503	15,348	21,722	5.4	594,285	1,641	153,304	2,368,189	10,661,580
Madera	3	385	17,866	108,175	170,552	297	467	6.1	14,721	10	1,740	75,716	329,017
Merced	1	160	10,924	43,000	71,797	118	197	3.9	6,456	24	2,938	42,386	144,864
Modesto	4	1,138	51,422	327,657	460,602	898	1,262	6.4	35,966	68	9,875	202,311	433,221
Napa	2	326	14,402	86,593	130,180	237	357	6.0	9,054	12	1,273	32,580	302,493
Oakland-Fremont-Hayward	18	4,552	222,805	1,220,376	1,829,942	3,344	5,013	5.5	113,640	266	28,922	786,114	3,785,065
Oxnard-Thousand Oaks-Ventura. .	6	1,314	58,860	325,255	480,806	891	1,317	5.5	36,462	108	10,073	263,955	1,061,489
Redding	3	496	21,637	128,625	202,973	352	556	5.9	12,222	13	2,260	68,733	114,216
Riverside-San Bernardino-Ontario .	33	6,165	347,375	1,674,868	2,423,042	4,591	6,638	4.8	196,907	442	44,270	1,027,143	3,095,245
Sacramento—Arden-Arcade—Roseville	15	3,479	185,739	899,018	1,340,196	2,463	3,671	4.8	136,031	297	34,095	562,892	6,037,376
Salinas	4	684	36,737	167,119	237,158	457	649	4.5	24,397	55	6,913	120,242	436,756
San Diego-Carlsbad-San Marcos .	19	5,492	274,164	1,545,865	2,220,007	4,236	6,079	5.6	194,557	361	44,511	671,411	2,909,087
San Francisco-San Mateo-Redwood City	19	4,697	182,589	1,283,805	1,988,612	3,519	5,450	7.0	137,358	161	16,200	776,359	5,591,839
San Jose-Sunnyvale-Santa Clara .	12	3,171	165,291	839,834	1,277,005	2,300	3,498	5.1	99,306	317	31,790	461,760	4,674,106
San Luis Obispo-Paso Robles . . .	3	337	13,526	60,090	96,821	165	265	4.4	10,389	23	2,068	59,785	273,626
Santa Ana-Anaheim-Irvine	28	5,209	273,176	1,283,273	1,904,844	3,517	5,219	4.7	188,167	377	45,684	763,158	3,062,889
Santa Barbara-Santa Maria	6	912	35,842	222,426	346,299	610	948	6.2	26,631	86	6,684	115,466	475,870
Santa Cruz-Watsonville	3	383	21,669	101,039	137,843	277	378	4.7	11,283	37	1,951	37,085	220,496
Santa Rosa-Petaluma	7	799	37,873	188,339	317,401	516	869	5.0	24,591	51	5,700	153,570	826,046
Stockton	7	1,059	61,023	282,301	414,990	774	1,137	4.6	29,849	90	10,891	199,971	1,175,998
Vallejo-Fairfield	4	536	30,816	148,659	242,045	406	662	4.8	17,132	37	4,933	119,193	1,036,825
Visalia-Porterville	3	602	33,963	190,044	284,038	521	778	5.6	16,047	56	7,285	163,222	713,978
Yuba City	2	371	14,906	64,059	106,840	175	293	4.3	7,826	22	2,990	48,126	111,780
Hawaii	24	2,969	111,713	841,667	1,458,592	2,308	3,997	7.5	87,441	199	11,543	339,863	1,883,414
Nonmetropolitan	11	822	30,452	236,775	438,327	649	1,202	7.8	21,038	67	4,400	102,837	269,144
Metropolitan.	13	2,147	81,261	604,892	1,020,265	1,659	2,795	7.4	66,403	132	7,143	237,026	1,614,270
Honolulu	13	2,147	81,261	604,892	1,020,265	1,659	2,795	7.4	66,403	132	7,143	237,026	1,614,270
Oregon.	58	6,609	341,540	1,508,314	2,812,375	4,131	7,704	4.4	323,527	712	47,369	1,250,008	8,257,876
Nonmetropolitan	29	1,458	65,473	302,528	749,046	829	2,052	4.6	60,283	179	8,782	346,935	1,994,846
Metropolitan.	29	5,151	276,067	1,205,786	2,063,329	3,302	5,652	4.4	263,244	533	38,587	903,073	6,263,030
Bend.	2	265	14,835	57,755	95,824	158	263	3.9	15,725	21	2,198	49,324	199,949
Corvallis.	1	163	8,295	35,856	64,622	98	177	4.3	8,467	24	1,059	18,663	234,377
Eugene-Springfield	4	654	35,155	141,038	211,239	386	578	4.0	27,934	70	3,552	112,166	237,252
Medford	3	452	22,314	100,242	157,184	274	431	4.5	20,644	34	2,281	73,286	624,836
Portland-Vancouver-Beaverton . . .	15	3,106	171,430	770,442	1,347,422	2,111	3,690	4.5	174,111	314	23,927	524,287	4,285,364
Salem	4	511	24,038	100,453	187,038	275	513	4.2	16,363	70	5,570	125,347	681,252

TABLE 8

U.S. CENSUS DIVISION 9, PACIFIC

U.S. Community Hospitals
(Nonfederal, short-term general and other special hospitals)

2006 Utilization, Personnel and Finances

FULL-TIME EQUIVALENT PERSONNEL					FULL-TIME EQUIV. TRAINEES			EXPENSES						
								LABOR				TOTAL		
Physicians and Dentists	Registered Nurses	Licensed Practical Nurses	Other Salaried Personnel	Total Personnel	Medical and Dental Residents	Other Trainees	Total Trainees	Payroll (in thousands)	Employee Benefits (in thousands)	Total (in thousands)	Percent of Total	Amount (in thousands)	Adjusted per Admission	Adjusted per Inpatient Day
82,249	1,138,633	112,897	2,419,268	4,343,480	85,320	7,428	92,748	$225,892,043	$57,781,527	$283,673,571	51.4	$551,835,328	$8,970.31	$1,612.23
9,876	143,037	32,484	356,147	641,178	1,422	280	1,702	27,189,409	7,290,060	34,479,464	53.5	64,488,354	5,979.83	914.81
72,373	995,596	80,413	2,063,121	3,702,302	83,898	7,148	91,046	198,702,635	50,491,466	249,194,107	51.1	487,346,974	9,605.99	1,793.12
10,209	146,449	12,074	298,192	535,136	9,648	698	10,346	31,292,116	9,043,246	40,335,365	52.8	76,421,526	10,825.60	2,077.60
551	7,943	1,047	19,799	34,630	17	10	27	1,765,349	554,713	2,320,062	56.1	4,133,107	8,200.71	1,370.90
9,658	138,506	11,027	278,393	500,506	9,631	688	10,319	29,526,767	8,488,534	38,015,303	52.6	72,288,418	11,027.41	2,140.70
154	2,483	216	5,302	9,727	51	40	91	588,778	162,948	751,727	52.8	1,424,480	14,224.17	2,455.24
100	774	104	1,899	3,500	7	1	8	203,142	62,385	265,528	57.3	463,089	12,368.18	1,991.64
54	1,709	112	3,403	6,227	44	39	83	385,637	100,563	486,199	50.6	961,390	15,332.44	2,765.29
51	1,374	84	2,730	5,031	44	39	83	321,999	82,875	404,873	49.8	812,700	15,532.06	3,161.55
3	335	28	673	1,196	0	0	0	63,638	17,688	81,326	54.7	148,690	14,326.08	1,641.07
6,648	109,102	9,850	214,092	390,928	7,546	519	8,065	22,783,715	6,739,979	29,523,696	52.6	56,137,019	10,994.72	2,056.48
61	2,291	386	5,203	9,329	5	1	6	472,099	178,214	650,316	54.4	1,196,449	9,191.58	1,379.14
6,587	106,811	9,464	208,889	381,599	7,541	518	8,059	22,311,616	6,561,765	28,873,380	52.6	54,940,570	11,041.90	2,078.71
71	1,632	239	3,437	6,416	26	0	26	341,283	95,572	436,855	53.1	822,033	8,019.21	1,350.94
19	895	143	1,816	3,318	4	1	5	167,716	74,083	241,798	53.9	448,942	9,899.49	1,947.79
2	260	34	786	1,257	0	0	0	56,150	14,011	70,160	53.4	131,428	6,587.89	1,654.00
333	2,951	258	7,022	12,307	188	17	205	590,609	155,695	746,306	53.4	1,397,909	8,134.14	1,718.23
2	233	53	658	1,158	3	0	3	64,781	18,087	82,869	52.8	156,964	7,728.81	1,834.64
1,853	32,394	3,257	62,571	115,873	3,055	197	3,252	6,508,991	1,760,181	8,269,171	51.7	15,979,850	10,868.87	2,015.49
36	813	100	1,825	3,243	21	4	25	138,191	37,658	175,848	53.7	327,398	12,239.16	1,919.64
1	269	31	514	914	24	0	24	62,216	11,591	73,807	58.2	126,713	6,946.97	1,764.88
8	2,013	117	2,518	5,436	2	73	75	332,676	84,758	417,434	54.8	762,000	10,966.24	1,654.36
0	534	25	1,132	1,867	0	0	0	121,983	48,324	170,307	56.1	303,524	13,928.21	2,331.57
390	6,910	712	14,504	25,979	245	24	269	1,789,372	543,604	2,332,975	54.4	4,285,590	12,766.70	2,341.93
27	1,817	204	3,178	6,069	14	0	14	366,065	116,784	482,849	55.2	874,149	9,933.17	1,818.09
10	896	76	1,358	2,667	24	0	24	137,719	47,126	184,845	52.0	355,259	11,462.17	1,750.28
1,120	10,032	996	17,949	34,664	885	64	949	1,699,077	482,366	2,181,443	50.9	4,282,142	8,406.66	1,767.26
717	7,278	474	14,352	26,231	509	23	532	1,512,857	440,292	1,953,149	54.7	3,569,198	12,762.86	2,663.19
16	1,153	79	2,292	4,108	24	0	24	311,764	159,948	471,712	61.9	761,631	15,136.96	3,211.49
124	8,471	587	15,267	27,792	704	45	749	1,636,725	394,198	2,030,922	51.2	3,967,602	10,240.35	1,787.20
788	6,929	469	14,318	25,556	468	41	509	1,840,838	525,514	2,366,353	51.7	4,576,131	16,141.04	2,301.17
811	6,132	339	11,492	21,274	996	11	1,007	1,616,193	638,542	2,254,736	53.9	4,183,168	16,796.70	3,275.76
0	406	11	535	1,193	0	0	0	77,875	17,471	95,345	49.0	194,749	8,930.98	2,011.43
127	8,264	577	16,854	29,190	184	6	190	1,525,010	452,378	1,977,388	49.2	4,018,291	9,840.55	2,109.51
25	1,015	115	2,331	4,125	54	0	54	211,161	58,663	269,826	52.6	513,205	9,738.97	1,481.97
11	727	47	1,208	2,236	1	0	1	153,237	45,044	198,280	59.8	331,554	10,903.17	2,405.31
20	1,099	85	2,708	4,387	40	0	40	270,544	87,827	358,371	53.3	671,906	10,436.73	2,116.90
36	1,863	178	4,131	6,962	58	9	67	340,421	121,716	462,136	57.8	798,900	8,791.39	1,925.11
15	438	23	1,043	1,675	6	1	7	172,562	49,862	222,423	49.8	446,642	8,889.64	1,845.29
14	942	175	2,080	4,013	6	2	8	188,496	60,363	248,859	54.9	453,544	8,774.14	1,596.77
11	445	60	1,010	1,689	0	0	0	77,106	20,107	97,213	48.6	200,148	8,104.80	1,873.34
308	4,171	377	8,242	15,230	19	8	27	845,332	216,242	1,061,574	52.6	2,017,583	10,532.77	1,383.24
28	930	145	1,898	3,596	0	0	0	182,002	58,406	240,408	56.8	423,470	7,763.97	966.11
280	3,241	232	6,344	11,634	19	8	27	663,330	157,836	821,166	51.5	1,594,113	11,635.01	1,562.45
280	3,241	232	6,344	11,634	19	8	27	663,330	157,836	821,166	51.5	1,594,113	11,635.01	1,562.45
1,436	12,583	342	26,211	45,362	761	70	831	2,562,974	768,689	3,331,664	53.8	6,192,331	9,701.36	2,201.82
201	2,202	108	5,746	9,590	2	6	8	490,008	147,349	637,358	56.9	1,120,212	7,151.46	1,495.52
1,235	10,381	234	20,465	35,772	759	64	823	2,072,965	621,339	2,694,306	53.1	5,072,119	10,530.63	2,458.22
0	520	10	1,406	2,045	0	0	0	115,292	34,896	150,188	51.8	290,203	11,711.16	3,028.50
52	279	4	632	1,113	0	1	1	75,928	23,613	99,541	53.9	184,700	12,354.51	2,858.16
56	1,069	40	2,132	3,760	0	5	5	206,609	56,085	262,695	52.5	500,575	9,151.96	2,369.71
28	806	26	1,621	2,939	0	1	1	148,348	57,195	205,543	51.7	397,908	11,275.69	2,531.48
1,074	6,808	111	12,397	22,433	759	57	816	1,331,515	397,269	1,728,784	52.8	3,277,221	10,772.64	2,432.22
25	899	43	2,277	3,482	0	0	0	195,273	52,282	247,555	58.7	421,513	8,832.68	2,253.62

Table continues

MSAs

TABLE 8

U.S. CENSUS DIVISION 9, PACIFIC
CONTINUED

U.S. Community Hospitals
(Nonfederal, short-term general and other special hospitals)

2006 Utilization, Personnel and Finances

CLASSIFICATION	Hospitals	Beds	Admissions	Inpatient Days	Adjusted Patient Days	Average Daily Census	Adjusted Average Daily Census	Average Stay (days)	Surgical Operations	NEWBORNS Bassinets	NEWBORNS Births	OUTPATIENT VISITS Emergency	OUTPATIENT VISITS Total
Washington	88	10,927	556,700	2,486,577	4,634,784	6,835	12,729	4.5	410,877	1,027	78,272	2,147,309	10,384,164
Nonmetropolitan	35	1,462	46,554	264,067	727,466	725	1,992	5.7	52,744	156	7,240	277,493	1,534,176
Metropolitan	53	9,465	510,146	2,222,510	3,907,318	6,110	10,737	4.4	358,133	871	71,032	1,869,816	8,849,988
Bellingham	1	235	14,517	56,597	90,959	155	249	3.9	6,359	30	1,943	25,495	118,451
Bremerton-Silverdale	1	254	16,630	61,577	90,969	169	249	3.7	12,976	24	1,985	64,404	137,174
Kennewick-Richland-Pasco	4	379	18,811	80,142	191,205	219	525	4.3	14,343	39	4,206	109,206	315,122
Lewiston	1	25	1,576	6,584	18,350	18	50	4.2	1,753	0	0	7,822	66,238
Longview	1	202	9,670	38,235	61,449	105	168	4.0	2,221	27	1,221	46,743	217,167
Mount Vernon-Anacortes	3	193	12,922	44,597	104,141	122	285	3.5	11,966	27	1,603	56,209	272,787
Olympia	2	410	22,923	90,651	133,135	249	365	4.0	13,604	22	2,786	78,746	337,591
Portland-Vancouver-Beaverton . . .	2	495	25,007	98,151	169,933	290	498	3.9	14,617	70	4,655	97,117	346,902
Seattle-Bellevue-Everett	21	4,267	235,214	1,074,705	1,961,937	2,945	5,373	4.6	171,767	424	31,610	830,139	4,924,461
Spokane	6	1,283	57,209	286,731	427,214	785	1,172	5.0	44,945	71	6,551	153,579	449,444
Tacoma	5	1,077	63,073	263,120	467,241	720	1,280	4.2	43,438	71	8,567	238,367	1,011,487
Wenatchee	2	183	10,627	40,484	62,602	111	171	3.8	7,175	16	2,108	40,258	185,327
Yakima	4	462	21,967	80,936	128,183	222	352	3.7	12,969	50	3,797	121,731	467,837

MSAs

TABLE **8**

**U.S. CENSUS DIVISION 9, PACIFIC
CONTINUED**

U.S. Community Hospitals
(Nonfederal, short-term general and other special hospitals)

2006 Utilization, Personnel and Finances

FULL-TIME EQUIVALENT PERSONNEL					FULL-TIME EQUIV. TRAINEES			EXPENSES						
								LABOR				TOTAL		
Physicians and Dentists	Registered Nurses	Licensed Practical Nurses	Other Salaried Personnel	Total Personnel	Medical and Dental Residents	Other Trainees	Total Trainees	Payroll (in thousands)	Employee Benefits (in thousands)	Total (in thousands)	Percent of Total	Amount (in thousands)	Adjusted per Admission	Adjusted per Inpatient Day
1,663	18,110	1,289	44,345	73,889	1,271	61	1,332	4,511,316	1,155,388	5,666,704	53.2	10,650,112	10,405.33	2,297.87
161	1,746	304	5,053	8,615	3	2	5	418,098	108,357	526,452	56.6	929,886	7,427.21	1,278.25
1,502	16,364	985	39,292	65,274	1,268	59	1,327	4,093,219	1,047,031	5,140,252	52.9	9,720,226	10,820.39	2,487.70
28	509	40	1,077	1,894	18	3	21	95,878	25,128	121,005	52.1	232,098	9,948.05	2,551.68
0	0	0	1,374	1,374	0	0	0	93,075	27,852	120,927	57.3	211,077	8,591.54	2,320.32
41	695	43	1,416	2,460	0	0	0	134,431	35,847	170,278	51.9	328,300	7,836.44	1,717.00
2	96	5	141	290	0	0	0	11,549	3,163	14,713	44.0	33,438	7,613.45	1,822.25
18	324	26	703	1,224	11	1	12	71,836	18,827	90,663	52.1	173,899	11,189.70	2,829.98
5	358	11	854	1,395	0	1	1	74,581	17,730	92,311	49.2	187,706	6,340.36	1,802.42
14	568	41	1,432	2,188	1	6	7	132,056	37,359	169,415	52.5	322,464	9,542.35	2,422.09
41	970	35	1,930	3,210	19	2	21	180,327	48,689	229,016	55.5	412,885	9,567.04	2,429.69
1,004	8,788	428	21,392	35,460	995	26	1,021	2,234,012	563,965	2,797,977	53.6	5,224,047	12,091.67	2,662.70
126	1,606	106	3,641	6,302	163	11	174	378,003	97,345	475,349	52.4	907,736	10,412.80	2,124.78
169	1,475	146	3,203	5,701	41	5	46	486,027	121,123	607,150	50.3	1,208,226	10,771.76	2,585.87
24	269	11	680	1,119	0	2	2	72,652	18,507	91,160	57.9	157,411	9,903.80	2,514.47
30	706	93	1,449	2,657	20	2	22	128,792	31,496	160,288	49.9	320,938	9,229.79	2,503.75

MSAs

Statistics for Multihospital Health Care Systems and their Hospitals

The following tables describing multihospital health care systems refer to information in section B of the 2008 *AHA Guide*.

Table 1 shows the number of multihospital health care systems by type of control. Table 2 provides a breakdown of the number of systems that own, lease, sponsor or contract manage hospitals within each control category. Table 3 gives the number of hospitals and beds in each control category as well as total hospitals and beds. Finally, Table 4 shows the percentage of hospitals and beds in each control category.

For more information on multihospital health care systems, please write to the Section for Health Care Systems, One North Franklin, Chicago, Illinois 60606–3401 or call 312/422–3000.

Table 1. Multihospital Health Care Systems, by Type of Organizaton Control

Type of Control	Code	Number of Systems
Catholic (Roman) church–related	CC	41
Other church–related	CO	12
Subtotal, church–related		53
Other not–for–profit	NP	245
Subtotal, not–for–profit		298
Investor Owned	IO	78
Federal Government	FG	5
Total		381

Table 2. Multihospital Health Care Systems, by Type of Ownership and Control

Type of Ownership	Catholic Church–Related (CC)	Other Church–Related (CO)	Total Church–Related (CC + CO)	Other Not–for–Profit (NP)	Total Not–for–Profit (CC, CO, + NP)	Investor–Owned (IO)	Federal Govern–ment	All Systems
Systems that only own, lease or sponsor	35	10	45	213	258	68	5	331
Systems that only contract–manage	0	0	0	0	0	2	0	2
Systems that manage, own, lease, or sponsor	6	2	8	32	40	8	0	48
Total	41	12	53	245	298	78	5	381

Table 3. Hospitals and Beds in Multihospital Health Care Systems, by Type of Ownership and Control

Type of Ownership	Catholic Church–Related (CC) H	B	Other Church–Related (CO) H	B	Total Church–Related (CC + CO) H	B	Other Not–for–Profit (NP) H	B	Total Not–for–Profit (CC, CO, + NP) H	B	Investor–Owned (IO) H	B	Federal Govern–ment H	B	All Systems H	B
Owned, leased or sponsored	515	102,525	101	21,536	616	124,061	1,144	263,670	1,760	387,731	1,175	138,413	220	47,730	3,155	573,874
Contract–managed	37	1,805	2	308	39	2,113	88	6,915	127	9,028	185	12,928	0	0	312	21,956
Total	552	104,330	103	21,844	655	126,174	1,232	270,585	1,887	396,759	1,360	151,341	220	47,730	3,467	595,830

H = hospitals; **B** = beds.

Table 4. Hospitals and Beds in Multihospital Health Care Systems, by Type of Ownership and Control as a Percentage of All Systems

Type of Ownership	Catholic Church–Related (CC) H	B	Other Church–Related (CO) H	B	Total Church–Related (CC + CO) H	B	Other Not–for–Profit (NP) H	B	Total Not–for–Profit (CC, CO, + NP) H	B	Investor–Owned (IO) H	B	Federal Govern–ment H	B	All Systems H	B
Owned, leased or sponsored	16.3	17.9	3.2	3.8	19.5	21.6	36.3	45.9	55.8	67.6	37.2	24.1	7.0	8.3	100.0	100.0
Contract–managed	11.9	8.2	0.6	1.4	12.5	9.6	28.2	31.5	40.7	41.1	59.3	58.9	0.0	0.0	100.0	100.0
Total	15.9	17.5	3.0	3.7	18.9	21.2	35.5	45.4	54.4	66.6	39.2	25.4	6.3	8.0	100.0	100.0

H = hospitals; **B** = beds.
*Please note that figures may not always equal the provided subtotal or total percentages due to rounding.

Glossary

This glossary explains specific terms as they are used in the tables and text of AHA Hospital Statistics

Acute long term care: Providers specialized acute hospital care to medically complex patients who are critically ill, have multisystem complications and/or failure, and require hospitalization averaging 25 days, in a facility offering specialized treatment programs and therapeutic intervention on a 24 hour/7day a week basis.

Adjusted average daily census: An estimate of the average number of patients (both inpatients and outpatients) receiving care each day during the reporting period, which is usually 12 months. The figure is derived by dividing the number of inpatient day equivalents (also called adjusted inpatient days) by the number of days in the reporting period.

Adjusted inpatient days: An aggregate figure reflecting the number of days of inpatient care, plus an estimate of the volume of outpatient services, expressed in units equivalent to an inpatient day in terms of level of effort. The figure is derived by first multiplying the number of outpatient visits by the ratio of outpatient revenue per outpatient visit to inpatient revenue per inpatient day. The product (which represents the number of patient days attributable to outpatient services) is then added to the number of *inpatient days*. Originally, the purpose of this calculation was to summarize overall productivity and calculate a unit cost that would include both inpatient and outpatient activities.

Formula 1:

$$\frac{\text{total expenses}}{\text{inpatient days} + \text{outpatient visits}\left(\dfrac{\dfrac{\text{outpatient revenue}}{\text{per outpatient visit}}}{\dfrac{\text{inpatient revenue}}{\text{per inpatient day}}}\right)}$$

However, the value of this calculation has changed over the years as the outpatient share of total revenue has grown and third-party payers have exerted a greater influence on pricing.

Admissions: The number of patients, excluding newborns, accepted for inpatient service during the reporting period; the number includes patients who visit the emergency room and are later admitted for inpatient service.

Adult Cardiac Surgery: Includes minimally invasive procedures that include surgery done with only a small incision or no incision at all, such as through a laparoscope or an endoscope and more invasive major surgical procedures that include open chest and open heart surgery.

Adult day care program: Program providing supervision, medical and psychological care, and social activities for older adults who live at home or in another family setting, but cannot be alone or prefer to be with others during the day. May include intake assessment, health monitoring, occupational therapy, personal care, noon meal, and transportation services.

Adult Diagnostic/invasive catheterization: (also called coronary angiography or coronary arteriography) is used to assist in diagnosing complex heart conditions. Cardiac angiography involves the insertion of a tiny catheter into the artery in the groin then carefully threading the catheter up into the aorta where the coronary arteries originate. Once the catheter is in place, a dye is injected which allows the cardiologist to see the size, shape, and distribution of the coronary arteries. These images are used to diagnose heart disease and to determine, among other things, whether or not surgery is indicated.

Adult Interventional cardiac catheterization: Non surgical procedure that utilizes the same basic principles as diagnostic catheterization and then uses advanced techniques to improve the heart's function. It can be a less-invasive alternative to heart surgery.

Airborne infection isolation room: A single-occupancy room for patient care where environmental factors are controlled in an effort to minimize the transmission of those infectious agents, usually spread person to person by droplet nuclei associated with coughing and inhalation. Such rooms typically have specific ventilation requirements for controlled ventilation, air pressure and filtration.

Alcoholism-drug abuse or dependency inpatient care: Provides diagnosis and therapeutic services to patients with alcoholism or other drug dependencies. Includes care for inpatient/residential treatment for patients whose course of treatment involves more intensive care than provided in an outpatient setting or where patient requires supervised withdrawal.

Alcoholism-drug abuse or dependency outpatient services: Organized hospital services that provide medical care and/or rehabilitative treatment services to outpatients for whom the primary diagnosis is alcoholism or other chemical dependency.

Alzheimer Center: Facility that offers care to persons with Alzheimer's disease and their families through an integrated program of clinical services, research, and education.

Ambulance services: Provision of ambulance services to the ill and injured who require medical attention on a scheduled or unscheduled basis.

Ambulatory Surgery Center: Facility that provides care to patients requiring surgery who are admitted and discharged on the same day. Ambulatory surgery centers are distinct from same day surgical units within the hospital outpatient departments for purposes of Medicare payments.

Arthritis treatment center: Specifically equipped and staffed center for the diagnosis and treatment of arthritis and other joint disorders.

Assisted living: A special combination of housing, supportive services, personalized assistance and health care designed to respond to the individual needs of those who need help in activities of daily living and instrumental activities of daily living. Supportive services are available, 24 hours a day, to meet scheduled and unscheduled needs, in a way that promotes maximum independence and dignity for each resident and encourages the involvement of a resident's family, neighbor and friends.

Auxiliary: A volunteer community organization formed to assist the hospital in carrying out its purpose and to serve as a link between the institution and the community.

Average daily census: The average number of people served on an inpatient basis on a single day during the reporting period; the figure is calculated by dividing the number of inpatient days by the number of days in the reporting period.

Bariatric/weight control services: Bariatrics is the medical practice of weight reduction.

Beds: Number of beds regularly maintained (set up and staffed for use) for inpatients as of the close of the reporting period. Excludes newborn bassinets.

Bed-size category: Hospitals are categorized by the number of beds set up and staffed for use at the end of the reporting period. The eight categories in Hospital Statistics are: 6 to 24 beds; 25 to 49; 50 to 99; 100 to 199; 200 to 299; 300 to 399; 400 to 499; and 500 or more.

Birthing room-LDR room-LDRP room: A single-room type of maternity care with a more homelike setting for families than the traditional three-room unit(labor/delivery/recovery) with a separate postpartum area. A birthing room combines labor and delivery in one room. An LDR room accommodates three stages in the birthing process—labor, delivery, and recovery. An LDRP room accommodates all four stages of the birth process—labor, delivery, recovery, and postpartum.

Births: Total number of infants born in the hospital during the reporting period. Births do not include infants transferred from other institutions, and are excluded from admission and discharge figures.

Blood Donor Center: A facility that performs, or is responsible for the collection, processing, testing or distribution of blood and components.

Bone marrow transplant: See definition for Transplant on page 210.

Breast cancer screening/mammograms: Mammography screening - The use of breast x-ray to detect unsuspected breast cancer in asymptomatic women. Diagnostic mammography - The x-ray imaging of breast tissue in symptomatic women who are considered to have a substantial likelihood of having breast cancer already.

Burn care: Provides care to severely burned patients. Severely burned patients are those with any of the following: (1) second-degree burns of more than 25% total body surface area for adults or 20% total body surface area for children: (2) third-degree burns of more than 10% total body surface area; (3) any severe burns of the hands, face, eyes, ears, or feet; or (4) all inhalation injuries, electrical burns, complicated burn injuries involving fractures and other major traumas, and all other poor risk factors.

Cardiac intensive care: Provides patient care of a more specialized nature than the usual medical and surgical care, on the basis of physicians' orders and approved nursing care plans. The unit is staffed with specially trained nursing personnel and contains monitoring and specialized support or treatment equipment for patients who, because of heart seizure, open-heart surgery, or other life-threatening conditions, require intensified, comprehensive observation and care. May include myocardial infarction, pulmonary care, and heart transplant units.

Cardiac Rehabilitation: A medically supervised program to help heart patients recover quickly and improve their overall physical and mental functioning. The goal is to reduce risk of another cardiac event or to keep an already present heart condition from getting worse. Cardiac rehabilitation programs include: counseling to patients, an exercise program, helping patients modify risk factors such as smoking and high blood pressure, providing vocational guidance to enable the patient to return to work, supplying information on physical limitations and lending emotional support.

Case management: A system of assessment, treatment planning, referral and follow-up that ensures the provision of comprehensive and continuous services and the coordination of payment and reimbursement for care.

Chaplaincy/pastoral care services: A service ministering religious activities and providing pastoral counseling to patients, their families, and staff of a health care organization.

Chemotherapy: An organized program for the treatment of cancer by the use of drugs or chemicals.

Children wellness program: A program that encourages improved health status and a healthful lifestyle of children through health education, exercise, nutrition and health promotion.

Chiropractic services: An organized clinical service including spinal manipulation or adjustment and related diagnostic and therapeutic services.

Closed physician-hospital organization (Closed PHO): A joint venture between the hospital and physicians who have been selected on the basis of cost-effectiveness and/or high quality. The PHO can act as a unified agent in managed care contracting, own a managed care plan, own and operate ambulatory care centers or ancillary services projects, or provide administrative services to physician members.

Community hospitals: All nonfederal, short-term general, and special hospitals whose facilities and services are available to the public. (Special hospitals include obstetrics and gynecology; eye, ear, nose, and throat; rehabilitation; orthopedic; and other individually described specialty services.) Short-term general and special childrens hospitals are also considered to be community hospitals.

A hospital may include a nursing-home-type unit and still be classified as short-term, provided that the majority of its patients are admitted to units where the average length of stay is less than 30 days. Therefore, statistics for community hospitals often include some data about such nursing-home-type units. An example is furnished by Montana, where in 1995 63.6 percent of all hospitals classified as community hospitals include nursing-home-type units. Expense, revenue, utilization, and personnel data for these hospitals include data about their nursing-home-type units. Thus, total admissions to Montana community hospitals in 1995 were 96,154; total inpatient days, 997,759; total expenses, $791,806,393; and total payroll expenses, $352,583,331. If nursing-home-type unit data were excluded, these same items would be 94,034; 457,340; 752,567,865; and $328,911841, respectively.

Note that before 1972, hospital units of institutions such as prison and college infirmaries were included in the category of community hospitals. Including these units made this category equivalent to the short-term general and other special hospitals category. Although these hospital units are few in number and small in size, this change in definition should be taken into consideration when comparing data.

Community outreach: A program that systematically interacts with the community to identify those in need of services, alerting persons and their families to the availability of services, locating needed services, and enabling persons to enter the service delivery system.

Complementary Medicine Services:
Organized hospital services or formal arrangements to providers that provide care or treatment not based solely on traditional western allopathic medical teachings as instructed in most U.S. medical schools. Includes any of the following: acupuncture, chiropractic, homeopathy, osteopathy, diet and lifestyle changes, herbal medicine, message therapy, etc.

Computer assisted orthopedic surgery (CAOS): Orthopedic surgery using computer technology, enabling three-dimensional graphic models to visualize a patient's anatomy.

Control: The type of organization responsible for establishing policy concerning the overall operation of hospitals. The three major categories are government (including federal, state, and local); nongovernment (nonprofit); and investor-owned (for-profit).

Crisis prevention: Services provided in order to promote physical and mental well being and the early identification of disease and ill health prior to the onset and recognition of symptoms so as to permit early treatment.

CT scanner: Computed tomographic scanner for head or whole body scans.

Deduction from revenue: The difference between revenue at full established rates (gross) and the payment actually received from payers (net).

Dental Services: An organized dental service or dentists on staff, not necessarily involving special facilities, providing dental or oral services to inpatients or outpatients.

Diagnostic radioisotope facility: The use of radioactive isotopes (Radiopharmaceuticals) as tracers or indicators to detect an abnormal condition or disease.

Electron beam computed tomography (EBCT): A high tech computed tomography scan used to detect coronary artery disease by measuring coronary calcifications. This imaging procedure uses electron beams which are magnetically steered to produce a visual of the coronary artery and the images are produced faster than conventional CT scans.

Emergency department: Hospital facilities for the provision of unscheduled outpatient services to patients whose conditions require immediate care.

Emergency room visits: The number of visits to the emergency unit. When emergency outpatients are admitted to the inpatient areas of the hospital, they are counted as emergency room visits and subsequently, as inpatient admissions.

Enabling services: A program that is designed to help the patient access health care services by offering any of the following: linguistic services, transportation services, and/or referrals to local social services agencies.

End of Life: Services offered to patients suffering from chronic, severe, and life-threatening diseases including comprehensive services that give patients and caregivers the resources and the confidence to manage symptoms, avoid emergency room admissions and frequent hospitalization, and remain in familiar and comfortable settings.

Enrollment assistance services: A program that provides enrollment assistance for patients who are potentially eligible for public health insurance programs such as Medicaid, State Children's Health Insurance, or local/state indigent care programs. The specific services offered could include explanation of benefits, assist applicants in completing the application and locating all relevant documents, conduct eligibility interviews, and/or forward applications and documentation to state/local social service or health agency.

Equity model: An arrangement that allows established practitioners to become shareholders in a professional corporation in exchange for tangible and intangible assets of their existing practices.

Expenses: Includes all expenses for the reporting period including payroll, non-payroll, bad debt, and all nonoperating expenses. *Payroll expenses* include all salaries and wages. *Non-payroll expenses* are all professional fees and those salary expenditures excluded from payroll. *Labor related expenses* are defined as payroll expenses plus employee benefits. *Non-labor related expenses* are all other non-payroll expenses. *Bad debt* has been reclassified from a "reduction in revenue" to an expense in accordance with the revised AICPA Audit Guide. However, for purposes of historical consistency, the expense total that appears throughout *AHA Hospital Statistics does not include "bad debt" as an expense item.* Note: Financial data may not add due to rounding.

Extracorporeal shock wave lithotripter (ESWL): A medical device used for treating stones in the kidney or ureter. The device disintegrates kidney stones noninvasively through the transmission of acoustic shock waves directed at the stones.

Fertility Clinic: A specialized program set in an infertility center that provides counseling and education as well as advanced reproductive techniques such as: injectable therapy, reproductive surgeries, treatment for endometriosis, male factor infertility, tubal reversals, in vitro fertilization (IVF), donor eggs, and other such services to help patients achieve successful pregnancies.

Fitness center: Provides exercise, testing, or evaluation programs and fitness activities to the community and hospital employees.

Foundation: A corporation, organized as a hospital affiliate or subsidiary, that purchases both tangible and intangible assets of one or more medical group practices. Physicians remain in a separate corporate entity but sign a professional services agreement with the foundation.

Freestanding/Satellite Emergency Department: A facility owned an operated by the hospital but physically separate from the hospital for the provision of unscheduled outpatient services to patients whose conditions require immediate care.

Full-field digital mammography (FFDM): Combines the x-ray generators and tubes used in analog screen-film mammography (SFM) with a detector plate that converts the x-rays into a digital signal.

Full time equivalent employees (FTE): Full time personnel on payroll plus one half of the part time personnel on payroll. For purposes of *AHA Hospital Statistics*, full time and part time medical and dental residents/interns and other trainees are excluded from the calculation.

General medical-surgical care: Provides acute care to patients in medical and surgical units on the basis of physicians' orders and approved nursing care plans.

Genetic testing/counseling: A service equipped with adequate laboratory facilities and directed by a qualified physician to advise parents and prospective parents on potential problems in cases of genetic defects. A genetic test is the analysis of human DNA, RNA, chromosomes, proteins, and certain metabolites in order to detect heritable disease-related genotypes, mutations, phenotypes, or karyotypes for clinical purposes. Genetic tests can have diverse purposes, including the diagnosis of genetic diseases in newborns, children, and adults; the identification of future health risks; the prediction of drug responses; and the assessment of risks to future children.

Geriatric services: The branch of medicine dealing with the physiology of aging and the diagnosis and treatment of disease affecting the aged. Services could include: Adult day care; Alzheimer's diagnostic-assessment services; Comprehensive geriatric assessment; Emergency response system; Geriatric acute care unit; and/or Geriatric clinics.

Government, nonfederal, state, local: Controlled by an agency of state, county, or city government.

Gross inpatient revenue: Revenue from services rendered to inpatients at full established rates (also known as "charges").

Gross outpatient revenue: Revenue from services rendered to outpatients at full established rates.

Group practice without walls: In this organization, the hospital sponsors the formation of a physician group or provides capital to physicians to establish one. The group shares administrative expenses, although the physicians remain independent practitioners.

Group Purchasing Organization: An organization whose primary function is to negotiate contracts for the purpose of purchasing for members of the group or has a central supply site for its members.

Health fair: Community health education events that focus on the prevention of disease and promotion of health through such activities as audiovisual exhibits and free diagnostic services.

Health information center: Education which is directed at increasing the information of individuals and populations. It is intended to increase the ability to make informed personal, family and community health decisions by providing consumers with informed choices about health matters with the objective of improving health status.

Health maintenance organization (HMO): A health care organization that acts as both insurer and provider of comprehensive but specified medical services in return for prospective per capita (capitation) payments.

Health screening: A preliminary procedure such as a test or examination to detect the most characteristic sign or signs of a disorder that may require further investigation.

Heart transplant: See definition for Transplant on page 210.

Hemodialysis: Provision of equipment and personnel for the treatment of renal insufficiency on an inpatient or outpatient basis.

HIV-AIDS services: (could include). *HIV-AIDS unit* - Special unit or team designated and equipped specifically for diagnosis, treatment, continuing care planning, and counseling services for HIV-AIDS patients and their families. *General inpatient care for HIV-AIDS* - Inpatient diagnosis and treatment for human immunodeficiency virus and acquired immunodeficiency syndrome patients, but dedicated unit is not available. *Specialized outpatient program for HIV-AIDS* - Special outpatient program providing diagnostic, treatment, continuing care planning, and counseling for HIV-AIDS patients and their families.

Home health services: Service providing nursing, therapy, and health-related homemaker or social services in the patient's home.

Hospice: A program providing palliative care, chiefly medical relief of pain and supportive services, addressing the emotional, social, financial, and legal needs of terminally ill patients and their families. Care can be provided in a variety of settings, both inpatient and at home.

Hospital unit: The hospital operation, excluding activity pertaining to nursing-home-type unit (as described below), for the following items: Admissions, Beds, FTEs (full-time, part-time, and total), Inpatient Days, Length of Stay, Net Revenue, and Total Expense.

Hospital unit of institutions: A hospital unit that is not open to the public and is contained within a nonhospital unit. An example is an infirmary that is contained within a college.

Hospitals in a network: Hospitals participating in a group that may include other hospitals, physicians, other providers, insurers, and/or community agencies that work together to coordinate and deliver a broad spectrum of services to the community.

Hospitals in a system: Hospitals belonging to a corporate body that owns and/or manages health provider facilities or health-related subsidiaries; the system may also own non-health-related facilities.

Image-guided radiation therapy (IGRT): Automated system for image-guided radiation therapy that enables clinicians to obtain high-resolution x-ray images to pinpoint tumor sites, adjust patient positioning when necessary, and complete a treatment, all within the standard treatment time slot, allowing for more effective cancer treatments.

Indemnity fee for service: The traditional type of health insurance, in which the insured is reimbursed for covered expenses without regard to choice of provider. Payment up to a stated limit may be made either to the individual incurring and claiming the expense, or directly to providers.

Independent practice association (IPA): An IPA is a legal entity that holds managed care contracts and contracts with physicians, usually in solo practice, to provide care either on a fee-for-services or capitated basis. The purpose of an IPA is to assist solo physicians in obtaining managed care contracts.

Inpatient days: The number of adult and pediatric days of care, excluding newborn days of care, rendered during the entire reporting period.

Inpatient surgeries: Surgical services provided to patients who remain in the hospital overnight.

Insurance product: In tables 3 through 6, insurance product refers to a hospital-owned insurance product.

Integrated salary model: In this arrangement, physicians are salaried by the hospital or other entity of a health system to provide medical services for primary care and specialty care.

Intensity-Modulated Radiation Therapy (IMRT): A type of three-dimensional radiation therapy, which improves the targeting of treatment delivery in a way that is likely to decrease damage to normal tissues and allows varying intensities.

Intermediate nursing care: Provides health-related services (skilled nursing care and social services) to residents with a variety of physical conditions or functional disabilities. These residents do not require the care provided by a hospital or skilled nursing facility, but do need supervision and support services.

Investor-owned, for-profit: Investor-owned, for-profit hospitals are those controlled on a for-profit basis by an individual, partnership, or profit-making corporation.

Kidney transplant: See definition for Transplant on page 210.

Labor-related expenses: Payroll expenses plus employee benefits. *Non-labor-related expenses refers* to all other nonpayroll expenses, such as interest depreciation, supplies, purchased services, professional fees, and others.

Length of stay (LOS): LOS refers to the average number of days a patient stays at the facility. Short-term hospitals are those where the average LOS is less than 30 days. Long-term hospitals are those where the average LOS is 30 days or more. The figure is derived by dividing the number of inpatient days by the number of admissions.

Note that this publication carries two LOS variables: *total facility length of stay and hospital unit length of stay. Total facility* includes admissions and inpatient days from nursing-home-type units under control of the hospital. In *hospital unit length of stay*, nursing home utilization is subtracted.

Licensed practical nurse (LPN): A nurse who has graduated from an approved school of practical (vocational) nursing and works under the supervision of registered nurses and/or physicians.

Liver transplant: See definition for Transplant on page 210.

Long-term: Hospitals are classified either short-term or long-term according to the average length of stay (LOS). A long-term hospital is one in which the average LOS is 30 days or more.

Lung transplant: See definition for Transplant on page 210.

Magnetic resonance imaging (MRI): The use of a uniform magnetic field and radio frequencies to study tissue and structure of the body. This procedure enables the visualization of biochemical activity of the cell in vivo without the use of ionizing radiation, radio-isotopic substances, or high-frequency sound.

Managed care: A term covering a broad spectrum of arrangements for health care delivery and financing, including managed indemnity plans (MIP), health maintenance organizations (HMO), preferred provider organizations (PPO), point-of-service plans (POS), and direct contracting arrangements between employers and providers.

Managed care contract: A contract between the hospital and a managed care organization.

Management services organization (MSO): A corporation owned by the hospital or a physician/hospital joint venture that provides management services to one or more medical group practices. As part of a full-service management agreement, the MSO purchases the tangible assets of the practices and leases them back, employs all non-physician staff, and provides all supplies/administrative systems for a fee.

Meals on wheels: A hospital sponsored program which delivers meals to people, usually the elderly, who are unable to prepare their own meals. Low cost, nutritional meals are delivered to individuals' homes on a regular basis.

Medical surgical intensive care: Provides patient care of a more intensive nature than the usual medical and surgical care, on the basis of physicians' orders and approved nursing care plans. These units are staffed with specially trained nursing personnel and contain monitoring and specialized support equipment for patients who, because of shock, trauma, or other life-threatening conditions, require intensified, comprehensive observation and care. Includes mixed intensive care units.

Mobile health services: Vans and other vehicles used to deliver primary care services.

Multi-slice spiral computed tomography (<64 slice CT): A specialized computed tomography procedure that provides three-dimensional processing and allows narrower and multiple slices with increased spatial resolution and faster scanning times as compared to a regular computed tomography scan.

Multi-slice spiral computed tomography (64+ slice CT): Involves the acquisition of volumetric tomographic x-ray absorption data expressed in Hounsfield units using multiple rows of detectors. 64+ systems reconstruct the equivalent of 64 or greater slices to cover the imaged volume.

Neonatal intensive care: A unit that must be separate from the newborn nursery providing intensive care to all sick infants including those with the very lowest birth weights (less than 1500 grams). NICU has potential for providing mechanical ventilation, neonatal surgery, and special care for the sickest infants born in the hospital or transferred from another institution. A full-time neonatologist serves as director of the NICU.

Neonatal intermediate care: A unit that must be separate from the normal newborn nursery and that provides intermediate and/or recovery care and some specialized services, including immediate resuscitation, intravenous therapy, and capacity for prolonged oxygen therapy and monitoring.

Net patient revenue: The estimated net realizable amounts from patients, third-party payers, and others for services rendered. The number includes estimated retroactive adjustments called for by agreements with third-party payers; retroactive adjustments are accrued on an estimated basis in the period the related services are rendered and then adjusted later as final settlements are determined.

Net total revenue: Net patient revenue plus all other revenue, including contributions, endowment revenue, governmental grants, and all other payments not made on behalf of individual patients.

Neurological services: Services provided by the hospital dealing with the operative and nonoperative management of disorders of the central, peripheral, and autonomic nervous system.

Nongovernment, nonprofit: Hospitals that are nongovernment, nonprofit are controlled by not-for-profit organizations, including religious organizations (Catholic hospitals, for example), fraternal societies, and others.

Nursing-home-type unit/facility: A unit/facility that primarily offers the following type of services to a majority of all admissions:

- *Skilled nursing*: The provision of medical and nursing care services, health-related services, and social services under the supervision of a registered nurse on a 24-hour basis.

- *Intermediate care*: The provision, on a regular basis, of health-related care and services to individuals who do not require the degree of care or treatment that a skilled nursing unit is designed to provide.

- *Personal care*: The provision of general supervision and direct personal care services for residents who require assistance in activities of daily living but who do not need nursing services or inpatient care. Medical and nursing services are available as needed.

- *Sheltered/residential care*: The provision of general supervision and protective services for residents who do not need nursing services or continuous personal care services in the conduct of daily life. Medical and nursing services are available as needed.

Nutrition programs: Those services within a health care facility which are designed to provide inexpensive, nutritionally sound meals to patients.

Obstetrics: Levels should be designated: (1) unit provides services for uncomplicated maternity and newborn cases; (2) unit provides services for uncomplicated cases, the majority of complicated problems, and special neonatal services; and (3) unit provides services for all serious illnesses and abnormalities and is supervised by a full-time maternal/fetal specialist.

Occupational health services: Includes services designed to protect the safety of employees from hazards in the work environment.

Oncology services: An organized program for the treatment of cancer by the use of drugs or chemicals.

Open physician hospital organization (Open PHO): A joint venture between the hospital and all members of the medical staff who wish to participate. The open PHO can act as a unified agent in managed care contracting, own a managed care plan, own and operate ambulatory care centers or ancillary services projects, or provide administrative services to physician members.

Orthopedic services: Services provided for the prevention or correction of injuries or disorders of the skeletal system and associated muscles, joints and ligaments.

Osteopathic hospitals: Osteopathic medicine is a medical practice based on a theory that diseases are due chiefly to a loss of structural integrity, which can be restored by manipulation of the neuro-muscular and skeletal systems, supplemented by therapeutic measures (such as medicine or surgery).

Other Intensive Care: A distinct intensive care unit that is not one of the following types: medical/surgical, cardiac, pediatric and neonatal.

Other long term care: Provision of long term care other than skilled nursing care or intermediate care. This can include residential care-elderly housing services for those who do not require daily medical or nursing services, but may require some assistance in the activities of daily living, or sheltered care facilities for developmentally disabled.

Other special care: Provides care to patients requiring care more intensive than that provided in the acute area, yet not sufficiently intensive to require admission to an intensive care unit. Patients admitted to this area are usually transferred here from an intensive care unit once their condition has improved. These units are sometimes referred to as definitive observation, step-down, or progressive care units.

Other transplant: See definition for Transplant on page 210.

Outpatient care: Treatment provided to patients who do not remain in the hospital for overnight care. Hospitals may deliver outpatient care on site or through a facility owned and operated by the hospital, but physically separate from the hospital. In addition to treating minor illnesses or injuries, a free-standing center will stabilize seriously ill or injured patients before transporting them to a hospital. Laboratory and radiology services are usually available.

Outpatient care center (Freestanding): A facility owned and operated by the hospital, but physically separate from the hospital, that provides various medical treatments on an outpatient basis only. In addition to treating minor illnesses or injuries, the center will stabilize seriously ill or injured patients before transporting them to a hospital. Laboratory and radiology services are usually available.

Outpatient care center-services (Hospital-based): Organized hospital health care services offered by appointment on an ambulatory basis. Services may include outpatient surgery, examination, diagnosis, and treatment of a variety of medical conditions on a nonemergency basis, and laboratory and other diagnostic testing as ordered by staff or outside physician referral.

Outpatient surgeries: Scheduled surgical services provided to patients who do not remain in the hospital overnight. In the AHA Annual Survey, outpatient surgery may be performed in operating suites also used for inpatient surgery, specially designated surgical suites for outpatient surgery, or procedure rooms within an outpatient care facility.

Outpatient visit: A visit by a patient who is not lodged in the hospital while receiving medical, dental, or other services. Each visit an outpatient makes to a discrete unit constitutes one visit regardless of the number of diagnostic and/or therapeutic treatments that the patient receives. Total outpatient visits should include all clinic visits, referred visits, observation services, outpatient surgeries, and emergency room visits.

Pain management: A hospital wide formalized program that includes staff education for the management of chronic and acute pain based on guidelines and protocols like those developed by the Agency for Health Care Policy Research, etc.

Palliative care program: An organized program providing specialized medical care, drugs or therapies for the management of acute or chronic pain and/or the control of symptoms administered by specially trained physicians and other clinicians; and supportive care services, such as counseling on advanced directives, spiritual care, and social services, to patients with advanced disease and their families.

Patient Controlled Analgesia (PCA). Patient-controlled Analgesia (PCA) is intravenously administered pain medicine under the patient's control. The patient has a button on the end of a cord than can be pushed at will, whenever more pain medicine is desired. This button will only deliver more pain medicine at pre-determined intervals, as programmed by the doctor's order.

Patient education center: Written goals and objectives for the patient and/or family related to therapeutic regimens, medical procedures, and self care.

Patient representative services: Organized hospital services providing personnel through whom patients and staff can seek solutions to institutional problems affecting the delivery of high-quality care and services.

Payroll expenses: Includes all salaries and wages. All professional fees and salary expenditures excluded from payroll, such as employee benefits, are defined as nonpayroll expenses and are included in total expenses.

Pediatric Cardiac Surgery: Includes minimally invasive procedures that include surgery done with only a small incision or no incision at all, such as through a laparoscope or an endoscope and more invasive major surgical procedures that include open chest and open heart surgery.

Pediatric Diagnostic/invasive catheterization: (also called coronary angiography or coronary arteriography) is used to assist in diagnosing complex heart conditions. Cardiac angiography involves the insertion of a tiny catheter into the artery in the groin then carefully threading the catheter up into the aorta where the coronary arteries originate. Once the catheter is in place, a dye is injected which allows the cardiologist to see the size, shape, and distribution of the coronary arteries. These images are used to diagnose heart disease and to determine, among other things, whether or not surgery is indicated.

Pediatric intensive care: Provides care to pediatric patients that is of a more intensive nature than that usually provided to pediatric patients. The unit is staffed with specially trained personnel and contains monitoring and specialized support equipment for treatment of patients who, because of shock, trauma, or other life-threatening conditions, require intensified, comprehensive observation and care.

Pediatric Interventional cardiac catheterization: Non surgical procedure that utilizes the same basic principles as diagnostic catheterization and then uses advanced techniques to improve the heart's function. It can be a less-invasive alternative to heart surgery.

Pediatric medical-surgical care: Provides acute care to pediatric patients on the basis of physicians' orders and approved nursing care plans.

Personnel: Number of persons on the hospital payroll at the end of the reporting period. Personnel are recorded in *Hospital Statistics* as full-time equivalents (FTEs), which are calculated by adding the number of full-time personnel to one-half the number of part-time personnel, excluding medical and dental residents, interns, and other trainees. *Per 100 adjusted census* indicates the ratio of personnel to adjusted average daily census, calculated on a per-100 basis.

Physical rehabilitation inpatient care: Provides care encompassing a comprehensive array of restoration services for the disabled and all support services necessary to help patients attain their maximum functional capacity.

Physical rehabilitation outpatient services: Outpatient program providing medical, health-related, therapy, social, and/or vocational services to help disabled persons attain or retain their maximum functional capacity.

Population: Population refers to the residential population of the United States. This includes both civilian and military personnel. Note that population is being used to calculate the values *for community health indicators per 1000 population.*

Positron emission tomography/CT (PET/CT): Provides metabolic functional information for the monitoring of chemotherapy, radiotherapy and surgical planning.

Positron emission tomography scanner (PET): A nuclear medicine imaging technology which uses radioactive (positron emitting) isotopes created in a cyclotron or generator and computers to produce composite pictures of the brain and heart at work. PET scanning produces sectional images depicting metabolic activity or blood flow rather than anatomy.

Preferred provider organization (PPO): A pre-set arrangement in which purchasers and providers agree to furnish specified health services to a group of employees/patients.

Primary care department: A unit or clinic within the hospital that provides primary care services (e.g. general pediatric care, general internal medicine, family practice, gynecology) through hospital-salaried medical and/or nursing staff, focusing on evaluating and diagnosing medical problems and providing medical treatment on an outpatient basis.

Psychiatric child-adolescent services: Provides care to emotionally disturbed children and adolescents, including those admitted for diagnosis and those admitted for treatment.

Psychiatric consultation-liaison services: Provides organized psychiatric consultation/liaison services to nonpsychiatric hospital staff and/or departments on psychological aspects of medical care that may be generic or specific to individual patients.

Psychiatric education services: Provides psychiatric educational services to community agencies and workers such as schools, police, courts, public health nurses, welfare agencies, clergy, and so forth. The purpose is to expand the mental health knowledge and competence of personnel not working in the mental health field and to promote good mental health through improved understanding, attitudes, and behavioral patterns.

Psychiatric emergency services: Services of facilities available on a 24-hour basis to provide immediate unscheduled out-patient care, diagnosis, evaluation, crisis intervention, and assistance to persons suffering acute emotional or mental distress.

Psychiatric geriatric services: Provides care to emotionally disturbed elderly patients, including those admitted for diagnosis and those admitted for treatment.

Psychiatric inpatient care: Provides acute or long-term care to emotionally disturbed patients, including patients admitted for diagnosis and those admitted for treatment of psychiatric problems, on the basis of physicians' orders and approved nursing care plans. Long-term care may include intensive supervision to the chronically mentally ill, mentally disordered, or other mentally incompetent persons.

Psychiatric outpatient services: Provides medical care, including diagnosis and treatment, of psychiatric outpatients.

Psychiatric partial hospitalization program: Organized hospital services of intensive day/evening outpatient services of three hours of more duration, distinguished from other outpatient visits of one hour.

Radiology, diagnostic: The branch of radiology that deals with the utilization of all modalities of radiant energy in medical diagnoses and therapeutic procedures using radiologic guidance. This includes, but is not restricted to, imaging techniques and methodologies utilizing radiation emitted by x-ray tubes, radionnuclides, and ultrasonographic devices and the radiofrequency electromagnetic radiation emitted by atoms.

Radiology, therapeutic: The branch of medicine concerned with radioactive substances and using various techniques of visualization, with the diagnosis and treatment of disease using any of the various sources of radiant energy. Services could include:

megavoltage radiation therapy; radioactive implants; stereotactic radiosurgery; therapeutic radioisotope facility; X-ray radiation therapy.

Registered nurse (RN): A nurse who has graduated from an approved school of nursing and who is currently registered by the state. RNs are responsible for the nature and quality of all nursing care that patients receive. In these tables, the number of RNs does not include those registered nurses more appropriately reported in other occupational categories, such as facility administrators, which are listed under *all other personnel* (Tables 1 and 2).

Rehabilitation services: A wide array of restoration services for disabled and recuperating patients, including all support services necessary to help them attain their maximum functional capacity.

Retirement housing: A facility which provides social activities to senior citizens, usually retired persons, who do not require health care but some short-term skilled nursing care may be provided. A retirement center may furnish housing and may also have acute hospital and long-term care facilities, or it may arrange for acute and long term care through affiliated institutions.

Robotic surgery: The use of mechanical guidance devices to remotely manipulate surgical instrumentation.

Rural: A rural hospital is located outside a Metropolitan Statistical Area (MSA), as designated by the U.S. Office of Management and Budget (OMB) effective June 6, 2003. An urban area is a geographically defined, integrated social and economic unit with a large population nucleus. Micropolitan areas, which are new to the OMB June 6, 2003 definitions, continue to be classified as rural for purposes of this publication.

Shaped beam radiation system. A precise, non-invasive treatment that involves targeting beams of radiation that mirror the exact size and shape of a tumor at a specific area of a tumor to shrink or destroy cancerous cells. This procedure delivers a therapeutic dose of radiation that conforms precisely to the shape of the tumor, thus minimizing the risk to nearby tissues.

Single photon emission computerized tomography (SPECT): A nuclear medicine imaging technology that combines existing technology of gamma camera imaging with computed tomographic imaging technology to provide a more precise and clear image.

Skilled nursing care: Provides non-acute medical and skilled nursing care services, therapy, and social services under the supervision of a licensed registered nurse on a 24-hour basis.

Sleep Center: Specially equipped and staffed center for the diagnosis and treatment of sleep disorders.

Social work services (could include): Organized services that are properly directed and sufficiently staffed by qualified individuals who provide assistance and counseling to patients and their families in dealing with social, emotional, and environmental problems associated with illness or disability, often in the context of financial or discharge planning coordination.

Sports medicine: Provision of diagnostic screening and assessment and clinical and rehabilitation services for the prevention and treatment of sports-related injuries.

Stereotactic radiosurgery: Stereotactic radiosurgery (SRS) is a radiotherapy modality that delivers a high dosage of radiation to a discrete treatment area in as few as one treatment session. Includes gamma knife, cyberknife, etc.

Support groups: A hospital sponsored program which allows a group of individuals with the same or similar problems who meet periodically to share experiences, problems, and solutions in order to support each other.

Surgical operations: Those surgical operations, whether major or minor, performed in the operating room(s). A surgical operation involving more than one surgical procedure is still considered only one surgical operation.

Swing bed services: A hospital bed that can be used to provide either acute or long-term care depending on community or patient needs. To be eligible a hospital must have a Medicare provider agreement in place, have fewer than 100 beds, be located in a rural area, do not have a 24 hour nursing service waiver in effect, have not been terminated from the program in the prior two years, and meet various service conditions.

Teen outreach services: A program focusing on the teenager which encourages an improved health status and a healthful lifestyle including physical, emotional, mental, social, spiritual and economic health through education, exercise, nutrition and health promotion.

Tissue transplant: See definition for Transplant on page 210.

Tobacco treatment/cessation program: Organized hospital services with the purpose of ending tobacco-use habits of patients addicted to tobacco/nicotine.

Transplant services. The branch of medicine that transfers an organ or tissue from one person to another or from one body part to another to replace a diseased structure or to restore function or to change appearance. Services could include: Bone marrow transplant program; heart, lung, kidney, intestine, or tissue transplant. The other transplant services include transplant services other than bone marrow, heart, kidney, liver, lung, tissue and heart/lung or other multi-transplant surgeries.

Transportation to health facilities: A long-term care support service designed to assist the mobility of the elderly. Some programs offer improved financial access by offering reduced rates and barrier-free buses or vans with ramps and lifts to assist the elderly or handicapped; others offer subsidies for public transport systems or operate mini-bus services exclusively for use by senior citizens.

Trauma center (certified): A facility to provide emergency and specialized intensive care to critically ill and injured patients. **Level 1:** A regional resource trauma center, which is capable of providing total care for every aspect of injury and plays a leadership role in trauma research and education. **Level 2:** A community trauma center, which is capable of providing trauma care to all but the most severely injured patients who require highly specialized care. **Level 3:** A rural trauma hospital, which is capable of providing care to a large number of injury victims and can resuscitate and stabilize more severely injured patients so that they can be transported to Level 1 or 2 facilities.

Ultrasound: The use of acoustic waves above the range of 20,000 cycles per second to visualize internal body structures.

Urban: An urban hospital is located inside a Metropolitan Statistical Area (MSA), designated by the U.S. Office of Management and Budget effective June 6, 2003. An urban areas is a geographically defined, integrated social and economic unit with a large population base. Micropolitan areas, which are new to the OMB June 6, 2003 definitions, are not considered to be urban for purposes of this publication.

E. TOTAL FACILITY BEDS, UTILIZATION, FINANCES, AND STAFFING (continued)

3. FINANCIAL

* a. Net patient revenue .... .00   .00
* b. Tax appropriations .... .00
* c. Other operating revenue .... .00
* d. Nonoperating revenue .... .00
* e. TOTAL REVENUE (add 3a thru 3d) .... .00   .00
  f. PAYROLL EXPENSES (only) .... .00   .00
  g. Employee benefits .... .00   .00
  h. Depreciation expense (for reporting period only) .... .00
  i. Interest expense .... .00
  j. **TOTAL EXPENSES** (Payroll plus all non-payroll expenses, including bad debt) .00   .00

*4. REVENUE BY TYPE

a. Total gross inpatient revenue .... .00
b. Total gross outpatient revenue .... .00
c. Total gross patient revenue .... .00

*5. UNCOMPENSATED CARE

a. Bad debt expense .... .00
b. Charity (Revenue forgone at full-established rates. Include in gross revenue) .... .00

*6. REVENUE BY PAYOR (report total facility gross and net figures)
(E.6a(2a) should include Medicaid disproportionate payments in the net column (2)

		(1) Gross	(2) Net
*a. GOVERNMENT	(1) Medicare:		
	a) Routine patient revenue	.00	.00
	b) Managed care revenue	.00	.00
	c) **Total (a + b)**	**.00**	**.00**
	(2) Medicaid:		
	a) Routine patient revenue	.00	.00
	b) Managed care revenue	.00	.00
	c) **Total (a + b)**	**.00**	**.00**
	(3) Other government:	.00	.00
*b. NONGOVERNMENT	(1) Self-pay	.00	.00
	(2) Third-party payors:		
	a) Managed care (includes HMO and PPO)	.00	.00
	b) Other third-party payors	.00	.00
	c) **Total third-party payors (a + b)**	**.00**	**.00**
	(3) All Other nongovernment:	.00	.00
*c. TOTAL		**.00**	**.00**

(Total gross should equal 4c on page 9. Total net should equal 3a on page 9.)

Are the financial data on pages 8 and 9 from your audited financial statement? .... YES ☐   No ☐

E. TOTAL FACILITY BEDS, UTILIZATION, FINANCES, AND STAFFING (continued)

7. FIXED ASSETS

a. Property, plant and equipment at cost .... _____.00

b. Accumulated depreciation .... _____.00

c. Net property, plant and equipment (a-b) .... _____.00

d. Total gross square feet of your physical plant used for or in support of your healthcare activities .... _____

8. TOTAL CAPITAL EXPENSES

Include all expenses used to acquire assets, including buildings, remodeling projects, equipment, or property. _____.00

9. INFORMATION TECHNOLOGY

*a. IT operating expense.._____.00

*b IT Capital expense..._____.00

*c. Number of employed IT staff (in FTEs) ...._____

*d. Number of outsourced IT staff (in FTEs)..._____

e. Does your hospital have an electronic health record (see definition)?

☐ Yes, fully implemented   ☐ Yes, partially implemented   ☐ No (If no, please skip to Question g)

f. Does your electronic health record include:	Yes, fully implemented	Yes, partially implemented	No
1. Patient-level health information and data (such as medications, orders, and clinical notes)?	☐	☐	☐
2. Results management (such as results from laboratory tests, radiology studies, and other tests)?	☐	☐	☐
3. Order entry management (such as orders for laboratory tests, radiology studies, and other tests)?	☐	☐	☐
4. Decision support (such as knowledge sources, drug alerts, reminders, and clinical guidelines and pathways)?	☐	☐	☐

g. What percentage of treating physicians in your hospital:	0%	1-24%	25-49%	50-74%	75-100%
1. Routinely order medications electronically?	☐	☐	☐	☐	☐
2. Routinely order laboratory or other tests electronically?	☐	☐	☐	☐	☐

E. TOTAL FACILITY BEDS, UTILIZATION, FINANCES, AND STAFFING (continued)

10. STAFFING

Report full-time (35 hours or more) and part-time (less than 35 hours) personnel who were on the hospital/facility **payroll at the end of your reporting period.** Include members of religious orders for whom dollar equivalents were reported. Exclude private-duty nurses, volunteers, and all personnel whose salary is financed entirely by outside research grants. Exclude physicians and dentists who are paid on a fee basis. FTE is the total number of hours worked by all employees over the full (12 month) reporting period divided by the normal number of hours worked by a full-time employee for that same time period. For example, if your hospital considers a normal workweek for a full-time employee to be 40 hours, a total of 2,080 would be worked over a full year (52 weeks). If the total number of hours worked by all employees on the payroll is 208,000, then the number of Full-Time Equivalents (FTE) is 100 (employees). The FTE calculation for a specific occupational category such as Registered nurses is exactly the same. The calculation for each occupational category should be based on the number of hours worked by staff employed in that specific category.

	(1) Full-Time (35 hr/wk or more) On Payroll	(2) Part-Time (Less than 35hr/wk) On Payroll	(3) FTE
a. Physicians and dentists..	_____	_____	_____
b. Medical and dental residents/interns.......................................	_____	_____	_____
c. Other trainees..	_____	_____	_____
d. Registered nurses...	_____	_____	_____
e. Licensed practical (vocational) nurses....................................	_____	_____	_____
f. Nursing assistive personnel..	_____	_____	_____
g. Radiology technicians..	_____	_____	_____
h. Laboratory technicians..	_____	_____	_____
i. Pharmacists, licensed..	_____	_____	_____
j. Pharmacy technicians..	_____	_____	_____
k. All other personnel..	_____	_____	_____
l. Total facility personnel (add 10a through 10k).........................	_____	_____	_____

(Total facility personnel should include hospital plus nursing home type unit/facility personnel reported in 10 m and 10 n.)

m. Nursing home type unit/facility Registered Nurses..................	_____	_____	_____
n. **Total nursing home type unit/facility personnel**.......................	_____	_____	_____

o. Do hospitalists provide care for patients in your hospital?......................... **YES** ☐   **NO** ☐

p. If yes, please report the number of full time and part time hospitalists? _____Full-time _____Part-time

q. If yes, please select the category below that best describes the employment model for your hospitalists?
☐ Independent provider group   ☐ Employed by your hospital
☐ Employed by a physician group   ☐ Employed by a university or school program   ☐ Other

F. SUPPLEMENTAL INFORMATION

1. Does your hospital provide services through a satellite facility(s)? .... YES ☐   NO ☐

2. Use this space or an additional sheet if more space is required for comments or to elaborate on any of the information supplied on this survey. Refer to the response by page, section, and item name. Also, use this space to describe your community benefit activities.

_____

_____

_____

_____

_____

2006 AHA ANNUAL SURVEY

As declared previously, hospital specific revenue data are treated as confidential. AHA's policy is not to release these data without written permission from your institution. The AHA will however, share these data with your respective state hospital association and if requested with your appropriate metropolitan/regional association.

On occasion, the AHA is asked to provide these data to external organizations, both public and private, for their use in analyzing crucial health care policy or research issues. The AHA is requesting your permission to allow us to release your confidential data to those requests that we consider legitimate and worthwhile. In every instance of disclosure, the receiving organization will be prohibited from releasing hospital specific information.

Please indicate below whether or not you agree to these types of disclosure:

[ ] I hereby grant AHA permission to release my hospital's revenue data to external users that the AHA determines have a legitimate and worthwhile need to gain access to these data subject to the user's agreement with the AHA not to release hospital specific information.

_____
Chief Executive Officer   Date

[ ] I do not grant AHA permission to release my confidential data.

_____
Chief Executive Officer   Date

Does your hospital or health system have an Internet or Homepage address?   Yes ☐   No ☐

If yes, please provide the address: http:// _____

Thank you for your cooperation in completing this survey. If there are any questions about your responses to this survey, who should be contacted?

_____   _____   _____
Name (please print)   Title   (Area Code) Telephone Number

_____/_____/_____   _____   (____) _____
Date of Completion   Chief Executive Officer   Hospital's Main Fax Number

NOTE: PLEASE PHOTOCOPY THE INFORMATION FOR YOUR HOSPITAL FILE BEFORE RETURNING THE ORIGINAL FORM TO THE AMERICAN HOSPITAL ASSOCIATION. ALSO, PLEASE FORWARD A PHOTOCOPY OF THE COMPLETED QUESTIONNAIRE TO YOUR STATE HOSPITAL ASSOCIATION.

THANK YOU

ANNUAL SURVEY

2006 AHA ANNUAL SURVEY

SECTION A
REPORTING PERIOD
Instructions

INSTRUCTIONS AND DEFINITIONS FOR THE 2006 ANNUAL SURVEY
HOSPITAL. For purposes of this survey, a hospital is defined as the organization or corporate entity licensed or registered as a hospital by a state to provide diagnostic and therapeutic patient services for a variety of medical conditions, both surgical and nonsurgical.
1. **Reporting period used (beginning and ending date):** Record the beginning and ending dates of the reporting period in an eight-digit number: for example, January 1, 2006 should be shown as 01/01/2006. Number of days should equal the time span between the two dates that the hospital was open. If you are reporting for less than 365 days, utilization and finances should be presented for days reported only.
2. **Were you in operation 12 full months at the end of your reporting period?** If you are reporting for less than 365 days, utilization and finances should be presented for days reported only.
3. **Number of days open during reporting period:** Number of days should equal the time span between the two dates that the hospital was open.

SECTION B
ORGANIZATIONAL STRUCTURE
Instructions and Definitions

1. **CONTROL**
   Check the box to the left of the type of organization that is responsible for establishing policy for overall operation of the hospital.
   Government, nonfederal.
   State. Controlled by an agency of state government.
   County. Controlled by an agency of county government.
   City. Controlled by an agency of municipal government.
   City-County. Controlled jointly by agencies of municipal and county governments.
   Hospital district or authority. Controlled by a political subdivision of a state, county, or city created solely for the purpose of establishing and maintaining medical care or health-related care institutions.
   Nongovernment, not for profit. Hospitals controlled by not-for-profit organizations, including religious organizations (Catholic hospitals, for example), community hospitals, cooperative hospitals, hospitals operated by fraternal societies, and so forth.
   Investor owned, for profit. Hospitals controlled on a for profit basis by an individual, partnership, or a profit making corporation.
   Government, federal. Hospitals controlled by an agency or department of the federal government.
2. **SERVICE**
   Indicate the ONE category that best describes the type of service that your hospital provides to the majority of admissions.
   General medical and surgical. Provides diagnostic and therapeutic services to patients for a variety of medical conditions, both surgical and nonsurgical.
   Hospital unit of an institution. Provides diagnostic and therapeutic services to patients in an institution.
   Hospital unit within an institution for the mentally retarded. Provides diagnostic and therapeutic services to patients in an institution for the mentally retarded.
   Surgical. An acute care specialty hospitals where 2/3 or more of its inpatient claims are for surgical/diagnosis related groups.
   Psychiatric. Provides diagnostic and therapeutic services to patients with mental or emotional disorders.
   Tuberculosis and other respiratory diseases. Provides medical care and rehabilitative services to patients for whom the primary diagnosis is tuberculosis or other respiratory diseases.
   Cancer. Provides medical care to patients for whom the primary diagnosis is cancer.
   Heart. Provides diagnosis and treatment of heart disease.
   Obstetrics and gynecology. Provides medical and surgical treatment to pregnant women and to mothers following delivery. Also provides diagnostic and therapeutic services to women with diseases or disorders of the reproductive organs.
   Eye, ear, nose, and throat. Provides diagnosis and treatment of diseases and injuries of the eyes, ears, nose, and throat.
   Rehabilitation. Provides a comprehensive array of restoration services for the disabled and all support services necessary to help them attain their maximum functional capacity.
   Orthopedic. Provides corrective treatment of deformities, diseases, and ailments of the locomotive apparatus, especially affecting the limbs, bones, muscles, and joints.
   Chronic disease. Provides medical and skilled nursing services to patients with long-term illnesses who are not in an acute phase, but who require an intensity of services not available in nursing homes.
   Institution for the mentally retarded. Provides health-related care on a regular basis to patients with psychiatric or developmental impairment who cannot be treated in a skilled nursing unit.
   Acute long term care hospital. Provides high acuity interdisciplinary services to medically complex patients that require more intensive recuperation and care than can be provided in a typical nursing facility.
   Alcoholism and other chemical dependency. Provides diagnostic and therapeutic services to patients with alcoholism or other drug dependencies.
3. **OTHER**
   a. **Children admissions.** A hospital whose primary focus is the health and treatment of children and adolescents.
   b. **Subsidiary.** A company that is wholly controlled by another or one that is more than 50% owned by another organization.
   c. **Contract managed.** General day-to-day management of an entire organization by another organization under a formal contract. Managing organization reports directly to the board of trustees or owners of the managed organization; managed organization retains total legal responsibility and ownership of the facility's assets and liabilities.
   d. **Network.** A group of hospitals, physicians, other providers, insurers and/or community agencies that voluntarily work together to coordinate and deliver health services
   e. **Group Purchasing Organization.** An organization whose primary function is to negotiate contracts for the purpose of purchasing for members of the group or has a central supply site for its members.

AHA Hospital Statistics © 2008 Health Forum LLC, an affiliate of the American Hospital Association **225**

SECTION C
FACILITIES AND SERVICES
Definitions

Owned/Provided by the hospital or its subsidiary. All patient revenues, expenses and utilization related o the provision of the service are reflected in the hospital's statistics reported elsewhere in this survey.

Provided by my Health System (in my local community). Another health care provider in the same system as your hospital provides the service and patient revenue, expenses, and utilization related to the provision of the service are recorded at the point where the service was provided and would n be reflected in your hospital's statistics reported elsewhere in this survey.

Provided by my network (in my local community). Another health care provider in the same network as your hospital provides the service and patient revenue, expenses and utilization related to the provision of the service are recorded at the point where the service was provided and would not be reflected in your hospital's statistics reported elsewhere in this survey.

Provided through a formal contractual arrangement or joint venture with another provider that is not in my system or network. All patient revenues and utilization related to the provision of the service are recorded at the site where the service was provided and would not be reflected in your hospital statistics reported elsewhere in this survey.

1. **General medical-surgical care.** Provides acute care to patients in medical and surgical units on the basis of physicians' orders and approved nursing care plans.
2. **Pediatric medical-surgical care.** Provides acute care to pediatric patients on the basis of physicians' orders and approved nursing care plans.
3. **Obstetrics.** Levels should be designated: (1) unit provides services for uncomplicated maternity and newborn cases; (2) unit provides services for uncomplicated cases, the majority of complicated problems, and special neonatal services; and (3) unit provides services for all serious illnesses and abnormalities and is supervised by a full-time maternal/fetal specialist.
4. **Medical surgical intensive care.** Provides patient care of a more intensive nature than the usual medical and surgical care, on the basis of physicians' orders and approved nursing care plans. These units are staffed with specially trained nursing personnel and contain monitoring and specialized support equipment for patients who because of shock, trauma or other life-threatening conditions require intensified comprehensive observation and care. Includes mixed intensive care units.
5. **Cardiac intensive care.** Provides patient care of a more specialized nature than the usual medical and surgical care, on the basis of physicians' orders and approved nursing care plans. The unit is staffed with specially trained nursing personnel and contains monitoring and specialized support or treatment equipment for patients who, because of heart seizure, open-heart surgery, or other life-threatening conditions, require intensified, comprehensive observation and care. May include myocardial infarction, pulmonary care, and heart transplant units.
6. **Neonatal intensive care.** A unit that must be separate from the newborn nursery providing intensive care to all sick infants including those with the very lowest birth weights (less than 1500 grams). NICU has potential for providing mechanical ventilation, neonatal surgery, and special care for the sickest infants born in the hospital or transferred from another institution. A full-time neonatologist serves as director of the NICU.
7. **Neonatal intermediate care.** A unit that must be separate from the normal newborn nursery and that provides intermediate and/or recover care and some specialized services, including immediate resuscitation, intravenous therapy, and capacity for prolonged oxygen therapy and monitoring.
8. **Pediatric intensive care.** Provides care to pediatric patients that is of a more intensive nature than that usually provided to pediatric patients. The unit is staffed with specially trained personnel and contains monitoring and specialized support equipment for treatment of patients who, because of shock, trauma, or other life-threatening conditions, require intensified, comprehensive observation and care.
9. **Burn care.** Provides care to severely burned patients. Severely burned patients are those with any of the following: (1) second-degree burns of more than 25% total body surface area for adults or 20% total body surface area for children: (2) third-degree burns of more than 10% total body surface area; (3) any severe burns of the hands, face, eyes, ears, or feet; or (4) all inhalation injuries, electrical burns, complicated burn injuries involving fractures and other major traumas, and all other poor risk factors.
10. **Other special care.** Provides care to patients requiring care more intensive than that provided in the acute area, yet not sufficiently intensive to require admission to an intensive care unit. Patients admitted to this area are usually transferred here from an intensive care unit once their condition has improved. These units are sometimes referred to as definitive observation, step-down, or progressive care units.
11. **Other intensive care.** A specially staffed, specialty equipped, separate section of a hospital dedicated to the observation, care, and treatment of patients with life threatening illnesses, injuries, or complications from which recovery is possible. It provides special expertise and facilities for the support of vital function and utilizes the skill of medical nursing and other staff experienced in the management of these problems.
12. **Physical rehabilitation.** Provides care encompassing a comprehensive array of restoration services for the disabled and all support services necessary to help patients attain their maximum functional capacity.
13. **Alcoholism-drug abuse or dependency care.** Provides diagnosis and therapeutic services to patients with alcoholism or other drug dependencies. Includes care for inpatient/residential treatment for patients whose course of treatment involves more intensive care than provided in an outpatient setting or where patient requires supervised withdrawal.
14. **Psychiatric care.** Provides acute or long-term care to emotionally disturbed patients, including patients admitted for diagnosis and those admitted for treatment of psychiatric problems, on the basis of physicians' orders and approved nursing care plans. Long-term care may include intensive supervision to the chronically mentally ill, mentally disordered, or other mentally incompetent persons.
15. **Skilled nursing care.** Provides non-acute medical and skilled nursing care services, therapy, and social services under the supervision of a licensed registered nurse on a 24-hour basis.
16. **Intermediate nursing care.** Provides health-related services (skilled nursing care and social services) to residents with a variety of physical conditions or functional disabilities. These residents do not require the care provided by a hospital or skilled nursing facility, but do need supervision and support services.
17. **Acute long-term care.** Provides specialized acute hospital care to medically complex patients who are critically ill, have multisystem complications and/or failure, and require hospitalization averaging 25 days, in a facility offering specialized treatment programs and therapeutic intervention on a 24-hour/7 day a week basis.
18. **Other long term care.** Provision of long term care other than skilled nursing care or intermediate care. This can include residential care-elderly housing services for those who do not require daily medical or nursing services, but may require some assistance in the activities of daily living, or sheltered care facilities for developmentally disabled.
19. **Other care.** (specify) Any type of care other than those listed above.
    The sum of the beds reported in 1-19 should equal what you have reported in Section E(1b) for beds set up and staffed.
20. **Adult day care program.** Program providing supervision, medical and psychological care, and social activities for older adults who live at home or in another family setting, but cannot be alone or prefer to be with others during the day. May include intake assessment, health monitoring, occupational therapy, personal care, noon meal, and transportation services.
21. **Airborne infection isolation room.** A single-occupancy room for patient care where environmental factors are controlled in an effort to minimize the transmission of those infectious agents, usually spread person to person by droplet nuclei associated with coughing and inhalation. Such rooms typically have specific ventilation requirements for controlled ventilation, air pressure and filtration.

22. **Alcoholism-drug abuse or dependency outpatient services.** Organized hospital services that provide medical care and/or rehabilitative treatment services to outpatients for whom the primary diagnosis is alcoholism or other chemical dependency.
23. **Alzheimer Center.** Facility that offers care to persons with Alzheimer's disease and their families through an integrated program of clinical services, research, and education.
24. **Ambulance services.** Provision of ambulance service to the ill and injured who require medical attention on a scheduled and unscheduled basis.
25. **Ambulatory Surgery Center.** Facility that provides care to patients requiring surgery who are admitted and discharged on the same day. Ambulatory surgery centers are distinct from same day surgical units within the hospital outpatient departments for purposes of Medicare payment.
26. **Arthritis treatment center.** Specifically equipped and staffed center for the diagnosis and treatment of arthritis and other joint disorders.
27. **Assisted living.** A special combination of housing, supportive services, personalized assistance and health care designed to respond to the individual needs of those who need help in activities of daily living and instrumental activities of daily living. Supportive services are available, 24 hours a day, to meet scheduled and unscheduled needs, in a way that promotes maximum independence an dignity for each resident and encourages the involvement of a resident's family, neighbor and friends.
28. **Auxiliary.** A volunteer community organization formed to assist the hospital in carrying out its purpose and to serve as a link between the institution and the community.
29. **Bariactric/weight control services.** Bariatrics is the medical practice of weight reduction.
30. **Birthing room/LDR room/LDRP room.** A single-room type of maternity care with a more homelike setting for families than the traditional three-room unit (labor/delivery/recovery) with a separate postpartum area. A birthing room combines labor and delivery in one room. An LDR room accommodates three stages in the birthing process--labor, delivery, and recovery. An LDRP room accommodates all four stages of the birth process--labor, delivery, recovery, and postpartum.
31. **Blood Donor Center.** A facility that performs, or is responsible for the collection, processing, testing or distribution of blood and components.
32. **Breast cancer screening/mammograms.** Mammography screening - The use of breast x-ray to detect unsuspected breast cancer in asymptomatic women. Diagnostic mammography - The x-ray imaging of breast tissue in symptomatic women who are considered to have a substantial likelihood of having breast cancer already.
33. **Cardiology and cardiac surgery services.** Services which include the diagnosis and treatment of diseases and disorders involving the heart and circulatory system.
    a-b. Diagnostic/invasive catheterization. (also called coronary angiography or coronary arteriography) is used to assist in diagnosing complex heart conditions. Cardiac angiography involves the insertion of a tiny catheter into the artery in the groin then carefully threading the catheter up into the aorta where the coronary arteries originate. Once the catheter is in place, a dye is injected which allows the cardiologist to see the size, shape, and distribution of the coronary arteries. These images are used to diagnose heart disease and to determine, among other things, whether or not surgery is indicated.
    c-d. Interventional cardiac catheterization. Nonsurgical procedure that utilizes the same basic principles as diagnostic catheterization and then uses advanced techniques to improve the heart's function. It can be a less-invasive alternative to heart surgery.
    e-f. Cardiac surgery. Includes minimally invasive procedures that include surgery done with only a small incision or no incision at all, such as through a laparoscope or an endoscope and more invasive major surgical procedures that include open chest and open heart surgery.
    g. Cardiac rehabilitation. A medically supervised program to help heart patients recover quickly and improve their overall physical and mental functioning. The goal is to reduce risk of another cardiac event or to keep an already present heart condition from getting worse. Cardiac rehabilitation programs include: counseling to patients, an exercise program, helping patients modify risk factors such as smoking and high blood pressure, providing vocational guidance to enable the patient to return to work, supplying information on physical limitations and lending emotional support.
34. **Case management.** A system of assessment, treatment planning, referral and follow-up that ensures the provision of comprehensive and continuous services and the coordination of payment and reimbursement for care.
35. **Chaplaincy/pastoral care services.** A service ministering religious activities and providing pastoral counseling to patients, their families, and staff of a health care organization.
36. **Chemotherapy.** An organized program for the treatment of cancer by the use of drugs or chemicals.
37. **Children wellness program.** A program that encourages improved health status and a healthful lifestyle of children through health education, exercise, nutrition and health promotion.
38. **Chiropractic services.** An organized clinical service including spinal manipulation or adjustment and related diagnostic and therapeutic services.
39. **Community outreach.** A program that systematically interacts with the community to identify those in need of services, alerting persons and their families to the availability of services, locating needed services, and enabling persons to enter the service delivery system.
40. **Complementary medicine services.** Organized hospital services or formal arrangements to providers that provide care or treatment not based solely on traditional western allopathic medical teachings as instructed in most U.S. medical schools. Includes any of the following: acupuncture, chiropractic, homeopathy, osteopathy, diet and lifestyle changes, herbal medicine, massage therapy, etc.
41. **Computer assisted orthopedic surgery (CAOS).** Orthopedic surgery using computer technology, enabling three-dimensional graphic models to visualize a patient's anatomy.
42. **Crisis prevention.** Services provided in order to promote physical and mental well being and the early identification of disease and ill health prior to the onset and recognition of symptoms so as to permit early treatment.
43. **Dental Services.** An organized dental service or dentists on staff, not necessarily involving special facilities, providing dental or oral services to inpatients or outpatients.
44. **Emergency services.** Health services that are provided after the onset of a medical condition that manifests itself by symptoms of sufficient severity, including severe pain, that the absence of immediate medical attention could reasonably be expected by a prudent layperson, who possesses an average knowledge of health and medicine, to result in placing the patient's health in serious jeopardy.
    a. **Emergency department.** Hospital facilities for the provision of unscheduled outpatient services to patients whose conditions require immediate care.
    b. **Satellite Emergency Department. A facility owned and operated by the hospital but physically separate from the hospital for the provision of unscheduled outpatient services to patients whose conditions require immediate care. A freestanding ED is not physically connected to a hospital, but has all necessary emergency staffing and equipment on-site.**
    d. **Trauma center (certified).** A facility to provide emergency and specialized intensive care to critically ill and injured patients. Level 1: A regional resource trauma center, which is capable of providing total care for every aspect of injury and plays a leadership role in trauma research and education. Level 2: A community trauma center, which is capable of providing trauma care to all but the most severely injured patients who require highly specialized care. Level 3: A rural trauma hospital, which is capable of providing care to a large number of injury victims and can

resuscitate and stabilize more severely injured patients so that they can be transported to level 1 or 2 facilities. Please provide explanation on page 10 if necessary.

45. **Enabling services.** A program that is designed to help the patient access health care services by offering any of the following: transportation services and/or referrals to local social services agencies.
46. **End of life services.** Services offered to patients suffering from chronic, severe, and life-threatening diseases including comprehensive services that give patients and caregivers the resources and the confidence to manage symptoms, avoid emergency department admissions and frequent hospitalization, and remain in familiar and comfortable settings.
    a. **Hospice Program.** A recognized clinical program with specific eligibility criteria that provides palliative medical care focused on relief of pain and symptom control and other services that address the emotional, social, financial and spiritual needs of terminally ill patients and their families. Hospice care can be provided either at home, in a hospital setting, or a freestanding facility.
    b. **Pain management program.** A recognized clinical service or program providing specialized medical care, drugs or therapies for the management of acute or chronic pain and other distressing symptoms, administered by specially trained physicians and other clinicians, to patients suffering from an acute illness of diverse causes.
    c. **Palliative care program.** An organized program providing specialized medical care, drugs or therapies for the management of acute or chronic pain and/or the control of symptoms administered by specially trained physicians and other clinicians; and supportive care services, such as counseling on advanced directives, spiritual care, and social services, to patients with advanced disease and their families.
47. **Enrollment assistance services.** A program that provides enrollment assistance for patients who are potentially eligible for public health insurance programs such as Medicaid, State Children's Health Insurance, or local/state indigent care programs. The specific services offered could include explanation of benefits, assist applicants in completing the application and locating all relevant documents, conduct eligibility interviews, and/or forward applications and documentation to state/local social service or health agency.
48. **Extracorporeal shock wave lithotripter (ESWL).** A medical device used for treating stones in the kidney or urether. The device disintegrates kidney stones noninvasively through the transmission of acoustic shock waves directed at the stones.
49. **Fitness center.** Provides exercise, testing, or evaluation programs and fitness activities to the community and hospital employees.
50. **Freestanding outpatient care center.** A facility owned and operated by the hospital, that is physically separate from the hospital and provides various medical treatments and diagnostic services on an outpatient basis only. Laboratory and radiology services are usually available.
51. **Geriatric services.** The branch of medicine dealing with the physiology of aging and the diagnosis and treatment of disease affecting the aged. Services could include: Adult day care; Alzheimer's diagnostic-assessment services; Comprehensive geriatric assessment; Emergency response system; Geriatric acute care unit; and/or Geriatric clinics.
52. **Health fair.** Community health education events that focus on the prevention of disease and promotion of health through such activities as audiovisual exhibits and free diagnostic services.
53. **Health information center.** Education which is directed at increasing the information of individuals and populations. It is intended to increase the ability to make informed personal, family and community health decisions by providing consumers with informed choices about health matters with the objective of improving health status.
54. **Health screening.** A preliminary procedure such as a test or examination to detect the most characteristic sign or signs of a disorder that may require further investigation.
55. **Hemodialysis:** Provision of equipment and personnel for the treatment of renal insufficiency on an inpatient or outpatient basis.
56. **HIV-AIDS services** (could include). HIV-AIDS unit-Special unit or team designated and equipped specifically for diagnosis, treatment, continuing care planning, and counseling services for HIV-AIDS patients and their families. General inpatient care for HIV-AIDS-Inpatient diagnosis and treatment for human immunodeficiency virus and acquired immunodeficiency syndrome patients, but dedicated unit is not available. Specialized outpatient program for HIV-AIDS-Special outpatient program providing diagnostic, treatment, continuing care planning, and counseling for HIV-AIDS patients and their families.
57. **Home health services.** Service providing nursing, therapy, and health-related homemaker or social services in the patient's home.
58. **Hospital-based outpatient care center-services.** Organized hospital health care services offered by appointment on an ambulatory basis. Services may include outpatient surgery, examination, diagnosis, and treatment of a variety of medical conditions on a nonemergency basis, and laboratory and other diagnostic testing as ordered by staff or outside physician referral.
59. **Indigent care clinic.** Health care services for uninsured and underinsured persons where care is free of charge or charged on a sliding scale. This would include "free clinics' staffed by volunteer practitioners, but could also be staffed by employees with the sponsoring health care organization subsidizing the cost of service.
60. **Linguistic/translation services.** Services provided by the hospital designed to make health care more accessible to non- English speaking patients and their physicians.
61. **Meals on wheels.** A hospital sponsored program which delivers meals to people, usually the elderly, who are unable to prepare their own meals. Low cost, nutritional meals are delivered to individuals' homes on a regular basis.
62. **Mobile health services.** Vans and other vehicles used to delivery primary care services.
63. **Neurological services.** Services provided by the hospital dealing with the operative and nonoperative management of disorders of the central, peripheral, and autonomic nervous system.
64. **Nutrition programs.** Those services within a health care facility which are designed to provide inexpensive, nutritionally sound meals to patients.
65. **Occupational health services.** Includes services designed to protect the safety of employees from hazards in the work environment.
66. **Oncology services.** Inpatient and outpatient services for patients with cancer, including comprehensive care, support and guidance in addition to patient education and prevention, chemotherapy, counseling and other treatment methods.
67. **Orthopedic services.** Services provided for the prevention or correction of injuries or disorders of the skeletal system and associated muscles, joints and ligaments.
68. **Outpatient surgery.** Scheduled surgical services provided to patients who do not remain in the hospital overnight. The surgery may be performed in operating suites also used for inpatient surgery, specially designated surgical suites for outpatient surgery, or procedure rooms within an outpatient care facility.
69. **Patient Controlled Analgesia (PCA).** Patient-controlled Analgesia (PCA) is intravenously administered pain medicine under the patient's control. The patient has a button on the end of a cord than can be pushed at will, whenever more pain medicine is desired. This button will only deliver more pain medicine at pre-determined intervals, as programmed by the doctor's order.
70. **Patient education center.** Written goals and objectives for the patient and/or family related to therapeutic regimens, medical procedures, and self care.
71. **Patient representative services.** Organized hospital services providing personnel through whom patients and staff can seek solutions to institutional problems affecting the delivery of high quality care and services.
72. **Physical rehabilitation outpatient services.** Outpatient program providing medical, health-related, therapy, social, and/or vocational services to help disabled persons attain or retain their maximum functional capacity.
73. **Primary care department.** A unit or clinic within the hospital that provides primary care services (e.g. general pediatric care, general internal

medicine, family practice, gynecology) through hospital-salaried medical and/or nursing staff, focusing on evaluating and diagnosing medical problems and providing medical treatment on an outpatient basis.

74. **Psychiatric services:** Services provided by the hospital that offer immediate initial evaluation and treatment to patients with mental or emotional disorders.
   a. **Psychiatric child-adolescent services.** Provides care to emotionally disturbed children and adolescents, including those admitted for diagnosis and those admitted for treatment.
   b. **Psychiatric consultation-liaison services.** Provides organized psychiatric consultation/liaison services to nonpsychiatric hospital staff and/or departments on psychological aspects of medical care that may be generic or specific to individual patients.
   c. **Psychiatric education services.** Provides psychiatric educational services to community agencies and workers such as schools, police, courts, public health nurses, welfare agencies, clergy, and so forth. The purpose is to expand the mental health knowledge and competence of personnel not working in the mental health field and to promote good mental health through improved understanding, attitudes, and behavioral patterns.
   d. **Psychiatric emergency services.** Services of facilities available on a 24-hour basis to provide immediate unscheduled out-patient care, diagnosis, evaluation, crisis intervention, and assistance to persons suffering acute emotional or mental distress.
   e. **Psychiatric geriatric services.** Provides care to emotionally disturbed elderly patients, including those admitted for diagnosis and those admitted for treatment.
   f. **Psychiatric outpatient services.** Provides medical care, including diagnosis and treatment, of psychiatric outpatients.
   g. **Psychiatric partial hospitalization program.** Organized hospital services of intensive day/evening outpatient services of three hours of more duration, distinguished from other outpatient visits of one hour.
75. **Radiology, therapeutic.** The branch of medicine concerned with radioactive substances and using various techniques of visualization, with the diagnosis and treatment of disease using any of the various sources of radiant energy. Services could include: megavoltage radiation therapy; radioactive implants; stereotactic radiosurgery; therapeutic radioisotope facility; X-ray radiation therapy.
   a. **Image-guided radiation therapy (IGRT).** Automated system for image-guided radiation therapy that enables clinicians to obtain high-resolution x- ray images to pinpoint tumor sites, adjust patient positioning when necessary, and complete a treatment, all within the standard treatment time slot, allowing for more effective cancer treatments.
   b. **Intensity-Modulated Radiation Therapy (IMRT).** A type of three-dimensional radiation therapy, which improves the targeting of treatment delivery in a way that is likely to decrease damage to normal tissues and allows varying intensities.
   c. **Shaped beam radiation system.** A precise, non-invasive treatment that involves targeting beams of radiation that mirrors the exact size and shape of a tumor at a specific area of a tumor to shrink or destroy cancerous cells. This procedure delivers a therapeutic dose of radiation that conforms precisely to the shape of the tumor, thus minimizing the risk to nearby tissues.
   d. **Stereotactic radiosurgery.** Stereotactic radiosurgery (SRS) is a radiotherapy modality that delivers a high dosage of radiation to a discrete treatment area in as few as one treatment session. Includes gamma knife, cyberknife, etc.
76. **Radiology, diagnostic.** The branch of radiology that deals with the utilization of all modalities of radiant energy in medical Diagnoses and therapeutic procedures using radiologic guidance. This includes, but is not restricted to, imaging techniques and methodologies utilizing radiation emitted by x-ray tubes, radionnuclides, and ultrasonographic devices and the radiofrequency electromagnetic radiation emitted by atoms.
   a. **CT scanner.** Computed tomographic scanner for head or whole body scans.
   b. **Diagnostic radioisotope facility.** The use of radioactive isotopes (Radiopharmaceuticals) as tracers or indicators to detect an abnormal condition or disease.
   c. **Electron beam computed tomography (EBCT).** A high tech computed tomography scan used to detect coronary artery disease by measuring coronary calcifications. This imaging procedure uses electron beams which are magnetically steered to produce a visual of the coronary artery and the images are produced faster than conventional CT scans.
   d. **Full-field digital mammography (FFDM).** Combines the x-ray generators and tubes used in analog screen-film mammography (SFM) with a detector plate that converts the x-rays into a digital signal.
   e. **Magnetic resonance imaging (MRI).** The use of a uniform magnetic field and radio frequencies to study tissue and structure of the body. This procedure enables the visualization of biochemical activity of the cell in vivo without the use of ionizing radiation, radioisotopic substances or high-frequency sound.
   f. **Multi-slice spiral computed tomography (<64+slice CT).** A specialized computed tomography procedure that provides three-dimensional processing and allows narrower and multiple slices with increased spatial resolution and faster scanning times as compared to a regular computed tomography scan.
   g. **Multi-slice spiral computed tomography (64+ slice CT).** Involves the acquisition of volumetric tomographic x-ray absorption data expressed in Hounsfield units using multiple rows of detectors. 64+ systems reconstruct the equivalent of 64 or greater slices to cover the imaged volume.
   h. **Positron emission tomography (PET).** A nuclear medicine imaging technology which uses radioactive (positron emitting) isotopes created in a cyclotron or generator and computers to produce composite pictures of the brain and heart at work. PET scanning produces sectional images depicting metabolic activity or blood flow rather than anatomy.
   i. **Positron emission tomography/CT (PET/CT).** Provides metabolic functional information for the monitoring of chemotherapy, radiotherapy and surgical planning.
   j. **Single photon emission computerized tomography (SPECT).** Single photon emission computerized tomography is a nuclear medicine imaging technology that combines existing technology of gamma camera imaging with computed tomographic imaging technology to provide a more precise and clear image.
   k. **Ultrasound.** The use of acoustic waves above the range of 20,000 cycles per second to visualize internal body structures.
77. **Reproductive health**
   a. **Fertility Clinic.** A specialized program set in an infertility center that provides counseling and education as well as advanced reproductive techniques such as: injectable therapy, reproductive surgeries, treatment for endometriosis, male factor infertility, tubal reversals, in vitro fertilization (IVF), donor eggs, and other such services to help patients achieve successful pregnancies.
   b. **Genetic testing/counseling.** A service equipped with adequate laboratory facilities and directed by a qualified physician to advise parents and prospective parents on potential problems in cases of genetic defects. A genetic test is the analysis of human DNA, RNA, chromosomes, proteins, and certain metabolites in order to detect heritable disease-related genotypes, mutations, phenotypes, or karyotypes for clinical purposes. Genetic tests can have diverse purposes, including the diagnosis of genetic diseases in newborns, children, and adults; the identification of future health risks; the prediction of drug responses; and the assessment of risks to future children.
78. **Retirement housing.** A facility that provides social activities to senior citizens, usually retired persons, who do not require health care but some short-term skilled nursing care may be provided. A retirement center may furnish housing and may also have acute hospital and long-term care facilities, or it may arrange for acute and long-term care through affiliated institutions.
79. **Robotic surgery.** The use of mechanical guidance devices to remotely manipulate surgical instrumentation.

80. **Sleep Center.** Specially equipped and staffed center for the diagnosis and treatment of sleep disorders.
81. **Social work services** (could include). Organized services that are properly directed and sufficiently staffed by qualified individuals who provide assistance and counseling to patients and their families in dealing with social, emotional, and environmental problems associated with illness or disability, often in the context of financial or discharge planning coordination.
82. **Sports medicine.** Provision of diagnostic screening and assessment and clinical and rehabilitation services for the prevention and treatment of sports-related injuries.
83. **Support groups.** A hospital sponsored program that allows a group of individuals with the same or similar problems who meet periodically to share experiences, problems, and solutions in order to support each other.
84. **Swing bed services.** A hospital bed that can be used to provide either acute or long-term care depending on community or patient needs. To be eligible a hospital must have a Medicare provider agreement in place, have fewer than 100 beds, be located in a rural area, do not have a 24 hour nursing service waiver in effect, have not been terminated from the program in the prior two years, and meet various service conditions.
85. **Teen outreach services.** A program focusing on the teenager which encourages an improved health status and a healthful lifestyle including physical, emotional, mental, social, spiritual and economic health through education, exercise, nutrition and health promotion.
86. **Tobacco Treatment/Cessation Program.** Organized hospital services with the purpose of ending tobacco-use habits of patients addicted to tobacco/nicotine.
87. **Transplant services.** The branch of medicine that transfers an organ or tissue from one person to another or from one body part to another to replace a diseased structure or to restore function or to change appearance. Services could include: Bone marrow transplant program; heart, lung, kidney, intestine, or tissue transplant. Please include heart/lung or other multi- transplant surgeries in other.
88. **Transportation to health facilities.** A long-term care support service designed to assist the mobility of the elderly. Some programs offer improved financial access by offering reduced rates and barrier-free buses or vans with ramps and lifts to assist the elderly or handicapped; others offer subsidies for public transport systems or operate mini-bus services exclusively for use by senior citizens.
89. **Urgent care center.** A facility that provides care and treatment for problems that are not life threatening but require attention over the short term.
90. **Virtual colonoscopy.** Noninvasive screening procedure used to visualize, analyze and detect cancerous or potentially cancerous polyps in the colon.
91. **Volunteer services department.** An organized hospital department responsible for coordinating the services of volunteers working within the institution.
92. **Women's health center/services.** An area set aside for coordinated education and treatment services specifically for and promoted to women as provided by this special unit. Services may or may not include obstetrics but include a range of services other than OB.
93. **Wound Management Services.** Services for patients with chronic wounds and nonhealing wounds often resulting from diabetes, poor circulation, improper seating and immunocompromising conditions. The goals are to progress chronic wounds through stages of healing, reduce and eliminate infections, increase physical function to minimize complications from current wounds and prevent future chronic wounds. Wound management services are provided on an inpatient or outpatient basis, depending on the intensity of **service needed.**
94. **Physician arrangements. An integrated healthcare delivery program implementing physician compensation and incentive systems for** managed care services.
    a. **Independent practice association (IPA).** AN IPA is a legal entity that holds managed care contracts. The IPA then contracts with physicians, usually in solo practice, to provide care either on a fee-for-services or capitated basis. The purpose of an IPA is to assist solo physicians in obtaining managed care contracts.
    b. **Group practice without walls**. Hospital sponsors the formation of, or provides capital to physicians to establish, a "quasi" group to share administrative expenses while remaining independent practitioners.
    c. **Open physician-hospital organization (PHO).** A joint venture between the hospital and all members of the medical staff who wish to participate. The PHO can act as a unified agent in managed care contracting, own a managed care plan, own and operate ambulatory care centers or ancillary services projects, or provide administrative services to physician members.
    d. **Closed physician-hospital organization (PHO).** A PHO that restricts physician membership to those practitioners who meet criteria for cost effectiveness and/or high quality.
    e. **Management services organization (MSO).** A corporation, owned by the hospital or a physician/hospital joint venture, that provides management services to one or more medical group practices. The MSO purchases the tangible assets of the practices and leases them back as part of a full-service management agreement, under which the MSO employs all non-physician staff and provides all supplies/administrative systems for a fee.
    f. **Integrated salary model.** Physicians are salaried by the hospital or another entity of a health system to provide medical services for primary care and specialty care.
    g. **Equity model.** Allows established practitioners to become shareholders in a professional corporation in exchange for tangible and intangible assets of their existing practices.
    h. **Foundation.** A corporation, organized either as a hospital affiliate or subsidiary, which purchases both the tangible and intangible assets of one or more medical group practices. Physicians remain in a separate corporate entity but sign a professional services agreement with the foundation.
95. **Joint venture.** A contractual arrangement between two or more parties forming an unincorporated business. The participants in the arrangement remain independent and separate outside of the ventures purpose.
98. **Percentage of hospital's net patient revenue.**
    a. **Capitation.** An at-risk payment arrangement in which an organization receives a fixed prearranged payment and in turn guarantees to deliver or arrange all medically necessary care required by enrollers in the capitated plan. The fixed amount is specified within contractual agreements between the payor and the involved organization. The fixed payment amount is based on an actuarial assessment of the services required by enrollees and the costs of providing these services, recognizing enrollees' adjustment factors such as age, sex, and family size.
    b. **Shared risk payments.** A payment arrangement in which a hospital and a managed care organization share the risk of adverse claims experience. Methods for sharing risk could include: capitation with partial refunds or supplements if billed hospital charges or costs differ from capitated payments, and service or discharge-based payments with withholds and bonus payouts that depend on expenditure targets.

SECTION D
COMMUNITY ORIENTATION
Definitions

1. **Mission statement**. A general statement that describes a company's reason for existence, its vision and direction, its areas of expertise and its goals.
4. **Health Status indicators.** A tool used to quantify various aspects of a populations health status.

9. **Self-assessment.** An evaluation of an organization's management system through achievements in areas such as: leadership, strategic planning, human resource management, information management, process management, customer focus and satisfaction, and business results.

SECTION E
TOTAL FACILITY BEDS, UTILIZATION, FINANCES, AND STAFFING

Instructions and Definitions

For the purposes of this survey, nursing home type unit/facility provides care for the elderly and chronic care in a non-acute setting in any of the following categories: *Skilled nursing care *Intermediate care *Other Long-term Care (*see page 13 definitions)**The nursing home type units/facilities are to be owned and operated by the hospital. Only one legal entity may be vested with title to the physical property or operate under the authority of a duly executed lease of the physical property.**

1a. **Total licensed beds** is the total number of beds authorized by the state licensing (certifying agency).

  b. Report the number of **beds** regularly available (those **set up and staffed for use**) at the end of the reporting period. Report only operating beds, not constructed bed capacity. Include all bed facilities that are set up and staffed for use by inpatients that have no other bed facilities, such as pediatric bassinets, isolation units, quiet rooms, and reception and observation units assigned to or reserved for them. Exclude newborn bassinets and bed facilities for patients receiving special procedures for a portion of their stay and who have other bed facilities assigned to or reserved for them. Exclude, for example, labor room, post anesthesia, or postoperative recovery room beds, psychiatric holding beds, and beds that are used only as holding facilities for patients prior to their transfer to another hospital.

  c. Report the number of normal newborn **bassinets**. Do not include neonatal intensive care or intermediate care bassinets. These should be reported on page 2, C6 and C7.

  d. Total **births** should exclude fetal deaths.

  e. Include the number of adult and pediatric **admissions** only (exclude births). This figure should include all patients admitted during the reporting period, including neonatal and swing admissions.

  f. Report the number of adult and pediatric **days of care** rendered during the entire reporting period. Do not include days of care rendered for normal infants born in the hospital, but do include those for their mothers. Include days of care for infants born in the hospital and transferred into a neonatal care unit. Also include swing bed inpatient days. **Inpatient day** of care (also commonly referred to as a **patient day** or a **census day**, or by some federal hospitals as an **occupied bed day**) is a period of service between the census-taking hours on two successive calendar days, the day of discharge being counted only when the patient was admitted the same day.

  g. **Emergency department visits** should reflect the number of visits to the emergency unit. Emergency outpatients can be admitted to the inpatient areas of the hospital, but they are still counted as emergency visits and subsequently as inpatient admissions.

  h. An **Outpatient visit** is a visit by a patient who is not lodged in the hospital while receiving medical, dental, or other services. Each appearance of an outpatient in each unit constitutes one visit regardless of the number of diagnostic and/or therapeutic treatments that the patient receives. Total outpatient visits should include all clinic visits, referred visits, observation services, outpatient surgeries, home health service visits, and emergency department visits.

  Clinic visits should reflect total number of visits to each specialized medical unit that is responsible for the diagnosis and treatment of patients on an outpatient, nonemergency basis (i.e., alcoholism, dental, gynecology, etc.). Visits to the satellite clinics and primary group practices should be included if revenue is received by the hospital.

  Referred visits should reflect total number of outpatient ancillary visits to each specialty unit of the hospital established for providing technical aid used in the diagnosis and treatment of patients. Examples of such units are diagnostic radiology, EKG, pharmacy, etc.

  Observation services are those services furnished on a hospital's premises, including use of a bed and periodic monitoring by a hospital's nursing or other staff, which are reasonable and necessary to evaluate an outpatient's condition or determine the need for a possible admission to the hospital as an inpatient. Observation services usually do not exceed 24 hours. However, there is no hourly limit on the extent to which they may be used.

  Home health service visits are visits by home health personnel to a patient's residence.

  Also include the number of outpatient surgeries reported on line E1j. and the emergency department visits reported on line E1g.

  i-j. Count each patient undergoing surgery as one surgical operation regardless of the number of surgical procedures that were performed while the patient was in the operating or procedure room.

  i. **Operating room.** A unit/room of a hospital or other health care facility in which surgical procedures requiring anesthesia are performed.
  For outpatient surgical operations, please record operations performed on patients who do not remain in the hospital overnight. Include all operations whether performed in the inpatient operating rooms or in procedure rooms located in an outpatient facility. Include an endoscopy only when used as an operative tool and not when used for diagnosis alone.

2a2. **Managed Care Medicare Discharges.** A discharge day where a Medicare Managed Care Plan is the source of payment.

2b2. **Managed Care Medicare Inpatient Days.** An inpatient day where a Medicare Managed Care Plan is the source of payment.

2c2. **Managed Care Medicaid Discharges.** A discharge day where a Medicaid Managed Care Plan is the source of payment.

2d2. **Managed Care Medicaid Inpatient Days.** An inpatient day where a Medicaid Managed Care Plan is the source of payment.

3a. **Net patient revenue.** Reported at the estimated net realizable amounts from patients, third-party payors, and others for services rendered, including estimated retroactive adjustments under reimbursement agreements with third-party payors. Retroactive adjustments are accrued on an estimated basis in the period the related services are rendered and adjusted in future periods, as final settlements are determined.

3b. **Tax appropriations.** A predetermined amount set aside by the government from its taxing authority to support the operation of the hospital.

  c. **Other operating revenue.** Revenue from services other than health care provided to patients, as well as sales and services to nonpatients. Revenue that arises from the normal day-to-day operations from services other than health care provided to patients. Includes sales and services to nonpatients, and revenue from miscellaneous sources (rental of hospital space, sale of cafeteria meals, gift shop sales). Also include operating gains in this category.

  d. **Nonoperating revenue.** Includes investment income, extraordinary gains and other nonoperating gains.

  e. **Total revenue.** Add net patient revenue, tax appropriations, other operating revenue and nonoperating revenue.

  f. **Payroll expenses.** Include payroll for all personnel including medical and dental residents/interns and trainees.

  g. **Employee benefits.** Includes social security, group insurance, retirement benefits, workman's compensation, unemployment insurance, etc.

  h. **Depreciation expense (for reporting period only)** report only the depreciation expense applicable to the reporting period. The amount also Should be included in accumulated depreciation(E 7-b).

  i. **Interest expense.** Report interest expense for the reporting period only.

  j. **Total expenses.** Includes all payroll and non-payroll expenses (including bad debt) as well as any nonoperating losses (including extraordinary losses).

4a. **Total gross inpatient revenue.** The hospitals full-established rates(charges) for all services rendered to inpatients.

4b. Total gross outpatient revenue. The hospitals full-established rates(charges) for all services rendered to outpatients.

4c. Total gross patient revenue. Total gross patient revenue (add total gross inpatient revenue and total gross outpatient revenue).

5. **Uncompensated care.** Care for which no payment is expected or no charge is made. It is the sum of bad debt and charity care absorbed by a hospital or other health care organization in providing medical care for patients who are uninsured or are unable to pay.

5a. **Bad debt expense.** The provision for actual or expected uncollectibles resulting from the extension of credit. Because bad debts are reported as an expense and not a deduction from revenue, the gross charges that result in bad debts will remain in net revenue (E3a).

5b. **Charity care.** Health services that were never expected to result in cash inflows. Charity care results from a provider's policy to provide health care services free of charge to individuals who meet certain financial criteria. For purposes of this survey, charity care is measured on the basis of revenue forgone, at full-established rates.

E. TOTAL FACILITY BEDS, UTILIZATION, FINANCES, AND STAFFING (continued)

6a1 Medicare. Should agree with the Medicare utilization reported in questions E2a1-Eb2.

6a1a Routine patient revenue. Include traditional Medicare fee-for-service.

6a1c.Total. Medicare revenue (add Medicare routine patient revenue and Medicare managed care revenue).

6a2. Medicaid. Should agree with Medicaid utilization reported in questions E2c1-E2d2.

6a2a.Routine patient revenue. Include Medicaid disproportionate payments under Medicaid routine patient care (2a), in the net column (2).

6a2c.Total Medicaid revenue (add Medicaid routine Patient revenue and Medicaid managed care revenue).

6c. Total revenue (gross should equal E4c and net should equal E3a).

7. **Fixed Assets.** Represent land and physical properties that are consumed or used in the creation of economic activity by the health care entity. The historical or acquisition costs are used in recording fixed assets. Net plant, property, and equipment represent the original costs of these items less accumulated depreciation and amortization.

7d. **Gross Square Footage:** Include all inpatient, outpatient, office, and support space used for or in support of your health care activities. Exclude exterior, roof, and garage space in the figure.

8. **Capital Expenses.** Expenses used to acquire assets, including buildings, remodeling projects, equipment, or property.

9. **Information Technology.**

   a. **IT Operating expense.** Exclude department depreciation and operating dollars paid against capital leases

   b. **IT Capital expense.** Include IT capital expense for the current year only. Any capital expense that is carried forward from the previous year should be excluded from this figure. Include IT related capital included in the budget of other departments. (i.e. lab, radiology, etc., if known or can be reasonably estimated.) Include the total value of capital leases to be signed in the current year.

   c. **Number of Employed IT staff (in FTEs).** Number of full-time equivalent (FTE) staff employed in the IT department/organization and on the hospital payroll

   d. **Total number of outsourced IT staff.** (i.e. contracted staff)

   f. **Electronic Health Record.** An electronic health record (EHR) integrates electronically originated and maintained patient-level clinical health information, derived from multiple sources, into one point of access. An EHR replaces the paper medical record as the primary source of patient information.

STAFFING

10 **Full-Time Equivalent (FTE)** is the total number of hours worked by all employees over the full (12 month) reporting period divided by the normal number of hours worked by a full-time employee for that same time period. For example, if your hospital considers a normal workweek for a full-time employee to be 40 hours, a total of 2,080 would be worked over a full year (52 weeks). If the total number of hours worked by all employees on the payroll is 208,000, then the number of Full-Time Equivalents (FTE) is 100 (employees). The FTE calculation for a specific occupational category such as Registered nurses is exactly the same. The calculation for each occupational category should be based on the number of hours worked by staff employed in that specific category.

   a. **Physicians and dentists.** Include only those physicians and dentists engaged in clinical practice and on the payroll. Those who hold administrative positions should be reported in "All other personnel."

   c. **Other trainees.** A trainee is a person who has not completed the necessary requirements for certification or met the qualifications required for full salary under a related occupational category. Exclude medical and dental residents/interns who should be reported on line 7b.

   d. **Registered nurses.** Nurses who have graduated from approved schools of nursing and who are currently registered by the state. They are responsible for the nature and quality of all nursing care that patients receive. Do not include any registered nurses more appropriately reported in other occupational categories, such as facility administrators, and therefore listed under "All other personnel."

   e. **Licensed practical (vocational) nurses.** Nurses who have graduated from an approved school of practical (vocational) nursing who work under the supervision of registered nurses and/or physicians.

   f. **Nursing assistive personnel.** Certified nursing assistant or equivalent unlicensed staff assigned to patient care units and reporting to nursing.

   g. **Radiology Technicians. Technical positions in imaging fields, including, but not limited to, radiology, sonography, nuclear medicine, radiation therapy, CT, MRI**

   h. **Laboratory professional/technical.** Professional and technical positions in all areas of the laboratory, including, but not limited to, histology, phlebotomy, microbiology, pathology, chemistry, etc.

   i. **Pharmacists, licensed.** Persons licensed within the state who are concerned with the preparation and distribution of medicinal products.

   i. **Pharmacy technicians.** Persons who assist the pharmacist with selected activities, including medication profile reviews for drug incompatibilities, typing labels and prescription packaging, handling of purchase records and inventory control.

   k. **All other personnel.** This should include all other personnel not already accounted for in other categories.

   l. **Total facility personnel.** This line is to include the total facility personnel - hospital plus nursing home type unit/facility personnel (for those hospitals that own and operate a nursing home type unit/facility).

   n. **Nursing home type unit/facility personnel.** This line should be filled out only by hospitals that own and operate a nursing home type   unit/ facility, where only one legal entity is vested with title to the physical property or operates under the authority of a duly executed   lease of the physical property. If nursing home type unit/facility personnel are reported on the total facility personnel line, but cannot be broken out, please write "cannot break out" on this line.

   o. **Hospitalist.** Physician whose primary professional focus is the care of hospitalized medical patients (through clinical, education, administrative and research activity).

   q. **Independent provider group.** A private practitioner or hospitalist only or a hospitalist management company.
       Employed by your hospital. Either as direct hospital employees or as employees of a hospital subsidiary corporation.
       Employed by a physician group. A multi-specialty group, a primary care group, an emergency physician group, or an IPA
       Employed by a university or school program. Either as a university/medical school employee or as an employee of a university-based group practice.
       Other. e.g., an insurance company, HMO.

SUPPLEMENTAL INFORMATION

1. **Does your hospital provide services through a satellite facility(s)?** Satellite Services are available at a facility geographically remote from the hospital campus.